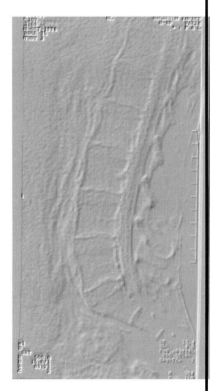

# The Nonsurgical Management of Acute Low Back Pain

*Cutting Through the AHCPR Guidelines*

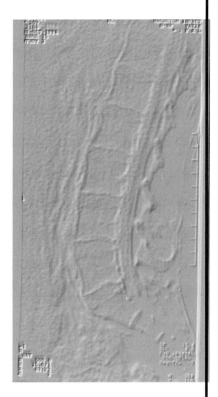

# The Nonsurgical Management of Acute Low Back Pain

*Cutting Through the AHCPR Guidelines*

EDITOR

## ERWIN G. GONZALEZ, M.D.

CO-EDITOR

## RICHARD S. MATERSON, M.D.

demos vermande

Demos Vermande, 386 Park Avenue South, New York, New York 10016

Library of Congress Cataloging-in-Publication Data
The nonsurgical management of acute low back pain : cutting through
    the AHCPR guidelines / Erwin G. Gonzalez, editor : Richard S.
    Materson, co-editor.
        p.   cm.
      Includes bibliographical references and index.
      ISBN 1-888799-13-7
      1. Backache—Treatment.   2. Backache—Diagnosis.   I. Gonzalez,
    Erwin G.   II. Materson, Richard.
      [DNLM: 1. Low Back Pain—therapy.   2. Low Back Pain—diagnosis.
    WE 755 N814 1997]
    RD771.B217N65   1997
    617.5'64—dc21
    DNLM/DLC
    for Library of Congress                                    97-45695
                                                                    CIP

Made in the United States of America

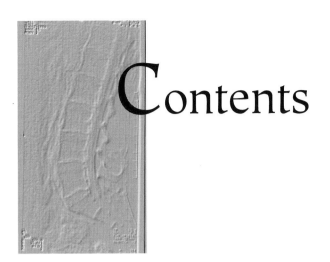

# Contents

*v*

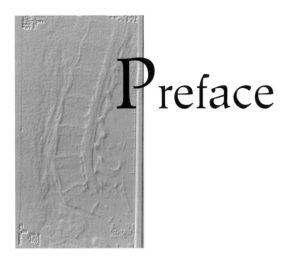

# Preface

True genius resides in the capacity for evaluation of uncertain and conflicting information.

*Winston Churchill*

With this quotation, the readers are challenged to formulate their own judgments on the materials presented in the book and weigh them against those of the Agency for Health Care Policy Research (AHCPR) guidelines on acute low back pain (LBP).

Acute low back pain has afflicted humanity throughout recorded history. Yet the problem remains as prevalent and without definitive solution. The AHCPR guidelines have attempted to present a rational, scientifically driven approach to guide primary care practitioners. Unfortunately, the reception they received was mired with angst and outright anger on the part of some spine care practitioners. Background information on the controversy is discussed in Chapter 1, and an overview of practice guidelines in general is reviewed in Chapter 2. The book is divided into several sections, detailing assessment and management. A significant portion of the book deals with diagnostic and therapeutic injection techniques in response to the growing popularity of these modalities.

The book is intended for all spine care practitioners but only touches on the nonsurgical management of LBP. All of the authors are physiatrists with expertise in the field of spine care. For the most part, they are eminent members of the Physiatric Association of Spine, Sports and Occupational Rehabilitation (PASSOR).

The book is an offshoot of a course sponsored by the Association of Academic Physiatrist (AAP) that I directed in February 1996. The course was a challenge from Robert Rondenelli, M.D., who was the AAP program chairman at the time, to put together a distinguished panel to rebut the AHCPR guidelines. While most of the materials were discussed in the symposium, and most of the speakers are contributing chapter authors, the book is not a written proceeding of the course. Many topics are added and the contents have been substantially updated to reflect the most recent literature.

The chapters are personal opinions of the individual authors, based on published scientific studies, their own writings, and, more importantly, their clinical experiences. The latter qualities may indeed be the striking difference between the book and the AHCPR guidelines. A major shortcoming of the AHCPR guidelines may lie in their rigid adherence to the scientific merit and methodology of the literature rather than their clinical relevance. As spine care practitioners, do we abandon the art of medicine in the name of pure science? Is the scientific evidence sufficient, and will our patients be better served by following the guidelines' algorithms?

Relying on statistical odds that most acute LBP will resolve on its own, the guidelines invoke a "wait and see" approach for the first 3 months, unless red flags exist. Because only a distinct minority of acute LBP patients present with frank radiculopathy and serious spinal conditions, patients with nonspecific LBP who comprise the majority of patients we see day to day, will fall into this category. Will this approach do more harms than good? Will adhering to the guidelines increase the likelihood of an acute episode of LBP turning into chronic LBP, at greater suffering and expense to the individual and society? Will patient satisfaction, a recognized outcome measure, erode because of this approach? Only time will tell.

I gratefully acknowledge the assistance of my co-editor, Richard Materson, M.D., and the contributing authors for their tolerance to my relentless request for rewrites and promptness in completing their manuscripts. They took to the task.

I am indebted to the staff of Demos Vermande, particularly Diana Schneider, Ph.D., for her encouragement in making the book a reality, and Joan Wolk, for her excellent editing. The editors and authors are thankful to all of our secretarial staff, without whom none of our writings would ever get published.

Our inspiration in putting together this body of work is our patients. They seek our care and we owe them their trust.

*Erwin G. Gonzalez, M.D.*

# Contributors

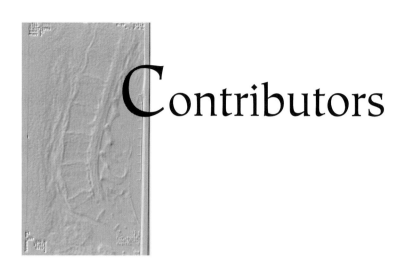

**James W. Atchison, D.O.**
Associate Professor of Physical Medicine
    and Rehabilitation
Department of Neurological Surgery
University of Florida College of Medicine
    *and*
Medical Director, Spine Care Program
Gainesville, Florida

**Krystal W. Chambers, M.D.**
Georgia Spine & Sports Physicians, P.C.
Marietta, Georgia

**Barbara J. de Lateur, M.D.**
Lawrence Cardinal Sheehan Professor and Chairman
Department of Physical Medicine and Rehabilitation
Johns Hopkins University
Baltimore, Maryland

**Brian A. Davis, M.D.**
Fellow, Sports Medicine
Kessler Instiutute for Rehabilitation
West Orange, New Jersey

**Timothy Dillingham, M.D.**
Assistant Professor
Department of Physical Medicine and Rehabilitation
Johns Hopkins University
Baltimore, Maryland

**Susan Dreyer, M.D.**
Assistant Professor
Department of Orthopedics and Physical
    Medicine and Rehabilitation
Emory University
Atlanta, Georgia
    *and*
Physiatrist, Emory Clinic Spine Center
Atlanta, Georgia

**Paul H. Dreyfuss, M.D.**
Associate Clinical Professor
Department of Rehabilitation medicine
University of Texas Health Science Center
San Antonio, Texas
    *and*
Spine Specialists, ETMC Neurological Institute
Tyler Texas

**Joseph H. Feinberg, M.D.**
Director, Sports Medicine
Kessler Institute for Rehabilitation
West Orange, New Jersey

**Erwin G. Gonzalez, M.D.**
Former Chairman, Department of Physical
    Medicine and Rehabilitation
Beth Israel Medical Center
New York, New York
    *and*
Professor of Rehabilitation Medicine
Albert Einstein College of Medicine
Bronx, New York

**Andrew J. Haig, M.D.**
Medical Director
University of Michigan Spine Center
*and*
Assistant Professor
Departments of Physical Medicine and Rehabilitation
and Surgery
University of Michigan Medical Center
Ann Arbor, Michigan

**Stanley A. Herring, M.D.**
Puget Sound Sports & Spine Physicians
Seattle, Washington
*and*
Clinical Associate Professor
Departments of Rehabilitation Medicine and
Orthopaedic Surgery
University of Washington
Seattle, Washington

**Christopher Huston, M.D.**
Physiatrist
Phoenix, Arizona

**Myron M. LaBan, M.D.**
Director, Department of Physical Medicine
and Rehabilitation
William Beaumont Hospital
Royal Oak, Michigan
*and*
Clinical Professor of Physical Medicine
and Rehabilitation
Wayne State University
Oakland University
Ohio State University

**Gerard A. Malanga, M.D.**
Assistant Professor
Department of Rehabilitation Medicine
and Rehabilitation
Kessler Institute for Rehabilitation
West Orange, New Jersey

**Richard S. Materson, M.D.**
Medical Vice President
Memorial Healthcare System
Houston, Texas
*and*
Clinical Professor of Physical Medicine
and Rehabilitation
Baylor College of Medicine
Houston, Texas
*and*
Clinical Professor, Physical Medicine
and Rehabilitation
University of Texas Health Science Center
Houston, Yexas

**Joel M. Press, M.D.**
Clinical Assistant Professor
Department of Physical Medicine
and Rehabilitation
Northwestern University Medical School
Chicago, Illinois
*and*
Medical Director
Sports Rehabilitation Program
Rehabilitation Institute of Chicago
Chicago, Illinois

**Edward S. Rachlin, M.D.**
Assistant Clinical Professor of Anesthesiology
Director, Myofascial Pain Program
UMDNJ - New Jersey Medical School
Newark, New Jersey
*and*
Assistant Professor of Clinical
Orthopedic Surgery
Robert Wood Johnson College of Medicine
Edison, New Jersey
*and*
Private physiatric practice
Watchung, New Jersey

**Jerrold N. Rosenberg, M.D.**
Assistant Clinical Professor
Department of Orthopedic Medicine
Brown University Medical School
Providence, Rhode Island

**Robert G. Schwartz, M.D.**
Clinical Instructor
Department of Physical Medicine
and Rehabilitation
Medical University of South Carolina
Greenville, South Carolina

**Curtis W. Slipman, M.D.**
Director, Penn Spine Center
Assistant Professor of Rehabilitation Medicine
Chief, Clinical Musculoskeletal Program
University of Pennsylvania Health System
Philadelphia, Pennsylvania

**Margaret A. Turk, M.D.**
Associate Professor of Physical Medicine
and Rehabilitation and Pediatrics
SUNY Health Science Center at Syracuse
Syracuse, New York

**Robert E. Windsor, Jr., M.D.**
Assistant Clinical Professor
Department of Physical Medicine
   and Rehabilitation
Emory University
Atlanta, Georgia
   *and*
Georgia Spine & Sports Physicians, P.C.
Marietta, Georgia

**Jeffrey L. Young, M.D.**
Assistant Professor of Rehabilitation Medicine
Albert Einstein College of Medicine
Bronx, New York
Assistant Director, Sports and Spine Rehabilitation
Beth Israel Medical Center
New York, New York

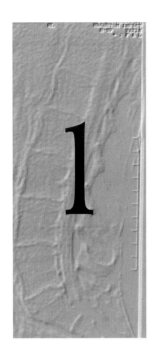

# The Guidelines, the Controversy, the Book

*Erwin G. Gonzalez, M.D., and Richard S. Materson, M.D.*

he Agency for Health Care Policy Research (AHCPR) was established in December 1989 under the Omnibus Budget Reconciliation Act of 1989. The agency was charged with enhancing the quality, appropriateness, and effectiveness of health care services and access to such services.

The AHCPR viewed itself as an agent for change. It identified those clinical areas with large resource costs and wide practice pattern variations but apparently similar outcomes. It particularly targeted the areas that are responsible for disproportionate government expenditures. A major portion of the AHCPR's agenda has been the development of practice guidelines. Since 1992, the agency has produced 19 clinical practice guidelines. One such guideline is Clinical Practice Guideline Number 14: Acute Low Back Problems in Adults (1).

The panel was chaired by an orthopedic surgeon, Stanley J. Bigos, M.D., of the University of Washington, who is recognized by his colleagues for his outstanding contributions to the literature, especially regarding industrial low back pain. Twenty-two other distinguished persons served on the panel, representing multiple medical specialties, physical and occupational therapy, research, nursing, psychology, chiropractic, and a consumer (1).

The AHCPR cited four principal reasons for developing the low back pain guidelines. First is the general yearly prevalence in the U.S. population of 15–20 percent (1). Among working-age people surveyed, 50 percent admit to back symptoms each year (2–3). The second reason springs from the enormous cost, amounting to $20–$50 billion annually (2,3,4,5). A third reason is the purported potentially harmful and probably unnecessary procedures being performed. (6,7) The rates of surgical interventions, diagnostic procedures, and pharmaceutical and therapy usage were all sufficiently varied to invite a review. The guidelines sought to establish the best practice model that was scientifically based.

A fourth reason for the guideline is a growing body of research on low back problems, allowing a systematic evaluation of commonly used assessment and treatment methods. Although the agency admitted to the shortcomings of existing literature, it claims that sufficient scientific evidence exists to support the conclusions of the guidelines. Several contributing authors of this book refute this supposition.

## THE CONTROVERSY

The AHCPR first set out for a change in paradigm by simply redefining acute low back problem as *activity limitations* due to symptoms in the low back and/or back-related leg symptoms (sciatica) of less than three months' duration (1). This definition of sciatica is considerably simpler, broader, and more general than previously accepted definitions, which often implied sacral-1 nerve root irritation as its cause.

The desire was to reduce the focus on pain associated with low back disorders and enhance attention to improving patient activity. The panel adopted this approach because of the perceived difficulty in properly diagnosing its cause and the generally favorable outcome with a *less is more* approach. This is in sharp contrast to what the general medical community and patients with low back pain would generally opine. Herein was the crux of the enormous counter-reaction to the guidelines, spewing considerable negative comments among spine care practitioners and the refusal by many professional organizations to endorse the guidelines.

Dr. Neil Kahanovitz, an orthopedic spine surgeon from Arlington, Virginia, read the AHCPR low back pain guidelines and got angry. And then he got even. Dr. Kahanovitz so objected to the contents of the guidelines, and to the central role played by a federal agency in writing the guidelines, that he formed the Center for Patient Advocacy. This organization raised money from Dr. Kahanovitz's former patients, friends, and others with similar beliefs. The advocacy group provided testimony before congressional committees charged with government oversight and appropriations. Dr. Kahanovitz testified that the AHCPR had, by the time of his testimony, produced 15 guidelines at an agency budget of $750 million. He contrasted that to the American Medical Association and similar professional organizations, which were successfully producing guidelines that are more acceptable to physicians at no cost to the taxpayers. Dr. Kahanovitz found little redeeming value to the guidelines. Perhaps, despite the guideline faults, that is an overzealous posture.

Most spine care practitioners are as disenchanted as Dr. Kahanovitz. There are lingering questions about the credibility of the U.S. government and our full faith in such federal guidelines. The AHCPR originally asserted that adhering to the guidelines is the prerogative of the practitioner, only to be followed shortly by subtle pressure for compliance. The controversy surrounding the guidelines has provided the impetus for increased attention to this important clinical complex. If for this reason alone, the document should be considered to be of value. The editors and contributors to this book urge you, as a practitioner caring for patients with acute low back pain, to thoroughly read these guidelines and decide which of the recommendations are agreeable and usable. To be sure, your colleagues, your patients, third-party carriers, and trial lawyers will know the contents of the guidelines, so you are well advised to be prepared.

As a result of overwhelming criticisms, Congress proposed to withdraw funding the AHCPR. The agency barely escaped total elimination but eventually survived with only a small portion of its then current budget. On August 23, 1996, Douglas Kamerow, M.D., Director of the Office of the Forum, AHCPR, announced that by 1997 the AHCPR would no longer be in the business of producing practice guidelines.

## DEVELOPING THE GUIDELINES

The literature reviewed in developing the guidelines was subjected to AHCPR standards as discussed in Chapter 2. The review relied principally on randomized controlled trials (RCTs) if possible, and otherwise on statistically significant, unbiased, reasonably well-designed trials and published meta-analysis results. As the reader will see, the frequency of RCTs or even highly acceptable unbiased articles upon which to base conclusions was unfortunately low despite the ubiquitousness of low back pain as a presenting symptom.

The AHCPR acute low back pain panel used the services of the National Library of Medicine to assist with their literature review. More than 10,000 abstracts (10,313) were identified. Of these, 38 percent (3,918) were thought to merit further review either because they were randomized controlled trials or because they seemed unbiased enough to be further studied. The Quebec Task Force on Spinal Disorders Report, last published in 1989, was added (9). Only 360 of the articles met their review criteria under meta-analyses for inclusion. The remainder were considered not well enough designed, biased, statistically insignificant, or lacking other qualities to be included. This left abundant room for panel interpretation of information that did not meet research-based evidence standards. The picking and choosing of data agreeable to the panel raised many complaints of panel bias when the guidelines were submitted for review. Some who were asked to be reviewers have stated that the materials they submitted and their opinions were ignored for the most part, and accused the panel of preparing press runs of the original document before assimilating the reviewers' comments and meaningfully considering them. This seeming insensitivity may well have added to the emotional state associated with the negative response to this work.

The AHCPR panel used grades to classify the literature upon which they based their conclusions (1):

A. Strong research-based evidence (multiple relevant and high quality articles).
B. Moderate research-based evidence (one relevant high quality scientific study or multiple adequate studies).
C. Limited research-based evidence (at least one adequate scientific study involving patients with low back pain).
D. Panel interpretation of information that did not meet inclusion criteria as research-based evidence.

Of the AHCPR recommendations, none had the literature grade of "A"; i.e., none had strong research-based evidence with multiple relevant and high quality scientific studies. Many of the conclusions were graded "C" and "D", with a few "Bs," again provoking a bias outcry from those who disagree.

The panel decided to limit their recommendations to acute back pain in adults, defined as activity intolerance of less than three months. Despite this, much of the available literature does not conform to this division of interest and fails to reflect only these "acute" patients but also adds in chronic patients, or does not define the cohort well by temporal terms. Nevertheless, the panel relied on these articles. Children with activity intolerance due to low back pain appear to be sufficiently different as to merit their own guidelines.

The reader should also become familiar with the classification of types of recommendations given by the panel (1):

*Recommend:*
The available evidence indicates that potential benefits outweigh potential harms.

*Optional:*
The available evidence indicates that potential benefits are weak or equivocal (inconsistency in some studies) but that potential harms and costs seem to be small.

*Not recommended:*
The available evidence indicates either that there is a lack of benefit or that potential harms outweigh potential benefits.

Because of the *optional* category, some items that are *recommended against* are there because they are perceived to cost too much. Note that economics drive this science. What procedure would be too costly and thus *not recommended* is surely subjective and would vary with various observers.

The recommendation language used, however, takes on a propagandizing function. For instance, the full text clinical guideline uses the term *not recommended* based on costs or weak evidence, yet in the Quick Reference Guide for Clinicians, the verbiage becomes *recommended against,* a much stronger and more coercive choice of words based on the very same data. This seems at a minimum disingenuous.

The reader should know that the guidelines are published in three booklets. Clinical Practice Guideline Number 14 is the full text intended for professionals. This version has an abstract, an executive summary, the full body of the report, references, and algorithms. Copies are available from the U.S. Department of Health and Human Services, Public Health Service, AHCPR Executive Office Center, Suite 501, 2101 East Jefferson Street, Rockville, MD 20852.. The consumer version, Understanding Acute Low Back Pain Problems, is reproduced in the appendix, as is the Quick Reference Guide for Clinicians. As pointed out, the different publications place different emphasis on the caveats of the study

## THE BOOK

The controversy surrounding the guidelines was the impetus for a course on this subject sponsored by the Association of Academic Physiatrists in February 1996, and subsequently for the writing of this book. Most of the contributors to this book were speakers at that conference.

The following chapters review the AHCPR's guidelines by topic. Each chapter's author indicates agreement or disagreement with the guidelines and provides literature and experience-based reasons for their position. Specific clarification of the references cited by the AHCPR is included where appropriate, and newer literature available since the AHCPR guidelines were written is provided. The reader is encouraged to attempt to understand the rationale of the guideline's authors and decide on the veracity of the guidelines versus the chapter author's or the reader's own information and experience. In this manner, a thoughtful re-examination of our thinking regarding the management of acute low back pain will occur, and the missions of both the AHCPR and the editors of this book will be fulfilled.

*R*eferences

1. Bigos S, Bowyer O, Braen G, et al. Acute Low Back Problems in Adults. Clinical Practice Guideline No. 14, AHCPR Publication No. 95–0642. Rockville, MD: Agency for Health Care Policy and Research, Public Health Service, U.S. Department of Health and Human Services, December 1994.

2. Spengler DM, Bigos SJ, Martin NA, Zeh J, Fisher L, Nachemson A. Back injuries in industry: A retrospective study. I. Overview and cost analysis. *Spine* 1986; 11:241–256.

3. Kelsey JL, White AA III. Epidemiology and impact of low-back pain. *Spine* 1980; 5:133–142.

4. Nachemson AL. Newest knowledge of low back pain. A critical look. *Clin Orthop* 1992; 279:8–20.

5. Deyo RA, Cherkln D, Conrad D, Volinn E. Cost, controversy, crisis: Low back pain and the health of the public. *Ann Rev Public Health* 1991; 12:141–156.

6. Keller RB, Soule DN, Wennberg JE, Hanley DF. Dealing with geographic variations in the use of hospitals: The experience of the Maine medical assessment foundation orthopaedic study group. *J Bone Joint Surg* 1990; 72A:286–293.

7. Volinn E, Mayer J, Diehr P, Van Koevering D, Connell FA, Leeser JD. Small area analysis of surgery for low-back pain. *Spine* 1992: 17:575–581.

8. Bigos S, Bowyer O, Braen G, et al. Acute Low Back Problems in Adults. Clinical Practice Guideline. Quick Reference Guide Number. 14. Rockville, MD: U.S. Department of Health and Human Services, Public Health Service, Agency for Health Care Policy and Research, AHCPR Pub. No. 95–0643, December 1994.

9. Quebec Task Force on Spinal Disorders. Scientific approach to the assessment and management of activity-related spinal disorders. A monograph for clinicians. Report of the Quebec Task Force on Spinal Disorders. *Spine* 1987; (Suppl 12):1S–9S.

# 2 Practice Guidelines

*Margaret A. Turk, M.D.*

P ractice guidelines have been available to physicians for over 50 years through medical textbooks and publications. Protocols for diagnosis and treatment have been developed and promoted by expert panels and individuals in the medical literature, specialty society courses and publications, and public health initiatives and advisories. However, practice guidelines have most recently become prominent as a response to rising health care costs, reported regional practice variations, and reports of "inappropriate" medical care (1).

Practice guidelines are therefore expected to meet a number of agendas, which include improvement of the quality of health care, protection of professional autonomy, reduction of litigation risk, minimization of practice variation, provision of standards for auditing medical records, reduction of health care costs (and thus health care premiums), defining areas of practice, improvement in efficiency of practice, and identification of inappropriate care, to name a few (1). It is obvious that all guidelines will not meet all expectations; clinicians are required to review each practice product and determine the applicability to and appropriateness for their own situations.

These practice products have been generally accepted as a part of health care policy. However, a number of issues remain uncertain in relationship to these products. Although these products are used as standards, benchmarks, or indicators for practice, they appear in a variety of formats and under a number of names (e.g., guidelines, parameters, algorithms, pathways, protocols, standards). Various methodologies are employed, and clinical and scientific rigor are inconsistent. Consequently, the validity of guidelines has not been established. Implementation is also variable and dependent on locale, practice situation, or other modifiers. Their use may be primarily educational for clinicians or may be punitive. In essence, the effectiveness of guidelines in improving patient outcomes has not been established.

This chapter serves as an overview regarding practice guidelines. It provides background for review of the AHCPR guideline "Acute Low Back Problems in Adults." The chapter describes the backdrop for the proliferation of guideline development from a historical perspective, outlines the methodologies used in development of guidelines, and discusses the effectiveness of guidelines in patient care and practice behaviors.

## HISTORICAL PERSPECTIVE

In the mid-1980s, health care expenditures were reported to be about 10 percent of the gross national product and rising. The federal government began to consider cost-containment strategies, specifically related to the Medicare program. Also at that time, there had been documentation of significant regional practice differences (2,3,4), and recommendations were made that practice guidelines might be useful in reducing the significant variation in practice and suspected inappropriate or unnecessary interventions and procedures (5).

Hence, an effectiveness initiative was introduced by the U.S. Department of Health and Human Services (6) to stimulate interest among academic and governmental health services researchers to obtain better information on the description and effectiveness of clinical practice. The Health Care Financing Administration (HCFA) responsible for the Medicare program spearheaded this initiative and promoted patient outcomes research. The U.S. Public Health Service (PHS) became involved when Congress established the Patient Outcome Assessment Research Program at the National Center for Health Services Research and Health Care Technology Assessment (NCHSR) in 1986. The federal government received a specific recommendation in 1988 to utilize practice guidelines as a review of medically necessary services to control costs and reduce practice variation, in a report to Congress (7) and the secretary of the U.S. Department of Health and Human Services (8) by the Physician Payment Review Commission (PPRC). By 1989, a role for the federal government in developing practice guidelines had achieved broad-based support.

A series of bills were introduced by Congress to expand the federal capacity in funding, development, and dissemination of practice guidelines in the Spring of 1989. The legislation received wide political support, including strong support from organized medicine. Also at this time, there were congressional plans to adopt PPRC recommendations to revise physician payment under Medicare with the use of a resource-based relative value scale (RBRVS) and national expenditure targets. The American Medical Association (AMA) actively campaigned against expenditure targets, arguing that such a plan would restrict medically necessary services and ration care for the aging and people with disabilities (9). Practice guidelines legislation benefited from this controversy, especially when a number of prominent physician organizations promoted guidelines as the means to control the delivery of unnecessary or inappropriate services (1).

The Omnibus Reconciliation Act of 1989, which established the Agency for Health Care Policy and Research (AHCPR) to replace NCHSR, was signed into law in December 1989. The guidelines legislation

achieved significant stature in national health policy, as noted by its elevation to a full PHS agency. The legislative mandate was to improve the quality, appropriateness, and effectiveness of health care and improve access to health services (10). Soon after its creation, AHCPR sought advice from the Institute of Medicine (IOM) regarding development of clinical practice guidelines. The key terminology, attributes, and guidelines generated by the IOM have been used in the creation of all 18 clinical practice guidelines developed, disseminated, and supported by AHCPR, and portions of this work have been adopted by other organizations developing guidelines. The first guideline was released in 1992, "Acute Pain Management: Operative or Medical Procedures and Trauma." Not all of the AHCPR-supported clinical practice guidelines have been accepted eagerly by organized medicine and other constituencies. Concern has been raised regarding methodology, expenditure, and utilization of these guidelines, particularly as they relate to influence on or modification of practice. In particular, the guideline "Acute Low Back Problems in Adults," the basis of this book, has engendered an overwhelming response from patients, practitioners, researchers, and policy analysts. In April 1997, Clifton R. Gaus, Sc.D., AHCPR Administrator, announced a major restructuring of the agency's clinical practice guidelines program to meet the changing needs of the health care system. The agency will serve as a "science partner" with private and public sector organizations by producing the scientific foundation to be used in guideline development. AHCPR will sponsor centers to develop literature reviews, evidence tables, decision analyses, meta-analyses, and other products; work with national organizations to develop a national guidelines database; and continue research and evaluation activities regarding guidelines development methodology through implementation strategies.

Aside from the federal government initiatives, practice guidelines have been developed by national medical specialty societies in a number of formats over a number of years. As early as 1938, the American Academy of Pediatrics began publishing its guidelines for the treatment of infectious diseases (11). The AMA supported guidelines development as an alternative to expenditure targets as noted, and therefore established an organizational structure for the development of clinically sound and relevant guidelines through the Forum on Practice Parameters in 1989. The Forum today comprises over 80 organizations. Later that year, the AMA formed a smaller committee, the AMA/Specialty Society Practice Parameters Partnership, which coordinates and guides medical profession activities in practice parameter projects. Go Guidelines developed in specialty organizations run the gamut from exclusively evidence-based products to exclusively expert-opinion-based products. They are presented in a variety of formats, for a variety of reasons. Guidelines on the same topic may provide the clinician with differing directions for diagnosis or treatment strategies, depending on the organizations or clinicians developing the guidelines and their objectives. Cost of development of guidelines can be overwhelming, particularly development of evidence-based products. Consequently, societies are formally or informally joining forces in guideline development. As an example, the Consortium for Spinal Cord Injury Medicine Clinical Practice Guidelines is composed of 15 specialty societies, involving health professionals who provide health care services to people with spinal cord injury. Nonphysician organizations are also developing guidelines and products, again with a variety of formats, methodologies, and contents. A strong need for evidence-based "best practices" is promoted by many of these organizations.

Other entities also have had an interest in practice product development over the past decade, and in particular over the past 5 years. Hospitals and their staffs are developing clinical or critical pathways to improve efficiencies, and through the Joint Commission on Accreditation of Healthcare Organizations, "clinical indicators" are being evaluated as marks of physician competence or privileging. Insurers are increasingly establishing pathways, algorithms, or other products to identify medical necessity of procedures or interventions. Managed care organizations and third-party payers are developing these products increasingly more often with clinician involvement. State and local governments are also participating in guideline development in response to malpractice issues and rising health care costs. More recently, voluntary and advocacy organizations are developing practice guidelines, usually by having notable consumer participation in the process. Practice guidelines that are of interest to the general public are now featured in popular magazines and broadcast media.

An unfinished aspect of guideline development is the evaluation and review process. AHCPR has adopted this mission as a part of their new three-pronged strategy. They have developed outcome and performance measures as a part of their initial mission. AHCPR has also reviewed the initially developed guidelines and reissued them in an updated form. The AMA Advisory Panel for the Evaluation of Practice Parameters has adopted evaluation instruments, used as self-assessment and through the panel, for voluntary review. Managed care organizations and third-party payers utilize their developed products for decision making, often in the area of cost-containment. However, information or medical literature based on use of practice products as they relate to patient outcomes or health care expenditures is limited at best and not universal in its conclusions.

## DEFINITIONS AND METHODOLOGY

Clinicians are increasingly being asked to remain current in aspects of clinical care and decision making by systematically gathering, analyzing, and combining evidence that links to outcomes. Overviews, clinical decision analyses, and economic analyses are more common in the medical literature. Yet these publications do not always link information in a direct way to clinical recommendations. Clinical practice guidelines, then, are "systematically developed statements to assist practitioner and patient decisions about appropriate health care for specific clinical circumstances."[1] Implicit in this statement developed by the IOM is that rigorous science-based procedures are a part of the development; decision making includes clinicians and patients; the focus is on specific clinical circumstances, without direction toward technology or procedures: and the guideline will be practical and definite (12). Guidelines refine the clinical question and balance tradeoffs, attempt to address issues relevant to the decision, and emphasize clinical contexts (13). Guidelines usually make specific recommendations. The AHCPR has accepted this definition of practice guidelines. The AMA uses the term *practice parameter* and defines these practice products as "strategies for patient management, developed to assist physicians in clinical decision making.... Practice parameters are highly variable in their content, format, degree of specificity, and method of development."[2] According to the AMA definition, all practice products, using all manner of development, and targeting a full range of topic areas, can be accepted into the AMA Directory of Practice Parameters

The methods that are used to develop practice guidelines vary among organizations and depend on objectives of the guideline and philosophic approach. Methods of development are classified as informal consensus development, formal consensus development, evidence-based guideline development, and explicit guideline development (14). The categories are a framework for comparing different approaches, and combinations of approaches may be utilized.

*Informal consensus development* has been the most common approach used by specialty societies, federal agencies, and task forces. Expert panels are convened, and through open discussion, agreement on recommendations may be produced. Guidelines are often of poor quality

---

[1] From Field MJ, Lohr KN, eds. *Guidelines for Clinical Practice: From Development To Use.* Washington DC: National Academy Press; 1990, p. 27 (Reference 25).

[2] From American Medical Association. *Attributes to Guide the Development of Practice Parameters.* Chicago, IL, American Medical Association: 1994, p. 1 (Reference 24).

because of limitations of opinion rather than scientific evidence in determining appropriateness, lack of formal consensus methods so group dynamics and dominant politics may rule, and absence of documented methodology to allow readers to judge panel biases. Conflicts of interest are raised if the methods and rationale are not documented. *Formal consensus development* provides greater structure to the analytic process by using defined methods of scoring techniques. Although the methods are standardized, there still exists an opinion basis for defining appropriateness. *Evidence-based guideline development* provides a linkage between the strength of recommendation and the quality of evidence. Although this approach has enhanced the scientific rigor of guideline development, neutral recommendations are often espoused because of the absence of acceptable scientific evidence. The AHCPR guidelines use a combination of evidence-based development and expert opinion. *Explicit guideline development* specifies benefits, harms, and costs of potential interventions and derives explicit estimates of the probability of outcomes (14,15,16). A "balance sheet" is derived using scientific evidence, expert opinion, and formal analytic methods, with all sources documented. The complex analytic method is often too costly and time-consuming to be practical.

There are a number of phases that are central to guideline development (Table 2–1), whatever methodologic approach is utilized. The methodologic approach defines the emphasis given at each phase. Depending on the method used, not all phases will be engaged before developing the final product. There are instructional manuals on guideline preparation (15,17). Each AHCPR guideline defines the development process and methods used in an initial "Overview" chapter. The following is a brief description of the process (14).

### 1. Introductory Decisions

Topic selection may be determined through formal methods, or may be driven by market or practice issues. Expert panels continue to be the technique utilized for guideline development. The size and composition greatly influences the product. Multidisciplinary representation is promoted. The target health problem, patient population, provider group/setting, and interventions are established by the panel.

### 2. Assessment of Admissible Evidence

Depending on methodology used, panels vary in the extent of their literature review. Reviews can be limited by type of published literature and research methodology utilized or can be quite broad. Literature search methods for admissible evidence should be documented. Individual studies are evaluated by study design, determin-

---

**TABLE 2–1**
*Guideline Development Process\**

1. Introductory Decisions
   Selection of topic
   Selection of panel members
   Clarification of purpose

2. Assessment of Admissible Evidence
   Assessment of scientific evidence
       Determination of retrieval strategies
       Evaluation of individual studies
       Synthesis of scientific evidence
   Assessment of expert opinion
   Summary of benefits and harms
   Determination of recommendations

3. Assessment of Public Policy Issues
   Identification of resource limitations
   Identification of feasibility issues

4. Document Development and Dissemination
   Drafting of document
   Peer review
   Dissemination plan development
   Evaluation plan development
   Updating plan development

\* Woolf, SH. Practice guidelines, a new reality in medicine. II. Methods of developing guidelines. *Arch Intern Med* 1992;152:946–52 (14).

---

ing internal (related to the reported study) and external (generalizability outside the study) validity. The evidence is then synthesized by comparing and combining evidence from multiple studies to reach conclusions about the strength of evidence on the topic. Formal analytic methods and models can enhance study results. Meta-analysis is one of those methods, which combines evidence by pooling data from multiple studies (18,19,20). This pooling can increase the sample size to allow conclusions about benefits and harms. However, improper analysis using noncomparable or inadequate studies can produce false conclusions. Expert opinion is important in the process, and documentation of formal or informal methods allows the clinician better understanding of the guideline. A summary of benefits and harms using these assessments can be portrayed in a balance sheet approach (15) or can use more sophisticated analyses.

The greatest challenge in developing guidelines is proposing the recommendations regarding appropriateness of care. Panels determine a strength of evidence classification for research-based evidence; expert opinion classifications or documentation of methodology can also be helpful to the clinician reading the guideline. Typically,

**TABLE 2–2**
*Guideline Recommendations Terminology**

| STANDARDS | Rigid application<br>Rare exceptions<br>Known consequences |
| GUIDELINES | Flexible application<br>Common deviations<br>Some known outcomes |
| OPTIONS | Neutral statements<br>Outcomes unknown or<br>dependent on variety of<br>preferences |

*Eddy DM. Designing a practice policy. Standards, guide-lines, and options. *JAMA* 1990;263:3077, 3081, 3084 (21).

**TABLE 2–3**
*Evidence Rating for*
*"Low Back Pain Problems in Adults"**

| A—STRONG | Research-based evidence with multiple relevant and high quality scientific studies |
| B—MODERATE | Research-based evidence with at least one relevant high quality scientific studies, or multiple adequate scientific studies |
| C—LIMITED | Research-based evidence with at least one adequate scientific study in patients with low back pain |
| D | Information did not meet inclusion criteria as research-based evidence |

The guideline was based on published scientific evidence as a priority over panel opinion. The acceptable method for establishing the efficacy of treatment methods was randomized controlled trials that focused on patient-oriented clinical outcome measures. Evidence about efficacy of assessment methods was felt to be adequate if results of the diagnostic test studied were compared to an independent reference to determine specificity and sensitivity. When strong evidence was not available, panel clinical judgment and expert opinion were used for interpretation.

*Bigos S, Bowyer O, Braen G, et al. Acute low back pain problems in adults. Clinical practice guidelines No. 14. AHCPR Publication No. 95–0642. Rockville, MD: Agency for Health Care Policy and Research, Public Health Service, U.S. Department of Health and Human Services. December 1994 (23).

randomized controlled trials are accepted as the "gold standard" for rigorous scientific evidence. When these studies are not well represented in the topic area or are of poor quality, more description is required. Weaker evidence is considered to be from observational studies with cohort or case-control designs. Often, the terminology standards, guidelines, or options are utilized (Table 2–2) (21). Choice of language, particularly in uncertain areas of practice (e.g., variability of patients and responses, differences in patient and practitioner preferences about outcomes, uncertainty of benefits and harms especially over a prolonged time) is important (22). In the "Acute Low Back Problems in Adults" guideline, evidence is rated on a scale of A through D (Table 2–3), then balanced against potential harms and costs.

### 3. Assessment of Public Policy Issues

The guidelines try to identify the most appropriate strategies for patient care and define the ideal management, issues of resource limitations, and practicality. Often these issues are best addressed by panel members who represent patients, "typical" practitioners, health economists, attorneys, government workers, and industry.

### 4. Document Development and Dissemination

The guideline should provide clear recommendations and document justification for these recommendations. The latter should be clearly identified through description of process and methods used, as outlined previously. The purpose of the document and process, as well as the supporting or endorsing organizations, can help to clarify any possible biases in the document. Specific attributes have been defined by the IOM and AMA (Table 2–4), discussing content and process, to guide the development of practice guidelines. Research priorities are often identified through the identified gaps in scientific evidence. Draft guidelines are usually reviewed by relevant content experts, process experts, and organizations that may have a content or policy interest. Some groups have used a pretesting strategy among clinicians and modified their guidelines based on suggestions. Guidelines are then published, with attempts at wide dissemination. However, affecting clinician behavior often requires more than publication. Some groups have attempted building consensus and evaluating changes in patient outcome or practitioner behavior, with minimal success. Guidelines require regular updating, and a plan must be established and implemented.

---

**TABLE 2–4**
*Attributes of Practice Guidelines*

AMERICAN MEDICAL ASSOCIATION MODEL*

Attribute I:      Practice guidelines should be developed by or in conjunction with physician organizations.

Attribute II:     Reliable methods that integrate relevant research findings and appropriate clinical expertise should be used to develop practice guidelines.

Attribute III:    Practice guidelines should be as comprehensive and specific as possible.

Attribute IV:     Practice guidelines should be based on current information.

Attribute V:      Practice guidelines should be widely disseminated.

INSTITUTE OF MEDICINE MODEL*

| ATTRIBUTES FOR GUIDELINE CONTENT | ATTRIBUTES FOR GUIDELINE DEVELOPMENT |
|---|---|
| Validity | Clarity |
| Reliability/reproducibility | Multidisciplinary process |
| Clinical applicability | Scheduled review |
| Clinical flexibility | Documentation |

*American Medical Association. Office of Quality Assurance. Attributes to guide the development of practice parameters. Chicago: American Medical Association, 1994 (24).

---

## EFFECTIVENESS OF GUIDELINES

Practice guidelines can have both positive and negative impact on patient care. Properly developed guidelines can provide clear information regarding clinical decisions, using current synthesized scientific information and expert opinion. However, if recommendations are impractical, poorly justified, biased, or otherwise flawed, rigid enforcement could interfere with appropriate health care decision making. A clinician must be able to review and evaluate the usefulness of guidelines in daily practice situations (Table 2–5) (26).

The guideline manuscript must document the purpose of the guideline and the target health problem, patients, and providers. The process and methodology must be reviewed. In particular, the extent and review of scientific literature should be noted, so the clinician can judge the usefulness of the guideline. It is important to recognize that determining strength of evidence from study design alone overlooks other important determinants in the study design such as sample size, recruitment bias, proxy measures, time interval, impractical settings, and other problems with internal and external validity (13). Expert opinion as the basis for guidelines is a much debated topic. Experts may have preeminent knowledge or distinguished direct clinical experience, but may be

**TABLE 2–5**
*Clinician Review of Guidelines*

Determine objectives and target audience

Review methodologies used
    Selection of topic and panel
    Assessment of evidence evaluation
        Scientific evidence
        Expert opinion
        Benefits, harms, costs
        Analysis and synthesis

Identify recommendations
    Clinical importance
    Strength of evidence
    Practicality
    Flexibility
    Research priorities identified

Determine review process
    Draft review process
    Sponsors and endorsers
    Update review process
    Dissemination and evaluation plan

biased by the direction of their research or locale of practice. Clinicians who have engaged in clinical trials or who participate in busy population-based practices may offer a different expertise, but also their own biases. It is infrequent that strength of expert opinion evidence is noted, and less frequent that a formal consensus method has been utilized. Differences in recommendations noted when comparing guidelines on the same topic may reflect differences in the relative value placed on various health practices, health outcomes, and economic outcomes (27). The description of the review process can also provide information about possible biases, as do the sponsors or endorsers of the guideline. Benefits, harms, and costs should be noted as they relate to implementation of the guideline. In particular, significant health and economic outcomes should be identified as the anticipated consequence of the practice strategies. The strength of the recommendations should be based on the presented evidence. If the underlying evidence is weak, despite the degree of opinion consensus of the panel or the review, the clinician's confidence in the guideline will be limited. The flexibility of the guideline recommendations will be indicated by the descriptive modifiers noted that require individualized decision making for certain patient characteristics. These modifiers may make the recommendations not useful for certain physician practices. In essence, a practice guideline will be clinically important if the clinician is convinced of the benefits to the patient by following the recommendations (27).

The larger issue is whether or not guidelines have an impact and in which spheres. In regard to physician practices, expanding medical knowledge is the most likely outcome (28). Changes in attitudes or behaviors are less likely to occur, in part because of the varied quality of the present practice guidelines or the scientific evidence on which they are based. Disclosure of the process and methodology used in the guideline development is an initial step in allowing clinicians, policy makers, and others to make informed choices about the quality of the guidelines and how they should be used (28). Physicians continue to express concern about "cookbook medicine" approaches to patient management and possible effects on autonomy of practice (29,30). Issues of implementation and enforcement have yet to be clarified. Guidelines, pathways, and audits have been used for quality assessment and physician performance measures in a variety of ways (31,32). Implementation strategies have been directed at local, regional, state, and national levels (28,33,34). Most success has been local or as a part of managed care organizations. What has become clear is that guidelines must be translated to the local environment to be accepted and effective. Having support from the health care system to change behaviors is also impor-

tant. Guidelines were also once touted as a means of liability protection; to date, reviews are mixed.

Issues of cost savings are also unclear. Practice products have both saved and increased spending (35). It has been reported that including patients in decision making with guidelines may decrease health costs (36). The goal of development and implementation of guidelines by insurers and other third-party payers must be to improve the quality of health care first, with elimination of interventions and procedures that have little or no value in a given clinical situation (37). The potential for savings in health care through voluntary or sanction-free guidelines has yet to be determined. Guidelines with sanctions do have the potential for savings, but the risk of a lower health outcome is possible, and uncertain at best (38). The physician does have a professional and ethical interest in providing the most appropriate care, taking into account issues of cost when possible.

Improvement in patient outcomes with use of guidelines is scattered. Certainly, measurement is an important issue in this endeavor. Rigorous evaluation of guidelines changing the process of care or patient outcomes has shown varied improvements (39). More importantly, the question of whether or not guidelines define optimal care has yet to be answered. If there were complete confidence in this approach, there would be no question regarding development and implementation of practice guidelines. The uncertainty is derived from the limitation of science defining optimal care with certainty, the imperfect process of analyzing evidence and opinion, and the fact that patients are not uniform.

Therefore, the question of effectiveness of guidelines has not been clearly determined.

# Summary

Practice guidelines and other practice products have been a part of medical education and practice for well over 50 years. They are developed for a variety of reasons, in a variety of formats, and with a variety of methods. The federal government has become particularly interested in guideline development and promotion of their development in the interest of rising health care costs and the extreme variation in medical practice noted nationally. Organized medicine has also embraced guideline development as a strategy to improve the quality of care for patients, and yet maintain some degree of flexibility in practice.

It is important for the practitioner to evaluate the usefulness of practice products on an individual basis.

Each guideline should be reviewed for the process and methodology used in its development. The recommendations must be clinically relevant and practical, well-supported, and convincing of the benefits to the patient. Issues of effectiveness remain unclear. Dissemination and evaluation strategies are part of ongoing research. The definition of optimal care remains elusive.

# References

1.  Woolf SH. Practice guidelines: a new reality in medicine. I. Recent developments. *Arch Intern Med* 1990; 150:1811–1818.
2.  Wennberg JE, Gittlesohn A. Small-area variation in health care delivery. *Science* 1973; 182:1102–1108.
3.  Wennberg JE, Freeman JL, Culp WJ. Are hospital services rationed in New Haven or over-utilized in Boston? *Lancet* 1987; 1:1185–1189.
4.  Perrin JM, Homer CJ, Berwick DM, Woolf AD, Freeman JL, Wennberg JE. Variations in rates of hospitalization of children in three urban communities. *N Engl J Med* 1989; 320:1183–1187.
5.  Chassin MR, Kosecoff J, Park RE. Does inappropriate use explain geographic variations in the use of health care services? A study of three procedures. *JAMA* 1987; 258:2533–2537.
6.  Roper WL, Winkenwerder W, Hackbarth GM, Krakauer H. Effectiveness in health care: an initiative to evaluate and improve medical practice. *N Engl J Med* 1988; 319:1197–1202.
7.  Physician Payment Review Commission. Annual Report to Congress. Washington, DC: Physician Payment Review Commission,1988:219–230.
8.  Prospective Payment Assessment Commission. Report and Recommendations to the Secretary, U.S. Department of Health and Human Services, March 1, 1988. Washington, DC: Prospective Payment Assessment Commission, 1988.
9.  American Medical Association. Statement of the American Medical Association to the Subcommittee on Health, Committee on Ways and Means. United States House of Representatives: RE: HR 1692: the 'Medical Care Quality Research and Improvement Act of 1989.' May 24, 1989. Chicago: American Medical Association, 1989
10. AHCPR Workgroup. *Using clinical practice guidelines to evaluate quality of care. Volume 1: Issues.* AHCPR Pub. No. 95–0045. Agency for Health Care Policy and Research, Public Health Service, U.S. Department of Health and Human Services. Rockville, MD: March 1995.
11. American Academy of Pediatrics. *Report of the Committee on Immunization Procedures of the American Academy of Pediatrics.* Evanston, IL: American Academy of Pediatrics, 1938.
12. Lohr KN. Guidelines for clinical practice: what they are and why they count. *J Law Med Ethics* 1995; 23:49–56.
13. Hayward SA, Wilson MC, Tunis SR, Bass EB, Guyatt G. Users' guides to the medical literature. VIII. How to use clinical practice guidelines. A. Are the recommendations valid? *JAMA* 1995; 274:570–574.
14. Woolf SH. Practice guidelines, a new reality. I medicine. II. Methods of developing guidelines. *Arch Intern Med* 1992; 152:946–952.
15. Eddy DM. Practice policies: guidelines for methods. *JAMA* 1990; 263:1839–1841.
16. Eddy DM. Guidelines for policy statements: the explicit approach. *JAMA* 1990; 263:2239–2243.
17. Eddy DM. *A Manual for Assessing Health Practices and Designing Practice Policies. The Explicit Approach.* Philadelphia: American College of Physicians, 1991.
18. Thacker SB. Meta-analysis: a quantitative approach to research integration. *JAMA* 1988; 259:1685–1689.
19. Sacks HS, Berrier J, Reitman D, Ancona-Berk VA, Chalmers TC. Meta-analyses of randomized controlled trials. *N Engl J Med* 1987; 316:450–455.
20. HasselkornJK, Turner JA, Diehr, PK, Ciol MA, Deyo RA. Meta-analysis. A useful tool for the spine researcher. *Spine* 1994; 19(185):2076S–82S.
21. Eddy DM. Designing a practice policy. Standards, guidelines, and options. *JAMA* 1990; 263:3077, 3081, 3084.
22. Spernak SM, Budetti PP, Zweig F. *Use of Language in Clinical Practice* Rockville, MD: Agency for Health Care Policy and Research, Public Health Service, U.S. Department of Health and Human Services, July 1992.
23. Bigos S, Bowyer O, Braen G, et al. *Acute low back pain problems in adults. Clinical practice guidelines No.14.* AHCPR Publication No. 95–0642. Rockville, Md: Agency for Health Care Policy and Research, Public Health Service, U.S. Department of Health and Human Services. December, 1994.
24. American Medical Association. *Attributes to guide the development of practice parameters.* Chicago: American Medical Association, 1994
25. Field MJ, Lohr KN (eds.). *Guidelines for clinical practice. From development to use.* Washington, DC: National Academy Press, 1992.
26. Hayward RSA, Wilson MC, Tunis SR, Bass EB, Rubin HR, Haynes RB. More informative abstracts of articles describing clinical practice guidelines. *Ann Intern Med* 1993; 118:731–737.
27. Wilson MC, Hayward RSA, Tunis SR, Bass EB, Guyatt G. Users' guides to the medical literature. VIII. How to use clinical practice guidelines. B. What are the recommendations and will they help you in caring for your patients? *JAMA* 1995; 274:1630–1632.
28. Woolf SH. Practice guidelines: a new reality in medicine. III. Impact on patient care. *Arch Intern Med* 1993; 153:2646–2655.
29. Harding J. Cookbook medicine. *Physician Executive* 1994; 20:3–6.
30. Tunis SR, Hayward RSA, Wilson MC, Rubin HR, Bass EB, Johnston M, Steinberg EP. Internists' attitudes about clinical practice guidelines. *Ann Intern Med* 1994; 120:956–963.
31. Parker, CW. Practice guidelines and private insurers. *J Law Med & Ethics* 1995; 23:57–61.
32. Wozniak GD. Profiles and feedback: how managed care organizations and others use physician performance measures. In: *Physician Marketplace Report.* Chicago: American Medical Association, Center for Health Policy Research, April 1995.
33. Gates PE. Think globally, act locally: An approach to implementation of clinical practice guidelines. *J Qual*

*Improve* 1995; 21:71–85.

34. Kaluzny AD, Konrad TR, McLaughlin CP. Organizational strategies for implementing clinical guidelines. *J Qual Improve* 1995; 21:347–351.

35. Gesensway D. Putting guidelines to work—lessons from the real world. *ACP Observer* 1995; 15(1):28–30.

36. Nease RF, Owens DK. A method for estimating the cost-effectiveness of incorporating patient preferences into practice guidelines. *Med Decision Making* 1994; 14:382–392.

37. Kanes RL. Creating practice guidelines: the dangers of over-reliance on expert judgment. *J Law Med & Ethics* 1995; 23:62–64.

38. Pauly MV. Practice guidelines: can they save money? Should they? *J Law Med & Ethics* 1995; 23:65–74.

39. Grimshaw JM, Russell IT. Effects of clinical guidelines on medical practice: a systematic review of rigorous evaluations. *Lancet* 1993; 342:1317–1322.

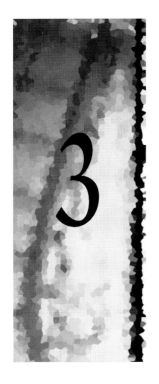

# 3 Initial Clinical Assessment

*Richard S. Materson, M.D.*

he AHCPR had eight initial assessment recommendations as follows (1):

1. Information about the patient's age, the duration and description of symptoms, the impact of the symptoms on activity, and the response to previous therapy are important in the care of back pain problems. (Strength of evidence = B). *I agree.*

2. Inquiries about history of cancer, unexplained weight loss, immunosuppression, intravenous drug use, history of urinary infection, pain increased by rest, and presence of fever are recommended to elicit "red flags" for possible cancer or infection. Such inquiries are especially important in patients over age 50. (Strength of evidence = B ). *I agree.*

3. Inquiries about signs and symptoms of cauda equina syndrome, such as bladder dysfunction and saddle anesthesia in addition to major limb motor weakness, are recommended to elicit "red flags" for severe neurologic risk to the patient. (Strength of evidence = C). *I agree.*

4. Inquiries about history of significant trauma relative to age (for example, a fall from a height or motor vehicle accident in a young adult or a minor fall or heavy lift in a potentially osteoporotic or older patient) are recommended to avoid delays in diagnosing fracture. (Strength of evidence = C). *I agree.*

5. Attention to psychological and socioeconomic problems in the individual's life is recommended since such nonphysical factors can complicate both assessment and treatment. (Strength of evidence = C). *I agree.*

6. Use of instruments such as a pain drawing or visual analogue scale is an option to augment the history. (Strength of evidence = D). *I agree.*

7. Recording the results of straight leg raising (SLR) is recommended in the assessment of sciatica in young adults. In older persons with spinal stenosis, SLR may be normal. (Strength of evidence = B). *I agree.*

8. A neurologic examination emphasizing ankle and knee reflexes, ankle and great toe dorsiflexion strength, and distribution of sensory complaints is recommended to document the presence of neurologic deficits. (Strength of evidence = B) *I partially agree.*

In addition to these eight recommendations in the executive summary the guidelines state:

> "...the primary purpose is to seek medical history responses or physical examination findings that suggest a serious underlying spinal condition such as fracture, tumor, infection, or cauda equina syndrome. The history and physical examination should also assess for nonspinal conditions (vascular, abdominal, urinary, or pelvic pathology) causing referred low back symptoms" (1).

Early in the Executive Summary appears:

> "...the panel agreed that the guideline should provide primary care clinicians with information on the detection of serious spinal pathology (such as tumor or infection, spinal fracture or cauda equina syndrome) as well as nonspinal pathology that could be causing limitations due to low back pain symptoms. ..."

The body of the report, the Quick Reference Guide (1,2), and the algorithm urge a very focused and (in my opinion) superficial history and physical examination because of the low frequency of serious disorders in this cohort. Diagnosis of visceral disorders unrelated to the spine, including diseases of the pelvic organs, kidneys, gastrointestinal tract, and aorta are not discussed in depth.

The casual reader is not alerted to the need for more extensive history and broader physical examination to discover the above save in small print and if one were to rely on the Quick Reference or algorithm alone, the history and examination might well be unsuitable. I believe this a great disservice to patients and practitioners alike.

Red flags were to alert clinicians to low back symptoms that may be related to a dangerous condition. However, the panel suggested that serious conditions presenting as low back problems are relatively rare, again seeming to excuse superficiality at least for a month.

The guidelines state that: "In the absence of red flags, special tests are usually not required in the first month of low back pain symptoms because most patients recover from their activity limitations within one month" (1).

"For over 95 percent of patients with acute low back problems, no special interventions or diagnostic tests would be required within the first month of symptoms" is a summary statement that seems optimistic and simple enough, but further exploration casts doubts on its pragmatism, especially when it can be misused and abused by third-party payers to deny or delay appropriate diagnostic workups thought necessary by the practitioner on the line.

The panel tended to look at the problem of acute low back pain as if it could be or should be appreciated in isolation. The panel states that the guidelines are aimed at the primary medical care practitioner. Perhaps the panel believed these practitioners needed the heavy hand of the government to put the brakes on their diagnostic enthusiasm or personal judgment because of perceived wastefulness in energy or procedures used by these practitioners in carrying out back pain investigations. The evidence for such wastefulness is lacking. Further, stating that in the end 95 percent do well (and therefore needed little or no workup save a screen for "red flags") is different from implying that nothing but the screening history and examination is (usually) worthwhile save red flag identification. Because of its ubiquitous nature, back pain may be the presenting complaint on the first visit to a primary care practitioner. Back pain has been identified as the second most common reason for primary care visits. The proposed problem-focused history and physical examination is likely inadequate in that setting. The opportunity for a full initial comprehensive history and physical examination should not be lost in the zeal to time and procedure limit this clinical interaction. Although comprehensiveness is mentioned as previously stated in the executive summary of the report, it is easily missed amongst the clamor for "less." Discovery of asymptomatic but prevalent disorders such as hypertension, anemia, obesity, chemical abnormalities such as endocrine disturbances or hyperlipidemia, and sexually transmitted diseases would be lost in this gun barrel vision haste and false economy. The issue is that humans with multiple adverse health possibilities present with back pain... not just another back pain case without human values seen as an opportunity to save dollars for the for-profit shareholders of a managed care entity or the government.

A hint of the bias of the panel comes from their use of the word *parsimonious* in their guidelines. R.A. Deyo, M.D., a major contributor to the panel, writes in his 1968 review of cancer as a cause of back pain, "...to develop a diagnostic approach that would identify malignancies while remaining parsimonious" (3). Similar verbiage is found in Report of the Quebec Task Force on Spinal Disorders first published in 1967 (4). Perhaps this is where Dr. Deyo became enamored of the adjective. I doubt that the American public would be as desirous of parsimonious medicine as is the panel if they knew the definition (Figure 3–1). The public, it seems to me, desires and deserves value, not parsimony.

Although the information presented in this portion of the guidelines is interesting and informative, suggesting the generally optimistic outcomes for these patients, it must be carefully considered by practitioners who consider reducing their full alertness to their general obligations as physicians in order to benefit from the cost and statistics driven parsimony. One missed or delayed diagnosis is one too many in my view. Given the choice, I would prefer to spend more time and be more comprehensive, and maybe to be less conserving of resources, if

"Parsimonious"

Parsi-mo-ni-ous (pär-sa-mo-ne-as). adj. Excessively sparing or frugal

Adjective: Ungenerously or pettily reluctant to spend money. Close, mean, cheap, tight, penurious, stingy, close-fisted, miserly.

**FIGURE 3–1**

Definition of "Parsimonious" (5).

it means a better outcome for even a single patient. While this is not current government or panel philosophy, it seems to me more consistent with my oath. I do not urge squandering resources or performing unnecessary procedures on wild goose chases. The issue is clearly one of emphasis and degree.

Now how much more history should one add? Obviously that depends on how well the physician knows the patient who presents with the back pain problem. If there is an already well-established general medical data base, it simply needs to be brought up to date and, in addition to the back protocol, complete whatever else is necessary for good prevention and general medical care.

In the case of a new patient or a former patient who has not been seen in over a year, a comprehensive new data base is highly desirable, including family, social, and detailed past medical history, a review of systems, and the focused back protocol. The physician must develop a positive relationship with the patient which will endure longer than most acute back pain symptoms and which will work toward the goal of appropriate total health care management. A patient who has had a thorough history and physical examination is likely one who will accept more readily an optimistic back prognosis with a watch and wait caveat.

Age and family history and review of systems will direct specific history and physical examination attention to rule out (6):

- vascular etiologies; i.e., aortic, hepatic, or other artery syndromes;
- gastrointestinal referred pain;
- renal/ureteral/genital referred pain (recall the most common young male tumor is seminoma); check for prostate disease;
- rheumatologic disorders (including spondyloarthropathies and myofascial pain)
- gynecological disorders; cervical, other uterine, ovarian, breast, and genital. If you have not done a timely PAP smear, breast exam, and appropriate mammograms, it is cancer until proven otherwise!
- hematologic; sickle cell, thallasemia, etc.

The Quick Reference Guide states, "a medical history suggestive of nonspinal pathology may warrant examination of pulses, abdomen, pelvis, or other areas" (2). However, in clinical presentations there is often little on history to distinguish "nonspinal pathologies" and a reader could be convinced thorough examination is optional. I strongly disagree with this. The patient has the right to expect—and the physician has the obligation to deliver—a thorough history and physical examination.

Physical examination features that this author would suggest adding to the algorithm (6):

▪ Voluntary muscle testing to include more proximal muscles. The guide deals with below knee muscles that can be weakened by a variety of other common causes other than radiculopathy to include but not limited to peripheral neuropathy, myopathy, central induced weakness (i.e., parasaggital meningiomas), and compartment syndromes. In a differential diagnosis of radiculopathy, more proximal muscles must also be observed for atrophy, shortening, fasiculation, and manual muscle testing. Tests of gluteus maximus (hip extensor) strength, hamstring (knee flexor), and gluteus medius/tensor fascia lata (hip abduction) all involve lumbar 5 (and some sacral 1 innervation muscles). Quadriceps for knee extension, and iliopsoas and sartorious and rectus femoris (hip flexors) look at lumbar 2,3,4 roots. The additional muscles also help rule out plexopathy and myopathy (such as muscular dystrophy) and diabetic multilumbar radiculopathy, which also contribute to their share of the population of low back pain patients. Extending the exam to the above the knee muscles gets the examiners thinking "outside the box" imposed by the guidelines so that less common diagnosis is not missed.

▪ Peripheral pulses; simple palpation and auscultation is little time-consuming but can rapidly point to such back pain provoking syndromes as aortic aneurysm and coarctation, and such leg symptom associated disorders as arteriosclerosis. As previously mentioned, the Quick Reference is permissive rather than directive about this additional exam.

▪ Abdominal exam; easy to do, allows discovery of intra-abdominal lesions such as hepatomegaly or splenomegaly or lymph node enlargement and is the prelude to observing the abdominals during the muscle testing of them and kinetics of spine motion. (How does one remediate abdominal weakness if it is not first measured?)

■ Vaginal and rectal exam; if the practitioner does not routinely perform these examinations, he or she should be certain to advise the patient to have them done by a competent practitioner with the results sent in writing for inclusion in the records of the back pain doctor. With cervical and ovarian pathology, frequent discoverable pathologies in women, it is cancer till proven not! "Pelvic deferred" is a contract to perform the examination later and should not be written in the chart when this examination is not performed. "Not examined" is a better word choice, especially if accompanied by a strategy to get the examination done or obtain a report from a more qualified other examiner.

■ Breast examination in women is critical. Breast disease is treatable if caught early. It is being discovered in ever younger women. Question about performance of breast self-examination. If the examiner does not routinely do such exams, he should assure that the patient has the exam done by a qualified practitioner and have a report made to him of the results. This is an opportunity to emphasize proper mammography scheduling as well. This opportunity to prevent should not be missed by any practitioner in the name of parsimony. A breast lesion may or may not be directly associated with the presenting back pain complaint, but the opportunity to find it cannot be missed.

■ Soft tissue flexibility—especially hamstring, triceps surae (calf), and lumbar fascia. Nearly all treatment programs focus on "normalization" of such flexibility despite lack of evidence that asymptomatic individuals differ little from symptomatic patients in their degree of flexibility. Symptomatic patients appear to benefit from soft tissue stretch to obtain range of motion levels consistent with the demands of their daily living activity. The physician who fails to examine and record such flexibility cannot possibly follow progress in gaining same. Further, the myofascial trigger point often is associated with soft tissue tightness in the affected muscle. If one does not look for it, it will not be found. And it can be a cause of nonneurogenic leg pain often mimicking radiculopathy.

■ Some version of Waddell's signs (7,8); which demonstrate nonphysiologic over-reaction to innocuous stresses, since over-reaction to pain stimuli or reaction greater than can be expected considering the objective findings may help with early identification of the cohort of patients who fail to respond to traditional treatment and who most often show up in low back loser status. For these patients early identification for appropriate behavioral modification is required. These patients cannot be assumed to be malingerers or "fakers" but rather are physiologic or psychological "maladaptors" who often

can be helped. There is credible evidence to suggest activation of secondary and tertiary soft tissue pain fiber neurons by a primary nociceptive stimulus in some patients. This may be the physiologic basis for allodynia and is likely associated with pain-induced movement fear known as kinesiophobia. Kinesiophobic patients do poorly in work hardening programs and require special desensitization procedures before physical therapy can work. These augmented behavioral reactions must be looked for and add little time to the exam. To allow this kind of patient to wait a month for the predictably bad outcome produces a difficult to reverse clinical course. The panel recognizes such in their behavioral recommendations, but comes up short in terms of wedding specific behavioral observations to potential remedies.

■ Babinski* and other upper motor signs should be searched for as spinal cord and intracranial disease can be associated with back and leg symptoms and in most cases much could be lost with a 1-month delay.

To be sure, the panel does not specifically preclude these additional history and physical examination features, but they press for the abridged examination based on the low yield of additional findings from their selected literature in their algorithms. In the body of the report Deyo and colleagues are quoted, ". . . summary of available data suggests that in the primary care setting for patients with leg symptoms, the neurologic examination can safely be limited to a few tests" (1,9). However, these data were collected on a back and leg pain population and did not include other patients with leg pain whose conditions might well call for a more complete and adequate examination. Further, no real justification is made for being skimpy except that one can usually get away with it on a statistical basis. In my opinion, this is poor medicine. If the whole cohort of patients with significant other pathology were studied, the value of these more comprehensive measures would be clear. They are buried among the much greater numbers of low back pain patients who do not have other pathology. But this cannot be used as an excuse for a 1-month delay for those who do have the pathology by spurning comprehensiveness as suggested by our pragmatic panel. I suggest that panel members would individually be less than pleased if one of their own family members or loved ones had an important diagnosis delayed a month by a practitioner relying on these guidelines and red flag thinking. I simply prefer to do the job right the first time, a generally good business principle.

If one reviews some of the literature sites provided to support the recommendations and adds some post

---

* Babinski is included in the Quick Reference Guide but does not appear in the Executive Summary or the body of the main guidelines.

1993 literature, additional support or another point of view can be appreciated.

Richard Deyo, M.D., M.P.H., was a member of the panel, as well as a contributor. A general internist, he was also principal investigator of the patient outcome research team (PORT). He was affiliated with the University of Texas, San Antonio, where his patient population consisted of mostly indigent Hispanics in a clinic setting when he wrote the article "Cancer as a Cause of Back Pain" (10), and later came to the Seattle Veterans Administration Center, where he wrote "What Can History and Physical Examination Tell Us About Low Back Pain?" (9). The cohort for the latter study was 833 patients with back pain at a walk-in clinic. Perhaps his interest in parsimony was dictated by his practice settings. He may lack appreciation for the sensitivities of patients usually seen in a primary care practitioner's private office. In the cancer study, for example, the few back pain patients with cancer were collected from a "100 percent report" tumor registry at the facility. However, there is no guarantee that all patients returned to the facility to be included. The mean age of his 1975 patients was 39.5 years (SD = 15.4) with 62 percent women 54 percent seeking care for back pain for the first time. In a subset of 833 subjects who had low back x-rays, 73.6 percent were Mexican American, 13.5 percent were white (non-Hispanic), and 12.9 percent were black. This population's data may or may not allow generalization to populations more commonly seen in primary care practices in the United States, which likely have slightly older, more white, more male, and more affluent characteristics. It is unclear from his physical examination article from where the population reported derived. For the latter article Deyo calculated the sensitivity and specificity of each of the physical examination findings he studied, leading him to the big ticket high yield history and physical examination findings which find themselves in recommendations 1–5 and 7–8. Many of the references given in the article refer to his own earlier work. Therefore, the transferability of statistics based on his cohorts to the general population remain to be proven by additional studies. If the clinic population was veterans, I am not surprised at the high order of diminished ankle jerk reflexes, particularly in the older patients, owing to the prevalence of peripheral neuropathy in that group.

Battie and Bigos (11) report on the lack of spine flexibility changes as a reliable indicator of future back pain problems, but found a statistically significant relationship between decreased flexibility and current or past back pain problems suggesting value in measuring same.

Christodoulides (12) points out the value of the femoral nerve stretch test in identifying patients with L4/5 disc protrusions when the patient experiences anterior ipsilateral thigh pain referral with the stretch. He considers this a pathognomonic sign of lateral L4/5 protrusion and states that L3/4 lesions never produce this sign.

Radiologist P.C. Milette and colleagues (13) demonstrate that some patients experience lower extremity referred pain during discography in which a radial tear through to the annulus is appreciated without frank bulge or herniation. The pain is relieved within one minute by the injection of lidocaine into the disc in 100 percent of the patients. He believes this is strong evidence for radial tears as one entity causing leg pain that might not be otherwise evident and certainly adds to the diagnostic dilemma. Should a strong suspicion lead to earlier than 1 month discography? Is the high incidence of discographic abnormalities that increase with age counter to this? And must one be certain to have the patient subjective component added to the discography to be valid? This will be further discussed in the imaging chapter. Also in that chapter is the issue of fatigue fracture of the pars interarticularis, which might be missed on standard x-rays yet deserves a different type of activity restriction than advocated by the algorithm with the less is more philosophy. These two potential additional diagnostic categories conflict with the desire to demedicalize the problem by classification into three broad categories (2): 1. *Potentially serious spinal condition,* i.e., tumor, infection, spinal fracture, or a major neurologic compromise, such as cauda equina syndrome, suggested by a red flag; 2. *Sciatica*—back-related lower limb symptoms suggesting lumbosacral nerve root compromise; 3. *Nonspecific back symptoms*—occurring primarily in the back and suggesting neither nerve root compromise nor a serious underlying condition. By ignoring the necessity of coming up with a specific diagnosis when it is possible to do so, at least for 4 weeks, the panel takes unwarranted risks with conditions that require more precise activity restrictions and therapies.

The use of pain drawings and visual analogue scales is highlighted in recommendation 6 (14,15,16). Researchers at LSU have studied pain mapping with provocative injection in the sacroiliac joint (17). These pain maps proved reliable in clinical use with blinded observers, correctly identifying patients with SI symptoms by comparison of their pain maps to the study pattern.

At the Karolinska Institute (18), computerized pain drawings were subjected to computer analysis of the pixel pattern and density and type of pain (indicated by different pixel shape) and were found to be highly localizing and helpful in predicting the grade of herniation. Communication with the patient about the drawing was considered most helpful and a good source of documentation.

At the Texas Back Institute (19), researchers explored the value of augmented pain drawing responses that predicted augmented pain responses on discography. This either warned against doing discography in the augmented cohort or at least warned of potential adverse complications so that precautions could be taken.

Hazard and colleagues (20) in Vermont conclude that chronic low back pain patients and their health care practitioners mutually set distinct pretreatment pain, impairment, and disability goals and judge outcomes accordingly. The guidelines proposed enhanced communication with the patient of the optimistic usual outcome in this condition and actually provide four timed patient information releases called Handouts, which are proposed for patient discussion (1, see appendix). I find these handouts misleading. Handout 2, for example, provides a table of diagnostic terms including annular tear, facet syndrome, and fibromyalgia, for which the statement is made that "...however scientific studies have not been able to show a connection between these diagnoses and back symptoms. In addition there is no evidence that these conditions benefit from surgery or other specialized forms of treatment." Of course, this is highly questionable propaganda. In the opinion of the panel, it may be true that they were unable to find evidence satisfactory to them. In no way do they acknowledge differing opinion among back pain practitioners and that these are highly disputed areas of knowledge. Nor do they imply that absence of proof of efficacy of a treatment for a specific diagnosis means that the proposed treatment does not have validity. The panel relies on poor studies and weak evidence to make very strong, highly contentious, and probably untrue statements, and thus richly deserves criticism for not leveling with the public in its desire to contain costs. Perhaps by telling the lie often enough they have come to believe it themselves. But patients are not so easily persuaded by this unbalanced information regardless of how often it is reinforced.

Guideline 5 refers to attention to psychological and socioeconomic problems in the individual's life, potentially complicating both assessment and treatment (8,21,22,23,24,25,26,27). An entire chapter is devoted to this subject regarding treatment implications, as this is an important part of the initial clinical assessment. I find Waddell's article (28) classic for putting the psychosocial factors in correct perspective. Waddell points out that there is good evidence that once a low back pain patient reaches a physician, medical assessment and treatment are more influenced by the patient's distress and illness behavior than by the actual physical disorder. Seeking health care appears to depend more on a patient's perception and interpretation of the significance of the symptoms, on the availability and expectations of treatment, and on learned and cultural patterns of illness behavior. A recent physician visiting from China expressed amazement at our statistics on lost days from work owing to low back pain. He assured me that the disease must be much rarer in China, or at least relatively few take off work for such complaints. In a similar example of cultural and societal influence, an important reinsurance company officer recently expressed to me great concern for the high order of permanent disability from upper extremity repetitive motion disorders experienced in a Scandinavian country where her company wished to write policies. Some people seem comfortable dealing with acute low back ache on their own while others with descriptions of the same intensity pain take much greater self-imposed activity restriction actions.

In acute pain, there is a relatively linear relation between the degree of injury to tissue and the perceived pain. In chronic pain, this relationship greatly diminishes and is replaced with an emotional component in which anxiety, fear, frustration, depression, projection, isolation, aggression, overprotection, and associated augmented illness behaviors can become the major disorders. While traditionalists use a 3-month division between acute and chronic, this is an artificial division. Pain that lasts longer than the usual healing course for the condition suspected of causing it can be considered chronic.

If one looks at cohorts of patients who are classified as "low back losers," those whose main characteristic is illness behavior despite all attempts at remediation, and whose health care costs are disproportionately high, can be recognized, at least in retrospect. Murphy and Cornish (29) identify them as having pain over a wider area of the body, deeper more central pain, highly anxious, and with lower activity levels. Nachemson (30) finds that psychosocial factors, including insurance benefits, have been demonstrated to be more important than biomechanical workload for both acute and chronic patients who are unable to work.

Common to the previously sited multiple references on this subject are the following most important psychosocial historical/physical features (red flags) that should alarm the evaluating physician:

- job dissatisfaction;
- job previous back pain history;
- substance abuse (alcohol, drugs, tobacco);
- previous poor treatment outcomes;
- family or job disharmonies;
- high levels of perceived stress;
- emotional content and amplitude of pain complaints;
- lurking lawyer.

The alarm previously mentioned must result in some beneficial reaction and not just anxiety increase on the physician's part. Presence of these psychological red flags means that you are going to have to spend more time getting to know this patient and establishing a mutually trusting relationship. In my practice recognizing these red flags has often helped me to assist the patient solve knotty life problems or develop coping strategies that make relieving the back pain shrink in relative importance to the patient's quality of life. In other words, the physician can be challenged with an opportunity to really help. Those who will get better anyway are not the tough cases that require the skills of a specialist who knows and recognizes the challenge of the pain augmenter. If the primary care physician is ill-equipped to deal with this kind of patient, he should be sure to refer to a medical specialist who is disposed by personality to deal with these more difficult patients. Surgery often fails in this kind of patient and if bad results are to be avoided, except in rare instances where neurologic deterioration is threatened, so too should surgical thinking be avoided.

In other related literature, Hultman and coworkers (31) identified that successful low back pain patient groups varied from those who do poorly in their perception of too difficult working tasks required and/or too great responsibility demanded of them. Others have observed that the perception of "too heavy loads" may be more important than the actual workload; i.e., perception becomes reality for these patients.

Hasenbring and colleagues (32) looked at biologic, psychological, and social predictors of therapy outcomes and found that the combination of the three helped predict outcomes with 86 percent accuracy. Early retirement at the 6-month follow-up was best predicted by depression and stress at work. Your evaluation must then pay attention to obtaining data about these factors.

Carosella aand colleagues (33) found that patients displaying the pattern of low return to work expectations, heightened perceived disability, pain, and somatic focus experience compliance problems in an intensive work rehabilitation program. Therefore, patients should be screened before being placed in such programs.

In an interesting related opinion sharing, two prominent pain experts have written recent editorials (34,35) regarding Back Pain in the Workplace I and II published in the lead issue of *Pain* for 1996 which come close to duplicating the AHCPR stance and reasoning. Patrick Wall states that "the report is an uncritical lurch back 150 years when chronic pain without lesions was already a major problem." He pointed out that Charcot considered angina and Parkinsonism to be neuroses because of unknown causative lesion. He further quotes Tate describing back pain without lesion as hysteria. Wall goes on to state that the authors of the task force "display no caution their certainty that there is no lesion" and "that there is nothing left to study." He criticizes the task force's consideration of low back pain as "a problem of activity intolerance, not a medical problem." He is particularly critical of the fact that the task force recommends abruptly at 6 weeks that "those still complaining of non-specific low back pain should be labeled activity intolerant and unemployed with removal of medical and wage benefits." He concludes that "Back Pain in the Workplace is at best an idiosyncratic, largely untested series of recommendations on how to treat the first 6 weeks of low back pain after which advice ends abruptly with the reassignment of the patient to the diagnosis of 'activity intolerance' which is not a 'medical problem'."

Loeser grudgingly admits, "malingering is rare; delusions of pain even rarer." He observes the enormous number of claims submitted for low back pain and the ubiquitous nature of the disorder, and opines that there is increasing evidence that treatments rendered to those with nonspecific back pain have no efficacy. He thinks the rate of surgery and chiropractic is more related to the number of surgeons and chiropractors than the number of citizens with back pain, and believes that health care is a social convention driven in only small part by anatomy, pathology, or physiology. He maintains that our current method for diagnosing, treating, and compensating claimants with nonspecific low back pain leads to increasing pain, suffering, impairment, disability, and costs. Patients are told things by their doctors that lead to inactivity and depression.

Thus we have a seemingly angry and negative group of medical experts who do not trust either patients or the rest of the medical community. We have patients who are more at risk if they have the misfortune of either being abused as children or adults, or who lack coping skills and suffer a disproportionate share of life's disharmonies; who suffer more and express their suffering and their own anger through perverse behaviors including depression and "work intolerance." However, recent work looking at central neurotransmitters (especially serotonin) encouragingly may lead to clusters of patients who are genetically more likely to experience pain, depression, sleep disturbance, easy fatigue, and activity intolerance. They may have stress reaction abnormalities in the pituitary adrenal axis. The entire neuropharmacological substrate of pain behavior and suffering is just beginning to evidence itself in the laboratories and with such imaging as PET scans. I believe that in 50 years we will laugh at our current ignorance and the somewhat nasty primarily dollar-driven decisions of these panels, made with an inexplicable degree of hostility toward these patients, as if the experts were personally charged with guarding the health care treasury. No one wants to waste precious dollars and services, but the physician's role is just that—a physician, and not a judge, prosecutor, and jury.

In the interim, with very short visits advocated for history and physical, and prejudging propaganda like material prepared for patients, these recommendations are not likely to facilitate the mutual trust and respect that will allow proper human relationships to develop between

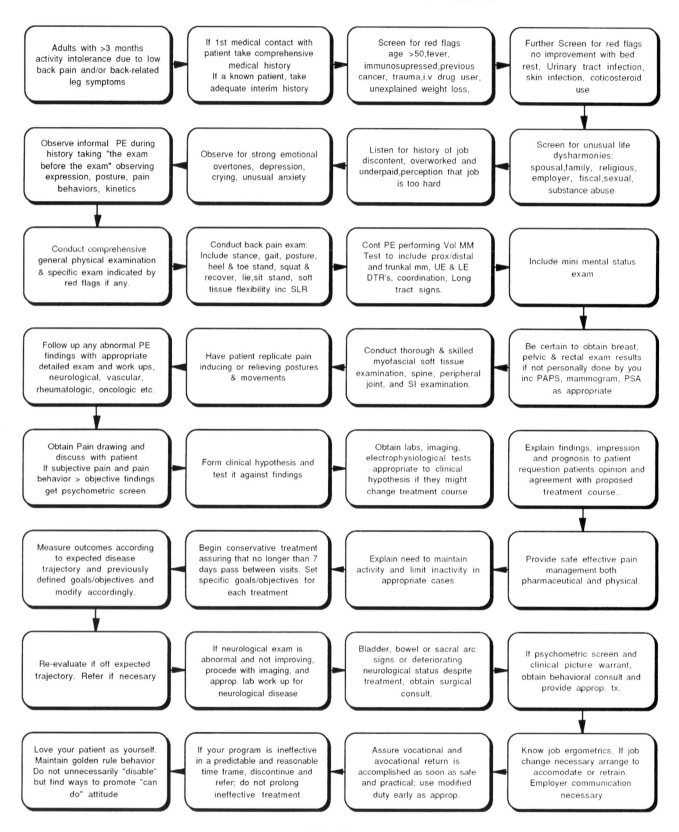

**FIGURE 3–2**

Acute back pain algorithm.

physician and patient and with it the sharing of sensitive, perhaps treatable, human conditions.

Physicians take an oath to "first do no harm." Both the overtreaters and undertreaters must look carefully at their behaviors if we are to be permitted to continue to earn the trust of our patients.

# Summary

We are indebted to the panel for giving us factual guidance such as the age of 50 as key to looking for higher frequency of severe spine problems, the role of higher than 50 sedimentation rate in warning of potential cancer or infection, and the highest yield physical examination features to identify neurologic deficits associated with radiculopathy. Readers are advised to glean the hard data and leave the less factual and more opinionated "hold the patient responsible" recommendations on the table for the time being. This author believes that back pain physicians have no more need to be in a hurry than they have to be efficient. You are encouraged to take appropriate time to get to know your patient and allow good two-way communications. Be thorough in history and physical examination and cognizant of psychosocial problems. Allow that we have a lot to learn about the causes of pain in general and back pain in particular. Do not allow our ignorance to create hostility toward our patients. Love your patients as yourself. Use golden rule behavior. The latter has stood the test of eternal time. A modified algorithm is provide in Figure 3–2.

# References

1. Bigos S, Bowyer O, Braen G, et al. Acute Low Back Problems in Adults. Clinical Practice Guideline No. 14, AHCPR Publication No. 95–0642. Rockville, MD: Agency for Health Care Policy and Research, Public Health Service, U.S. Department of Health and Human Services. December 1994.
2. Bigos S, Bowyer O, Braen G, et al. Acute Low Back Problems in Adults. Clinical Practice Guideline. Quick Reference Guide Number 14. Rockville, MD: U.S. Department of Health and Human Services, Public Health Service, Agency for Health Care Policy and Research, AHCPR Pub. No. 95–0643. December 1994.
3. Deyo RA, Diehl AK. Cancer as a cause of back pain: frequency, clinical presentation, and diagnostic strategies. *J Gen Intern Med* 1988 May-Jun; 3(3):230–238.
4. Quebec Task Force on Spinal Disorders. Scientific approach to the assessment and management of activity-related spinal disorders. A monograph for clinicians. Report of the Quebec Task Force on Spinal Disorders. *Spine* 1987; 12(7S):S1–S9.
5. *Webster's encyclopedic unabridged dictionary of the English language.* New rev ed. ISBN 0–517–11888–2. 1996 Random House Gramercy Books New Jersey.
6. Materson RS. Assessment and diagnostic techniques. Chapter 5 in Weiner RS, ed. *Innovations in pain management: A practical guide for clinicians.* Orlando: Deutsch Press, 1990: 1–25.
7. Quebec Task Force on Spinal Disorders. Scientific approach to the assessment and management of activity-related spinal disorders. A monograph for clinicians. Report of the Quebec Task Force on Spinal Disorders. *Spine* 1987; 12(7S):S1–S9.
8. Waddell G, Main CJ, Morris EW, Venner RM. Rae PS, Sharmy SH, Galloway H. Normality and reliability in the clinical assessment of backache. *Br Med J [Clin Res]* 1982 May; 22; 284(6328):1519–1523.
9. Deyo RA, Rainville J, Kent DL. What can history and physical examination tell us about low back pain? *JAMA* 1992 Aug; 12; 268(6):760–765
10. Deyo RA, Diehl AK. Cancer as a cause of back pain: frequency, clinical presentation, and diagnostic strategies. *J Gen Intern Med* 1988 May-Jun; 3(3):230–238.
11. Batlié MC, Bigos SJ, Fisher LD, Spengler DM, Hansson TH, Nachemson AL, Wortley MD. The role of spinal flexibility in back pain complaints within industry. A prospective study. *Spine* 1990 Aug; 15(8):768–773.
12. Christodoulides AN. Ipsilateral sciatica on femoral nerve stretch test is pathognomonic of an L4/5 disc protrusion. *J Bone Joint Surg [Br]* 1989 Jan; 71(1):88–89.
13. Milette PC, Fontaine S, Lepanto L, Breton G. Radiating pain to the lower extremities caused by lumbar disc rupture without spinal nerve involvement. *Am J Neuroradiol* 1995 Sept; 16(8)1605–13; discussion 1614–1615.
14. Ransford AO, Cairns D, Mooney V. The pain drawing as an aid to the psychologic evaluation of patients with low-back pain. *Spine* 1976 Jun; 1(2):127–134.
15. Udén A, Landin LA. Pain drawing and myelography in sciatic pain. *Clin Orthop Rel Res* 1987 Mar; 216:124–130.
16. Von Baeyer CL, Bergstrom KT, Brodwin MG, Brodwin SK. Invalid use of pain drawings in psychological screening of back pain patients. *Pain* 1983 May; 16(1):103–107
17. Sacroiliac joint: pain referral maps upon applying a new injection/arthrography technique. Part II: Clinical evaluation. Department of Rehabilitation, Louisiana State University, New Orleans. *Spine* 1994 Jul 1; 19(13): 1483–1489.
18. Vucetic N, Maattanen H, Svensson O. Pain and pathology in lumbar disc hernia. Department of Orthopedics, Karolinska Institute, Huddinge University Hospital, Sweden. *Clin Orthop* 1995 Nov; (320):65–72.
19. Ohnmeiss DD, Vanharanta H, Guyer RD. The association between pain drawings and computed tomographic/discographic pain responses. Texas Back Research Foundation. Plano, Texas. *Spine* 1995 Mar 15; 20(6):729–733.
20. Hazard RG, Haugh LD, Green PA, Jones PL. Chronic low back pain: the relationship between patient satisfaction and pain, impairment and disability outcomes. Spine Institute of New England, Williston, Vermont. *Spine* 1994 Apr 15; 19(8):881–887

21. Lacroix JM, Powell J, Lloyd GJ, Doxey NC, Mitson GL, Aldam CF. Low-back pain. Factors of value in predicting outcome. *Spine* 1990 Jun; 15(6):495–499.

22. McNeill TW, Sinkora G, Leavitt F. Psychologic classification of low-back pain patients: a prognostic tool. *Spine* 1986 Nov; 11(9):955–959.

23. Murphy KA, Cornish RD. Prediction of chronicity in acute low back pain. *Arch Phys Med Rehabil* 1984 Jun; 65(6):334–337.

24. Nehemkjs AM, Carver DW, Evanski PM. The predictive utility of the orthopedic examination in identifying the low back pain patient with hysterical personality features. *Clin Orthop* 1979 Nov–Dec; (145):158–162.

25. Nykvist F, Hurme M, Alaranta H, Miettinen ML. Social factors and outcome in a five-year follow-up study of 276 palients with sciatica. *Scand J Rehab Med* 1991; 23(1): 19–26.

26. Deyo RA, Diehl AK. Psychosocial predictors of disability in patients with low back pain. *J Rheumatol* 1988 Oct; 15(10):1557–1564.

27. Julkunen J, Hurri H, Kankainen J. Psychological factors in the treatment of chronic low back pain. Follow-up study of a back school intervention. *Psychother Psychosom* 1988; 50(4):173–181.

28. Waddell G. A new clinical model for the treatment of low-back pain. *Spine* 1987 Sep; 12(7):632–644.

29. Murphy KA, Cornish RD. Prediction of chronicity in acute low back pain. *Arch Phys Med Rehabil* 1984 Jun; 65(6):334–337.

30. Nachemson AL. Newest knowledge of low back pain. A critical look. *Clin Orthop* 1992:279:8–20.

31. Hultman G, Nordin M, Seraste H. Physical and psychological workload in men with and without low back pain. Dept. of Orthopedics. Karolinska Hospital, Stockholm, Sweden. *Scand J Rehab Med* 1995 Mar; 27(1):11–17.

32. Hasenbring M, Marienfeld G, Kuhlendahl D, Soyka D. Risk factors of chronicity in lumbar disc patients. A prospective investigation of biologic, psychologic, and social predictors of therapy outcome. Dept. of Med. Psych., University Hospital of Kiel, Germany. *Spine* 1994 Dec 15; 19(24):2759–2765

33. Carosella AM, Lackner JM, Fuerstein M. Factors associated with early discharge from a multidiciplinary work rehabilitation program for chronic low back pain. Center for Occupational Rehabilitation, University of Rochester School of Medicine and Dentistry, *NY Pain* 1994 Apr; 57(1):69–76.

34. Wall PD. Editorial comment: back pain in the workplace I. *Pain* 1996 65(1):5

35. Loeser J. Editorial comment: back pain in the workplace II. *Pain* 1996; 65(1):7–8

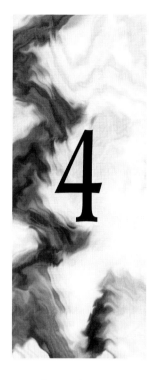

# 4 Assessment of Psychosocial Factors

*Richard S. Materson, M.D.*

s in many clinical settings, assessment of psychosocial factors was left for last and appears at the end of the AHCPR Acute Low Back Problems in Adults guideline. The panel had only two official findings and recommendations (1,2):

> Social, economic, and psychological factors can significantly alter a patient's response to back symptoms and to the treatment of those symptoms. (Strength of evidence = D) *I agree.*

> In a patient with acute low back symptoms and no evidence of serious underlying spinal pathology, the inability to regain tolerance of required activities may indicate unrealistic expectations or psychosocial factors need to be explored before considering referral for a more extensive evaluation or treatment program. (Strength of evidence = D). *I partly agree.*

The panel opined: "Social, economic, and psychological factors have been reported to be more important than physical factors in affecting the symptoms, response to treatment, and the long-term outcomes of patients with chronic low back problems (3). There are indications that such nonphysical factors may affect clinical outcomes for patients with acute low back symptoms.... A heightened awareness among clinicians to the way such factors may affect a patient's response to symptoms and treatment is therefore warranted."

Guideline readers are informed that none of the articles screened regarding psychosocial factors in the assessment and treatment of low back problems were controlled studies. Therefore, they did not meet the panel's criteria for adequate evidence about efficacy. The panel did agree that five articles provided useful information as they included prospective cohort studies (3,4,5,7,8,9).

Bigos and colleagues (4) in a large prospective study of "asymptomatic individuals at a worksite found premorbid nonphysical factors (i.e., measures of low work satisfaction and poor work performance reports) to be the best predictors of individuals reporting back problems at work."

Cats-Baril and Frymoyer (5) contrariwise found that "psychological variables measured early in the course of an acute low back pain episode did not predict outcome, although other nonphysical factors, such as educational level and perception of both job characteristics and 'fault' concerning the back problem were strong predictors of outcome."

In a more recent work, Burton and colleagues (6) reviewed 252 patients with low back pain with a structured clinical interview and a battery of psychosocial instruments. They found that discriminant models developed after multiple regression analysis could successfully allocate 76 percent of the patients to recovered/not recovered groups largely on the basis of psychosocial factors present at presentation. The previous history of low back pain was also highly discriminatory.

Skovron and colleagues (7) performed a population-based study in Belgian adults, which suggested that psychosocial issues affect how individuals with low back symptoms make decisions about working.

Two other articles were cited for their reference to psychosocial factors in predicting outcome for elective discectomy (8) and chemonucleolysis (9).

Based on the paucity of good literature and especially the lack of data regarding efficacious evaluation or intervention techniques, no specific tools or interventions were recommended. Rather the panel recommended that clinicians be aware of the role of psychosocial factors, especially in those patients whose recovery of activity tolerance following an acute low back problem is delayed. They suggested further research is needed to define specific methods of detection of nonphysical factors as well as interventions that might improve outcomes in such cases.

All back pain practitioners encounter patients who seem to have augmented pain behaviors typified by facial expressions such as grimacing, aberrant postures, and movement patterns such as kinesiophobia that do not well fit the pathophysiologic facts, and/or oral-aural manifestations such as moaning and groaning or crying out. At this level, detection of psychophysiologic factors that have a potential for changing outcome does not require any special expertise other than sensitivity to its presence.

In the pre-examination history format in which a patient fills out a pain questionnaire, the use of highly emotional terms to describe pain, i.e., "crucifying," or statements such as "my pain is so severe it is ruining the quality of my life," alert the examiner, as does the pain drawing in which extracorporeal pain is indicated or nonphysiologic patterns of referrals or overzealous pain markings. Finally, pain analogue scales in which the pain is rated at the highest or higher than a scale provides, i.e., 10+ on a scale of 10 with no indication of change with any position or intervention also alert the practitioner to a patient for whom the pain is a reality with which he or she cannot cope.

Finally, there is a cohort of patients whose physical examination findings indicate a significant or unusual amount of anxiety, including palmar and sole and axillary sweating, tachycardia, increased respiratory rate, nonphysiologic bizarre postures and movement disturbances usually with labored or slow movements, jerky movement where smooth movement would produce less painful afferent stimulation, curtailed range of motion where motion should not affect the painful tissues, or unusual pain behaviors in response to the examination. Waddell has described a series of signs depicting such behaviors (10). I recall the vivid poetic description provided by the Scottish neurologist McCrae at a grand rounds—"the patient demonstrates with feats of agility her inability to maintain stability"—to describe a hysterical ataxic woman. While these cases are not common, indeed they are also not rare.

In such cases, I do not believe that it is wise to attempt usual treatment algorithms as these patients are giving us a strong message demanding different attention. Many physicians consider such augmentation to be a sign of malingering. In my practice, I find anxiety, anger, hysteria, and fear but rarely malingering in the pejorative sense of that term. Further, we might cause some of the behavior we observe. Some patients learn from us that if they want our attention for leg pain, they must demonstrate a positive straight leg raising, for they are put off if the test is negative. In other words, we sometimes force a pain patient to demonstrate specific behaviors in order to to be rewarded with attention. So blaming patients for these behaviors is counterproductive and can never really solve the problem even though we can use the excuse to pass the problem along to others, not infrequently exacerbating the problem as we do so.

Therefore, whenever I discover augmented pain reporting and suffering beyond that which I would expect from the remainder of the history and physical examination, I waste no time obtaining a behavioral consultation (see Figure 3–2). How we refer the patient is critical. To avoid "he said it's all in my head" reactions, understanding verbiage such as "this really has made you anxious . . . or depressed, or angry . . . or frightened. . . . , hasn't it?" is useful. Be empathetic with the patient, explaining that fear and anxiety increase pain suffering and experience, and that investigation by professionals trained to do so will allow steps to be taken that will help the patient feel better and cope better regardless of the cause of the back pain. Simply demonstrating caring and interest and coaching in such relaxation techniques as deep breathing or contract/relax cycles enhances one's therapeutic relationship with the patient. How often I have heard language like "If I'm off any more, he'll fire me," or "I'm the third one to be hurt by that defective ladder and I'm afraid to return," or "I can't afford to be sick; I have a child with. . . . " All of this leads to the physician's being much better prepared to communicate fully with the patient and to help him or her as a human being as well as a "back case."

The choice between psychiatrist and psychologist (or others, i.e., psychiatric social worker or psychiatric nurse) is an individual one. The psychiatrist has the diagnostic expertise to more readily identify complicating medical factors such as hypothyroid-related depression, and to advise regarding pharmaceutical measures to assist anxiety or depression or obsessive compulsive disorders. Psychologists, augmented when necessary by psychiatrists, have worked well for me with reasonable time frames and costs. Interviews supplemented by selective psychometric testing are usually provided. Recent literature suggests that Hispanic versions of common psychometric instruments have validity in low back pain patients who are Hispanic (11). Special care is required in communicating sensitive information about mental hygiene and is a legal requirement in many states. Be certain to maintain rules of strict confidentiality in your own office. Allied health or nurse mental hygiene workers often lead individual, family, or group counseling sessions in a cost-effective manner. In chronic pain programs, learning and controlling the pain-stress-pain cycle, changing from an external to an internal locus of pain control, learning anxiety and stress control through relaxation techniques, often through imagery or various biofeedback techniques, and operant or respondent conditioning or cognitive pain control training techniques are effective. One might reason that they could be equally effective in the acute pain patient with augmented pain in the absence of specific literature saying so.

Viaeyen and coworkers (12 ) explored the different treatment technologies in chronic low back pain patients in the Netherlands. Seventy-one chronic low back pain patients were assigned to one of three behavioral rehabilitation treatments or to a waiting list. The first intervention consisted of an operative treatment aimed at increasing health behaviors and activity levels while reducing pain and illness behaviors. The second intervention was a cognitive treatment aimed at the reinterpretation of catastrophizing pain cognitions and enhancing self-control and was combined with the operant techniques. A third intervention consisted of the operant approach and a respondent treatment. During the respondent treatment, patients were taught to decrease muscle tension levels using applied relaxation techniques supported by EMG biofeedback and graded exposure to situations that elicit tension. A repeated measurements design included observer rating of pain behaviors, observer ratings of mood, self-reported depression, residual health behaviors, pain cognitions, and experienced pain intensity. Follow-up assessment occurred at 6 months and 1 year after termination of treatment. Results suggest that for the sample as a whole improvements are found on measures of pain behaviors, health behaviors, pain cognitions, and affective distress and that these improvements are maintained at 6 months and 1 year follow-up. During the treatment, all three groups improved

significantly more than the waiting list control group on most of the measures and showed better scores on outcome-efficacy than the controls. In general, the results suggest that behavioral rehabilitation programs for chronic low back pain are effective and that the effects of an operant treatment are magnified when self-control techniques are added.

Some observers have suggested that patients involved in litigation are particularly difficult to deal with and may have slow return of activity tolerance (4,10). Shofferman and Wasserman (13) looked at a cohort of low back and neck pain patients who had litigation pending using the McGill Pain Questionnaire (MPQ) and the Oswestry Low Back Pain Disability Questionnaire (OSW) to quantify function and interviewed them regarding medication use and work status at their initial and final visits. The results indicated that 33 patients completed the MPQ at initial and final visits. Pain decreased in 29 (88 percent) and increased in 4 (12 percent). Thirty-eight patients completed the OSW at initial and final visits. Function improved in 34 (89.5 percent) and worsened in four (10.5 percent). The authors observed statistically significant improvements in pain, function, and medication use. They concluded that patients with low back or neck pain resulting from a motor vehicle accident showed a statistically significant improvement with treatment despite ongoing litigation.

Back pain seems to be an equal opportunity disease. It can affect populations of patients who have premorbid psychosocial disorders. On the other hand, back pain that does not easily recover activity may be simply another face of a more generalized somatization disorder. Bacon and colleagues (14) studied this issue. They assessed somatization symptoms in a cohort of chronic low back pain patients not selected for psychiatric or pain clinic referral. Ninety-seven male chronic low back pain patients attending a primary care orthopedic clinic and 49 matched healthy controls were assessed using the Diagnostic Interview Schedule III-A (DIS), Beck Depression Inventory (BDI), Hamilton Rating Scale for Depression (HRSD), McGill Pain Questionnaire (MPQ), Sickness Impact Profile (SIP), and the Pain and Impairment Rating Scale (PAIRS). Although none of the subjects met strict DMS-III criteria for a lifetime diagnosis of somatization disorder, 25.8 percent of chronic low back pain patients reported a lifetime history of 12 or more somatic symptoms as compared to only 4.1 percent of controls. In the less symptomatic range, low back pain patients still generally reported more symptoms than controls with 51.5 percent of patients vs. 8.2 percent of controls reporting 7–11 symptoms and 87.2 percent of low back pain patients vs. 22.7 percent of controls reporting 0–6 symptoms. Major depression and alcohol dependence were significantly associated with increased severity of somatization. Lower mood state and increased impairment, but not pain intensity, were related to a greater number of somatic complaints. The authors conclude that while symptoms of somatization are prevalent but not universal, the pattern of these symptoms in chronic low back pain is not reminiscent of the spectrum of severity reported in other medical populations. This higher spectrum of somatization may lead to better treatment matching and better outcomes.

That treatment of one somatization disorder may lead to the emergence of another is discussed by Ford (15). He found that patients who communicate their psychosocial distress in the form of physical symptoms, i.e., somatisizers tend to overuse medical services. They present symptoms with indirect boundaries, and there tends to be some fluidity of their symptomatic presentations. He noted that underlying psychiatric disorders such as mood disorders, anxiety disorders (including obsessive-compulsive disorder), and personality disorders are frequently present. Once again, identification of such patients who will often have delayed return to activity tolerance is insufficient if it is only to inform them that there is no serious identifiable cause of their back problem, but rather demands proper referral and treatment. Some workers compensation case managers and some physicians divide the body, as did the French philosopher Rene Descartes, into psyche and soma. Then they allow treatment of the soma but somehow believe that dysfunction of the psyche is "not work-related" and uncovered. This is, of course, medical rubbish. We treat people.

Suffering appears to be unusually high in patients whose psychosocial issues interfere with activity return. Chapman and Gavrin (16) state that "suffering refers to a perceived threat to the integrity of the self, helplessness in the face of the threat, and exhaustion of psychosocial and personal resources for coping. The concepts of pain and suffering therefore share negative emotion as a common ground." They believe that the physiologic basis of suffering and the casual influences of persistent pain and other stressors are linked through central mechanisms that involve both limbic processing of aversive stimulation and disturbance of the hypothalamic-pituitary-adrenocortical axis with consequent biologic disequilibrium. They see treating potentially chronic pain and stress symptoms aggressively while also addressing suffering proactively and reactively to promote psychosocial well-being.

While depression and anxiety have been most frequently studied in dealing with chronic pain, anger stands out as the most salient emotional correlate of pain. This may be underestimated because it is often denied by patients. Dealing directly with the anger is discussed in an article from the Department of Psychology at Southern Methodist University (17) and seems to be a most important intervention.

There are many common beliefs about patients with low back pain. One is that they overanticipate pain experiences. Amtz and Peters (18) disprove this in a study of the chronic low back pain patient's tendency to overpredict or underpredict pain. In contrast to controls, these patients are shown to significantly underpredict pain, whereas controls tend to be accurate. This underprediction might then encourage such patients to overperform, or at least to be less safety-conscious than necessary, and thus experience repeated pain episodes.

The poverty of ideas on how to manage difficult patients is partially improved by an article by Borken from Israel (19). This author looks to understanding the patient's perceptions, beliefs, illness behaviors, and lived experiences. His research finds that low back pain subjects articulate a rich world of pain sensation, awareness, and meanings. He then uses subjects' own words and experiences to produce a patient-centered classification system of backache symptoms based on typical pain intensity, dysfunction, duration, and treatment. He presents an elaborate system of explanatory models of low back pain and a typology of dominant coping styles designed to either minimize pain or maximize function. Subjects are allowed to choose multiple conventional and alternative treatments based on "what works" and can articulate ample criticisms of and suggestions for the medical system. Considerable variation in the social construction of the back pain experience, which vary sharply, were discovered even between similar neighboring communities. In this model, attempts at better understanding patients' health beliefs, experiences, and behaviors pay dividends when the patient selects from an array of interventions acceptable to him. In my experience, such a smorgasbord is a good idea for patients who are discontent with already developed algorithms. Allowing a patient to choose "what works" for him not only facilitates patient autonomy but also is a first step toward activity increase, i.e., self-decision making, and can be portrayed as such to the patient.

While we await further research, we are faced with the dilemma of how to properly screen low back pain patients. Performing psychometric screens on all is overly taxing and expensive. Allowing that only a small percentage have psychosocial issues that are severe enough to prevent regain of activity, perhaps the screens on history and physical exam behavior previously suggested in this chapter are adequate. Obtaining accurate data on job satisfaction and performance upfront is not easy and may not be desirable, even if useful, as most patients and employers will be reluctant to share this sensitive information with a new physician. Better to apply the suggested screens and go for added data as the need arises with the display of psychological red flags.

We also need to discover which psychometric data are most useful and cost-effective. Do computer-based exams offer adequate data that might bypass professional interviews for more cost-effective screening? My bias is opposed as I find such patients reluctant to expose their innermost thoughts to a computer, and because the information gained at the interview level may be accumulated with verbiage and personal interaction that is in itself therapeutic. Does MMPI II do better than Derogatis or Millon or McGill or Oswestry, or is there a best combination? Do the Sickness Impact Profile or the Medical Outcome Study Short Form 36 (MOS SF36) or the MOS SF12 help identify cases for special attention, as they do in other medical settings? What is the proper role of such anxiety-reducing activity as meditation or Yoga or Tai Chi, or muscle tension-lowering training and other physiologic control systems as EMG or temperature biofeedback and electrogalvanic resistance measures? Will the computerized pain drawing assist both in diagnosis via specific pain referral patterns and in identification of pain augmenters? What is the appropriate role of axiolytics and antidepressants in psychosocially challenged people? Until we have further data, we must fly by the seat of our clinical pants, aware of and sensitive to psychosocial assessment and need.

Finally, we need to build an inventory of strategies, referral sources, and community agencies that might be of assistance to these patients. We must be prepared to spend the time necessary to adequately communicate with the patient, the family, the employer, and the treatment team to assure well-coordinated management and desirable outcomes.

# References

1. Bigos S, Bowyer O, Braen G, et al. Acute Low Back Problems in Adults. Clinical Practice Guideline No.14. AHCPR Publication No 95–0642. Rockville, MD.: Agency for Health Care Policy and Research, Public Health Service, U.S. Department of Health and Human Services. December 1994.

2. Bigos S, Bowyer O, Braen G, et al. Acute Low Back Problems in Adults. Clinical Practice Guideline, Quick Reference Guide Number 14. Rockville, MD: U.S. Department of Health and Human Services, Public Health Service, Agency for Health Care Policy and Research, AHCPR Pub No. 95–0643. December 1994.

3. Waddell G. Biopsychosocial analysis of low back pain. *Baillieres Clin Rheumatol* 1992 Oct; 6(3):523–557.

4. Bigos SJ, Battié MC, Spengler DM, Fisher LD, Fordyce WE, Hansson TH, Nachemson AL, Wortley MD. A prospective study of work perceptions and psychosocial factors affecting the report of back injury. *Spine* 1991; 16(1):1–6

5. Cats-Baril WL, Frymoyer JW. Identifying patients at risk of becoming disabled because of low-back pain. The Vermont Rehabilitation Engineering Center predictive model. *Spine* 1991 Jun; 16(6):605–607.

6. Burton AK, Tillotson KM, Main CJ, Hollis S. Psychosocial predictors of outcome in acute and subchronic low back trouble. *Spine* 1995 Mar 15; 20(6):722–728.

7. Skovron ML, Szpalski M, Nordin M, Melot C, Cukier D. Sociocultural factors and back pain. A population-based study in Belgian adults. *Spine* 1994 Jan 15; 19(2):129–137.

8. Spengler DM, Ouellette EA, Battié M, Zeh J. Elective discectomy for herniation of a lumbar disc. Additional experience with an objective method. *J Bone Joint Surg* [Am] 1990 Feb; 72(2):230–237.

9. Wiltse LL, Rocchio PD. Preoperative psychological tests as predictors of success of chemonucleolysis in the treatment of the low-back syndrome. *J Bone Joint Surg* [Am] 1975 Jun; 57(4):478–483.

10. Waddell G, Main CJ, Morris EW, Venner RM, Rae PS, Sharmy SH, Galloway H. Normality and reliability in the clinical assessment of backache. *Br Med J (Clin Res)* 1982 May 22; 284(6328):1519–1523.

11. Leavitt F, Gilbert NS, Mooney V. Development of the Hispanic Low Back Pain Symptom Check List. Department of Psychology and Social Services, Rush Medical College, Chicago, Illinois. *Spine* 1994 May 1; 9(9):1048–1052; discussion 1052–1053.

12. Viaeyen JW, Haazen IW, Schuerman JA, Kole-Snijders AM, van Eek H. Behavioural rehabilitation of chronic low back pain: comparison of an operant treatment, an operant-cognitive treatment and an operant-respondent treatment. Institute for Rehabilitation Research, Hoensbroek, The Netherlands. *Br J Clin Psychol* 1995 Feb; 34 (pt 1):95–118.

13. Schofferman J, Wasserman S. Successful treatment of low back pain and neck pain that resulted from a motor vehicle accident despite litigation. SpineCare Medical Group, San Francisco Spine Institute, Daly City, CA. *Spine* 1994 May 1; 19(9):1007–1010.

14. Bacon NM, Bacon SF, Atkinson JH, Slater MA, Patterson TL, Grant I, Garlin SR. Somatization symptoms in chronic low back pain patients. Psychiatry service, San Diego Veterans Affairs Medical Center, CA. *Psychosom Med* 1994 Mar–April; 56 (2):118–127.

15. Ford CV. Dimensions of somatization and hypochondriasis. Neuropsychiatry Clinic, University of Alabama at Birmingham, USA. *Neurol Clin* 1995 May; 13(2):241–253

16. Chapman CR, Gavrin J. Suffering and its relationship to pain. *J Palliat Care* 1993 Summer; 9(2):5–13. Comment in *J Palliat Care* 1993 Summer; 9(2):3–4.

17. Fernandez E, Turk DC. The scope and significance of anger in the experience of chronic pain. *Pain* 1995 May; 6(2):165–175

18. Amtz A, Peters M. Chronic low back pain and inaccurate predictions of pain: is being too tough a risk factor for the development and maintenance of chronic pain? *Behav Res Ther* 1995 Jan; 33(1):49–53.

19. Borken J, Reiss, Hermoni D, Biderman A. Talking about the pain: a patient centered study of low back pain in primary care. *Soc Sci Med* 1995 Apr; 40(7):977–988

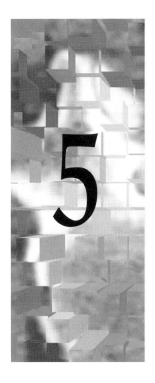

# 5 Anatomic Localization: Imaging Techniques

*Brian A. Davis, M.D., and Joseph H. Feinberg, M.D., M.S.*

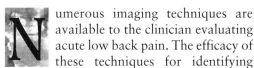umerous imaging techniques are available to the clinician evaluating acute low back pain. The efficacy of these techniques for identifying pathology often remains in question. All too often, imaging is used as part of a routine screening without understanding the efficacy, risks, or benefits of a particular technique. Additionally, imaging may help in diagnosis, but may not change patient management, and can therefore be eliminated to reduce cost of medical (patient) care and avoid possible untoward effects. As physicians, we must be keenly aware of the imaging techniques available for managing acute low back pain, as well as the efficacy, risks, and benefits of each. We must also understand when imaging will have a significant impact on patient man-

agement, and therefore reduce cost and risk. Recently, the Public Health Service's Agency for Health Care Policy and Research (AHCPR) published Acute Low Back Problems in Adults: Clinical Practice Guidelines (1). These guidelines made an attempt to address the need for obtaining imaging studies in patients with low back problems. The AHCPR guidelines reviewed the efficacy of standard radiography, bone scan scintigraphy, magnetic resonance imagery (MRI), myelography, discography, computed tomography (CT), CT–myelography, and CT–discography. Based on these reviews, the AHCPR established recommended practice guidelines for the clinician treating acute low back pain. This chapter addresses the AHCPR guidelines set forth and provides literature-based comments on the clinical relevance of these recommendations.

## STANDARD RADIOGRAPHY

Standard radiographs, or X-rays, are the oldest, most readily available, and most widely used of all forms of imaging for low back disorders (2). Traditional training has favored the use of standard radiographs as one of the initial steps in managing individuals with acute low back pain (2). X-rays are produced by bombarding a tungsten target with an electron beam. These rays are then passed through the object of interest and recorded on a photographic film. Areas of the film remain light where the rays have been obstructed by the object. The variations in film exposure are determined by the object's density and result in some areas of the film being exposed to a greater extent than others (3,4).

The most commonly used projections for viewing the low back include anteroposterior (AP), lateral, oblique (right and left), and lumbosacral junction coned views of the lumbosacral spine (2). AP views of the spine are best for visualizing alignment of the facet joints, lateral osteophytes, pedicle defects, and the transverse processes. AP views can also diagnose spina bifida and spina bifida occulta, lumbarization, and sacralization of the spine. Lateral projections evaluate height of the vertebral body, integrity of the endplate, disc space size, anterior margin osteophytosis, the spinous processes, canal width, and relationship of the vertebral bodies to one another (i.e., spondylolisthesis) and when there are bilateral pars interarticularis defects (see Figures 5–1 to 5–4). Oblique projections are most often used for observing defects in the pars interarticularis and ruling out spondylolysis. They also provide another view for evaluating vertebral body height, endplate integrity, and disc space size. The oblique view is the best for examining the facet joints (5). (Figures 5–5 and 5–6). Coned views are detailed images of the lumbosacral junction and are most often used to evaluate spondylolisthesis.

Standard radiographs can also provide the clinician with other pertinent information concerning intra-abdominal structures that may be a cause for referral of pain. Some examples would include aortic calcification and aneurysmal dilation, gallbladder calculi, bowel obstruction, and pancreatitis.

The AHCPR guidelines on standard radiographs recommend:

1. Standard radiographs not be ordered for routine evaluation within the first month of symptoms unless a "red flag" (any of the conditions listed in 2 or 3) is noted on examination;
2. Standard lumbar radiographs only be ordered for patients with significant trauma, recent mild trauma and age over 50, history of prolonged steroid use, osteoporosis, or age over 70 years old;

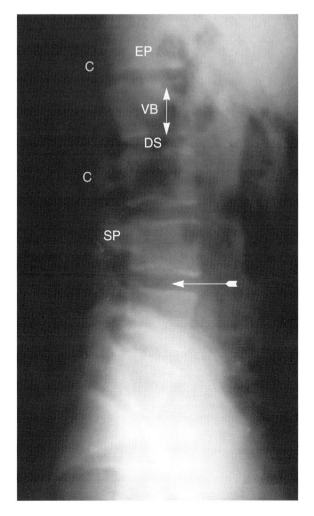

**FIGURE 5–1**

Standard lateral radiograph of the spine. Lateral projections evaluate height of the vertebral body (VB), integrity of the endplate (EP), disc space size (DS), the spinous processes (SP), canal width (C), and relationship of the vertebral bodies to one another. This radiograph was taken from a 30-year-old male with acute low back pain, and subsequently determined to have a disc herniation at the L5–S1 level. The disc space height is poorly maintained at this interspace *(arrow)*.

3. Use of complete blood count (CBC) and erythrocyte sedimentation rate (ESR) in conjunction with standard radiographs to rule out tumor or infection as the cause of low back pain when there is history of prior cancer or recent infection, fever greater than 100°F, intravenous drug abuse, prolonged use of steroids, low back pain with rest, or unexplained weight loss;
4. Use of other imaging technique if there are historical or physical signs of cancer, infection, or fracture

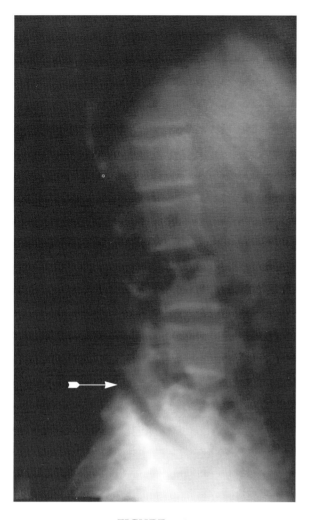

**FIGURE 5–2**

Lateral radiograph of the spine demonstrating spondylolis-thesis. This radiograph demonstrates bilateral pars interar-ticularis defects at L5–S1 *(arrow)*. There is evidence of mild slippage of the L5 vertebra on the S1 vertebra, resulting in a grade 1 (0–25 percent) spondylolisthesis.

even if standard radiographs are negative; and
5. Not ordering oblique views of the lumbosacral spine routinely due to increased radiation exposure to patients.

The authors are in agreement with many of these recommendations, but some deserve special discussion.

The AHCPR recommends not obtaining films prior to 1 month of symptoms, as long as no historical symp-toms or signs are suggestive of infection, fracture, or tumor (1). Specifically, they suggest that only low back pain patients with significant trauma at any age, mild trauma and age over 50, prolonged steroid use, osteoporosis, age

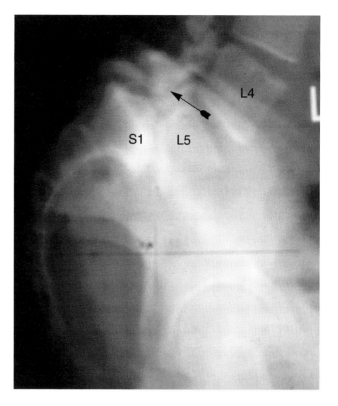

**FIGURE 5–3**

Lateral radiograph of the spine demonstrating spondylolis-thesis. This radiograph demonstrates bilateral pars interar-ticularis defects at L5–S1 *(arrow)*. There is evidence of mod-erate slippage of the L5 vertebra on the S1 vertebra, resulting in a grade 2 (26–50 percent) spondylolisthesis.

over 70, previous cancer, recent infection, temperature over 100° F, back pain worse with rest, or unexplained weight loss should receive standard radiographs. No men-tion is made of ordering standard radiographs in those with complaints of radiating pain to the buttock or extrem-ity or new or advancing neuromotor deficits. These symp-toms and signs are suggestive of either spinal canal encroachment, nerve root entrapment, or both. Standard radiographs can provide information regarding canal cal-iber, vertebral alignment, and foraminal aperture on lat-eral views, and, therefore, in our opinion should be con-sidered if any of these other neurologic signs or symptoms are present, regardless of the acuteness of injury. If an obvi-ous or suspicious lesion is present on radiographic exam-ination and thought to be responsible for the deficits noted on physical examination, an additional imaging procedure may not be necessary. For example, if a patient has no evi-dence of osteoarthritis, then referred pain or neurologic symptoms are likely to be disc-related. This would affect management. Additionally, it is our belief that any patient

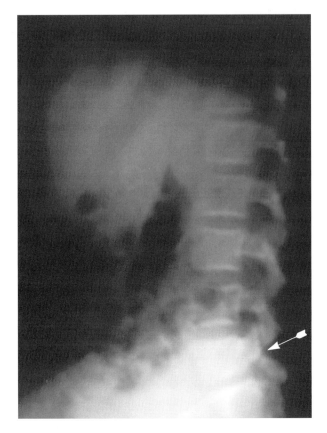

**FIGURE 5–4**

Lateral radiograph demonstrating bilateral pars interarticularis defects. This radiograph also demonstrates bilateral pars interarticularis defects at the L5–S1 level *(arrow)*. Relative loss of lumbar lordosis can also be detected by this view on this film.

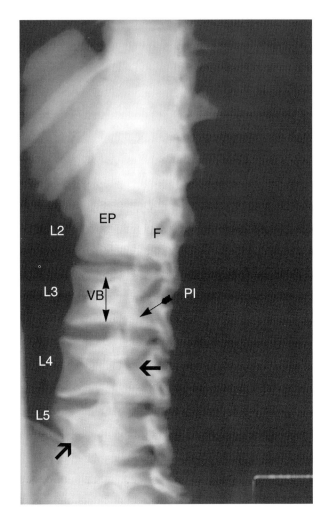

**FIGURE 5–5**

Standard oblique radiograph. Oblique projections offer the best view of the pars interarticularis (PI—normal pars, *small arrow*) for ruling out spondylolysis. Oblique radiographs can also evaluate vertebral body height (VB), end plate integrity (EP), disc space size (DS), and the facet joints (F). On this radiograph, spondylolysis is present at both the L4 and L5 levels *(large arrows)*. This radiograph uniquely depicts fragmentation of the pars interarticularis at the L4 level. The L5 level shows mild sclerosis across the pars interarticularis.

exhibiting pain to palpation or percussion of the spinous or transverse processes or deep palpation into the paravertebral gutters, with any trauma, even in the absence of the "red flags" listed previously, may require radiographic examination for fracture. The authors have seen cases in which simple falls have led to nonpathologic thoracic or lumbar vertebral body fractures in healthy young adults. Based on the recommendations of the AHCPR, radiographs and other imaging techniques should not be ordered when minor trauma causes low back pain (1). This may lead to undetected fractures that may require further evaluation and effect management in active young adults.

It has been well described that adolescent and young adult gymnasts and other athletes who undergo repetitive extension (e.g., football lineman, ballet dancers, and volleyball players) are at increased risk for developing spondylolysis (6–9). The AHCPR states in its guidelines that spondylolysis has not been documented to be associated with low back pain in adults and no special treatment is

required (1). Hall also states that evidence of spondylolysis does not necessarily change treatment plan (5). The authors disagree, as do others (10–12). Although often asymptomatic, when spondylolysis is present and symptomatic, specific management is required, both for pain reduction and for possible prevention of advancement to spondylolisthesis. Whether or not the spondylolysis will progress to spondylolisthesis is primarily determined by the stability of the remaining supporting structures of the

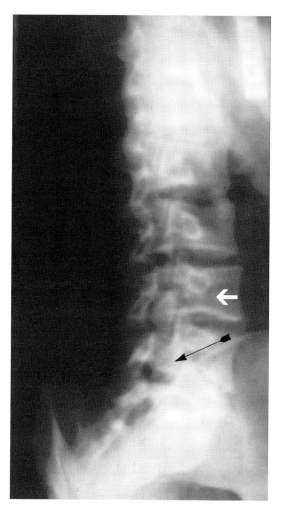

**FIGURE 5–6**

L4 spondylolysis on oblique radiograph. This oblique radiograph is a follow-up from that in Figure 5–5. This film demonstrates almost complete resorption of the fracture fragment seen at the L4 level in Figure 5–5 *(large arrow)*. There is also mild sclerosis at the L5 pars interarticularis *(small arrow)*.

lumbosacral spine, such as the discs, anterior longitudinal ligament, and the iliolumbar ligaments (13). Management of an individual with spondylolysis will be affected and a course of recovery can be better predicted. Spondylolisthesis results when these secondary structures fail, as can occur with repeated extension on an already weakened bony support system (14). Spondylolisthesis has been associated with low back pain in some studies (15–17), but not in others (18–22). Preventing progression requires diagnosis. Oblique views of the spine are the best of the standard radiographic views for detecting abnormalities within the pars interarticularis (23) that can be missed by AP and

lateral views alone (24), and so are indicated in those individuals with acute hyperextension injuries or those with repeated stress in extension, such as gymnasts, football lineman, ballet dancers, and volleyball players. Libson and colleagues recommend only imaging from L3–S1 to reduce overall radiation during oblique radiographs (10). Once diagnosis is made, treatment can be initiated. Others address spondylolysis through bracing (11,25) or surgery (26). Most individuals will respond to a program of physical therapy (9) that includes abdominal, gluteal, and paraspinal musculature strengthening to protect and properly support the posterior elements. The authors agree that oblique views should not be used routinely for evaluating patients with acute low back pain, yet we believe they are necessary in patients suspected of having spondylolysis. By identifying spondylolysis early and providing appropriate intervention at an earlier juncture, we may reduce the risk of progression to spondylolisthesis. The use of standing flexion and extension lateral views have not been addressed by the AHCPR, but may be of added value in assessing spondylolisthesis.

Deyo and Diehl recommend that lumbar radiographs be ordered for patients with neuromotor deficits, drug or alcohol abuse, a recent visit for the same problem without improvement after 4 weeks of symptoms, and legal claims for compensation (27). These criteria are in addition to those recommended by the AHCPR. Frazier and colleagues determined that the criteria proposed by Deyo and Diehl would actually have increased radiographs ordered as opposed to reducing usage (28).

To reduce the amount of unnecessary radiation and costs, the authors recommend that the clinician consider obtaining certain standard radiographic views based on the symptoms present (as discussed previously) or the suspected diagnosis, and correlating these with the physical findings (Tables 5–1 and 5–2) and known spinal biomechanics. This provides less of a "cookbook" for ordering films and requires that the clinician use his or her diagnostic skills before using diagnostic imaging techniques. This also assists the physician in designing an aggressive program of physical therapy. For spondylolisthesis, lateral views are sufficient (23,29). Coned view films of the lumbosacral spine and the L5–S1 junction in particular are not necessary (30). Oblique and lateral views will adequately demonstrate the pars interarticularis in cases of suspected spondylolysis (23). As suggested by Libson (10), obtaining views from L3–S1 may reduce irradiation to the individual. AP and lateral films alone will demonstrate spondylosis at the lateral, anterior, and posterior vertebral margins, show disc space narrowing and annular calcification, and provide basic information concerning involvement of the facets. Deyo and colleagues state that spinal stenosis may not be diagnosable by standard radiographs (2). AP and lateral views may not

**TABLE 5–1**
*Recommended Standard Radiographs Based on Suspected Diagnosis.*

| SUSPECTED CONDITION | RECOMMENDED STANDARD RADIOGRAPHS FOR DIAGNOSIS |
|---|---|
| Spondylolisthesis | Lateral View ± Standing Lateral Flexion and Extension Views |
| Spondylolysis | Oblique and Lateral Views |
| Spondylosis | Anteroposterior and Lateral Views |
| Facet Arthropathy | Oblique Views |
| Compression Fracture | Lateral View ± Anteroposterior View |
| Chance Fracture | Lateral View |
| Ankylosing Spondylitis or | Anteroposterior View ± Lateral View for |
| Other Inflammatory Arthropathy | Lumbosacral Spine |
| Metastatic Disease to Spine | Anteroposterior, Lateral, and Oblique Views |
| Osteoporosis | Lateral Views |

clearly diagnose stenosis but they can demonstrate those degenerative changes consistent with advanced osteoarthritic changes of the spine, including disc space narrowing and spondylosis, both of which have been correlated with the incidence of low back pain (31). Facet arthropathy is probably best detected on oblique views. Suspected compression fractures can best be identified on lateral views, but some additional information may be added by the AP view. Chance fractures are probably best identified on lateral radiographs (23). Ankylosing spondylitis can be detected by AP view alone (32), especially of the sacroiliac (SI) joint, and lateral views are not necessary unless more information is needed about the lumbosacral spine. Suspected metastatic disease to the spine should receive all views to assure that no malignancy is present. Osteoporosis can easily be diagnosed by lateral views once the disease is advanced enough for radiographic visualization.

Standard radiographs cost roughly $100 for one view and up to $300 for combined AP, lateral, and oblique views. Radiation exposure during an AP view ranges from approximately 200 to 400 mrad to the skin, 5 to 6 mrad to the testes, and 120 to 140 mrad to the ovaries. Lateral views subject the ovaries to 25 to 40 mrad and the testes to 1 to 2 mrad (33). Oblique view radiation dosage is probably up to double that of a standard AP view for the ovaries, with the testes again being subject to minimal doses (34). Clearly, radiographs are of greater concern for female patients, especially prior to the onset of menopause.

## BONE SCINTIGRAPHY

Bone scintigraphy, also known as bone scanning, is a form of imaging that uses a radioactive nuclide injected intra-

**TABLE 5–2**
*Recommended Standard Radiographs Based on Mechanism of Injury or Symptoms Present.*

| MECHANISM OF INJURY OR SYMPTOM | RECOMMENDED STANDARD RADIOGRAPHS FOR DIAGNOSIS |
|---|---|
| Axial load | Lateral View ± Anteroposterior View |
| Hyperextension—Acute or Repetitive | Oblique and Lateral Views |
| Deceleration | Lateral View |
| Pain with Oblique Extension | Oblique and Lateral Views |
| Pain with Forward Flexion | Lateral View |
| Pain with Palpation to Spine or Paravertebral Gutters | Anteroposterior, Lateral, and Oblique Views |

venously into the patient to identify areas of disease, primarily within the bone. Many varieties of radioactive substances have been used in the past, but the most commonly used compound used today is Technetium-99m ($^{99m}$Tc). Other radioactive compounds used include Strontium-85, Fluorine-18, and Indium-113 (35). After these radioactive compounds are in the patient's system, they can be detected by a gamma counter.

Technetium-99m combined with phosphorus may localize in bone, normal structures, soft tissue abnormalities, and the urinary system. Several factors affect localization within bone, the most important of which are bone blood flow, diffusion of tracer within the bone, and increased surface absorption to bone (35). Areas of increased intensity on scanning suggest increased bone turnover, and the reverse is true when activity is decreased (3). The usefulness of bone scintigraphy in low back pain is primarily to detect primary or metastatic bony tumors, primary or secondary metabolic bone disease, infection, inflammation, or stress reactions and fractures. Bone scintigraphy radiation is highest to the bladder, with the ovaries and testes encountering minimal doses of radiation (33). The cost of bone scintigraphy ranges from $300 to $500.

The AHCPR reviewed the use of bone scintigraphy for detection of stress fracture injuries of the pars interarticularis, inflammatory sacroiliitis, spine infections, metastatic cancer and other systemic disease, and symptomatic spondylolysis (1). The whole of the AHCPR guidelines established were based on the review of five articles (32,36–39). The main AHCPR guidelines recommend the use of bone scintigraphy when spinal tumor, infection, or occult fracture is suspected from "red flags" on medical history, physical examination, or suggestive laboratory data or standard radiographs (1). They found bone scan to be a moderately sensitive test in the detection of tumor, infection, or occult vertebral fracture in patients with low back pain, but not specific for diagnosis. Bone scan was also considered to be more sensitive than standard radiographic techniques. The AHCPR did not comment on the use of scintigraphy in patients with symptomatic spondylolysis.

Schütte and Park (38) retrospectively evaluated 176 patients with the complaint of low back pain to determine the value of bone scintigraphy in diagnosing systemic illness, and malignancy in particular. Thirty-eight patients had no previously known disease, and 138 had a previously diagnosed malignancy. In the group without previous disease, all those with negative radiographs and normal laboratory data (lactate dehydrogenase, alkaline phosphatase, white blood cell count, temperature, and erythrocyte sedimentation rate [ESR]) had normal bone scans (24/38—63 percent). Seven of 38 (18 percent) had normal radiographs, normal bone scans, but abnormal laboratory values and were found to have some type of systemic condition; 6 had elevations of the ESR. seven of 38 (18 percent) positive scans were found in patients with malignancy or infection, all of whom had elevations in the ESR. Seventy-four of 138 patients with a previous malignancy had positive scans (54 percent); 19 were from osteoporotic fractures and the other 55 from confirmed metastasis. They found a false-positive rate of 7 percent with no false-negatives. The authors concluded that bone scintigraphy is not likely to be positive in patients with "nonspecific" low back pain, normal radiographs, and normal laboratory data, especially ESR. Deyo and Diehl (40) also found that elevated ESR had a high correlation with incidence of cancer, especially if greater than or equal to 50 mm/hr. Schütte and Park determined that scans are very useful in detecting metastases in low back pain patients with previously diagnosed malignancies (38).

Whalen and colleagues (39) retrospectively evaluated the usefulness of indium-111 white blood cell ($^{111}$In WBC) scintigraphy in detecting vertebral osteomyelitis. A total of 22 patients had extensive workup for possible spinal infection, with 4 ultimately being negative based on open biopsy or aspirate culture. Indium-111 WBC scan specificity was 3/18 (17 percent), sensitivity was 4/4 (100 percent), positive predictive value was 3/3 (100 percent), and negative predictive value was 4/19 (21 percent). Twenty-one of the 22 patients also had $^{99m}$Tc scans, which revealed 82 percent (14/17) specificity, 0 percent (0/4) sensitivity, 78 percent (14/18) positive predictive value, and 0 percent (0/3) negative predictive value. Gallium scan was performed on four patients; one was falsely negative, and the remainder were correct in diagnosing infection. The authors concluded that $^{111}$In WBC scans had little to no usefulness in detecting vertebral osteomyelitis, and it is clear from this data that $^{99m}$Tc scans are superior to $^{111}$In WBC scans for detection of disease.

Miron and co-workers (37) evaluated the use of $^{99m}$Tc quantitative sacroiliac scintigraphy for the detection of sacroiliitis in 5 groups of patients: group A—90 controls (no history of low back pain); group B—18 with "active sacroiliitis" (ankylosing spondylitis—9, Crohn's associated sacroiliitis—4, psoriatic sacroiliitis—1); group C—4 with inactive chronic ankylosing spondylitis (no pain, sacroiliac joints ankylosed); group D—14 with "noninflammatory low back pain"; and group E—5 with rheumatoid arthritis without signs or symptoms of sacroiliitis. All groups underwent quantitative scanning to determine the sacroiliac index, SII (a measure of uptake at the sacroiliac joint), and all groups except group A underwent standard AP radiographs and computed tomography (CT) scans of the sacroiliac (SI) joints. Controls (group A) showed decreases in the SII with age (r = 0.503, p < 0.001). The control data served as the baseline counts for groups B, C, D, and E; an abnormal test was defined as any result outside of two standard deviations from age- and sex-specific norms. The results showed group B with eight abnormal and one "borderline" test, group C with no abnormal tests, group D with one abnormal test, and group E with one "borderline" test. Three of the eight positives in group A were HLA-B27 positive and had normal radiographs and CT scans. The one positive from group D and the one "borderline" from group E had normal radiographs and CT scans. None of the four patients under age 30 years with sacroiliitis had an abnormal scintigraphy scan. The authors concluded that quantitative sacroiliac scintigraphy was not a reliable screening method for detecting sacroiliitis as the test displayed low sensitivity (50 percent) even in the face of high specificity (93 percent). The authors also considered the test least useful for patients under the age of 30 years.

Esdaile and co-workers (32) also evaluated $^{99m}$Tc quantitative scintigraphy for detecting sacroiliitis in 34 patients with chronic active ankylosing spondylitis. Eighteen patients with nonarticular rheumatism were used as controls to establish a mean against which all patients were tested. No patient or control had side-to-side differences in activity. Eight of 12 (66 percent) patients with "probable ankylosing spondylitis" (New York grades 0, 1, and 2) and 10 of 22 (46 percent) with "definite ankylosing spondylitis" (grades 3 and 4) had abnormal scans. These authors concluded that quantitative sacral scintigraphy had low sensitivity (53 percent) and was not a useful technique for identifying inflammatory low back pain. The authors did note that overall counts of patients significantly decreased with anti-inflammatory treatment and that sequential scanning may help in following the course of disease. Additionally, they stated that patients in the early stages of disease (i.e., grades 0, 1, or 2) may be more readily detectable than those in the later stages (i.e., grades 3 or 4).

Lowe and colleagues (36) used $^{99m}$Tc scintigraphy to prospectively study 53 young (average age was 21 years old) military recruits with spondylolysis as documented by radiographs. Forty-three had persistent low back pain (8 with traumatic onset within last year, 15 with insidious onset within last year, and 23 with several years duration), and 7 were asymptomatic individuals imaged as part of a routine physical examination. Ten of 23 (43 percent) with symptoms less than 1 year, 3/23 (13 percent) with longstanding low back pain, and 0/7 asymptomatic individuals (0 percent) had positive scans. Fourteen of the 46 with back pain had spondylolisthesis, and 5/14 (36 percent) had positive scans. They concluded that bone scintigraphy is a useful tool for evaluating spondylolysis in a young individual to determine whether the injury is acute or not.

The AHCPR conclusions concerning these data appear reasonable, suggesting that $^{99m}$Tc bone scintigraphy can be helpful in searching for metastatic disease or vertebral osteomyelitis responsible for low back pain (1). From the papers reviewed, quantitative $^{99m}$Tc scintigraphy does not appear useful for screening for ankylosing spondylitis or other inflammatory spondylitides. This technique may, however, be useful in detecting early stages of disease or following the effect of anti-inflammatory therapy on the course of disease. In contrast to $^{99m}$Tc scintigraphy, $^{111}$In WBC scans had little to no usefulness in detecting vertebral osteomyelitis. The AHCPR did not discuss the study by Lowe and colleagues or its findings, but stated that bone scintigraphy can be helpful when searching for occult fractures.

An entity that requires comment is the pars interarticularis stress reaction. Deyo and colleagues state that bone scintigraphy is not indicated for patients with mechanical low back pain (2). It is not clear what diagnoses fall within this category, but we suspect that pars stress reactions would be one such condition. Spondylolysis is known to occur with greater frequency in individuals exposed to repeated lumbar extension stress (8,41), especially when combined with rotation (7,42). Early in the course of development of spondylolysis, the individual usually complains of a vague, diffuse low lumbar pain, especially with prolonged standing or overhead activities, as these can exaggerate lordosis and apply load on the posterior elements. In this early phase of disease, the pars interarticularis has not fully degenerated but has undergone a periosteal or "stress" reaction (12,42). On physical examination, the individual often exhibits localized pain with oblique extension to the affected side or on reverse straight leg raise. More often than not pain is present on palpation of the paravertebral gutter. Standard radiographs are often negative or may show a vertical oblique lucency or a sclerosis of the pars. This is when the authors find the triple-phase bone scan to be quite useful. Bone scan may detect the area with increased uptake when the injury is acute and not longstanding (43). A positive scan and a consistent history and physical examination would be suggestive of a recent stress injury to the pars interarticularis (Figure 5–7). Once the diagnosis of a stress reaction is made, treatment is directed toward reducing extension stress on the posterior spinal elements in the hopes of preventing a completed spondylolysis. In reference to the study discussed previously by Lowe and co-workers (36), it is not surprising that only 43 percent of those patients with "acute" low back injury (less than 1 year) demonstrated abnormal bone scans. As the injury becomes less acute, the chances of blood flow remaining increased to the area of fracture or stress reaction diminish; i.e., more acute injuries are more likely to be positive. Had Lowe and colleagues used more acutely injured patients, say 3–4 months post injury, there probably would have been a larger percentage of patients with abnormal scans. Another flaw of this study was that bone scintigraphy was being evaluated as a diagnostic tool for fracture identification. Diagnosis of spondylolysis was determined by standard radiographic examination, which cannot be considered the gold standard for diagnosis.

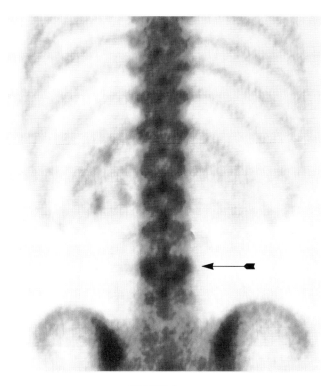

**FIGURE 5–7**

Spondylolysis as visualized by bone scintigraphy. This scan, taken from a 16–year-old gymnast, revealed recent bilateral spondylolysis at the L4 level *(arrow)*.

Athletes and other patients exposed to repetitive extension stresses or an acute hyperextension injury who develop low back pain may have spondylolysis or may be progressing toward spondylolysis. When examination is suggestive and standard radiographs are negative or equivocal, abnormal bone scintigraphy confirms the diagnosis of spondylolysis or stress reaction of the pars interarticularis. Once diagnosis is made, treatment can be initiated to halt progression from stress reaction to complete lysis or from lysis to spondylolisthesis

## ADVANCED IMAGING TECHNIQUES (MAGNETIC RESONANCE IMAGING, COMPUTED TOMOGRAPHY, COMPUTED TOMOGRAPHY–MYELOGRAPHY, AND MYELOGRAPHY)

The AHCPR guidelines reviewed literature on the efficacy of each of these imaging techniques for evaluating suspected nerve root compromise secondary to lumbar disc herniation and spinal stenosis. The guidelines also reviewed literature in asymptomatic individuals. Based on the reviews, the AHCPR made the following recommendations (1):

1. In the presence of symptoms suggestive of cauda equina syndrome, tumor, infection, fracture, or other space-occupying lesion causing spine compression or "major motor weakness," imaging studies such as MRI, computed tomography (CT), CT–myelography, or myelography should be ordered promptly in simultaneous consultation with a surgeon;
2. MRI with contrast is the imaging method of choice for individuals with low back pain and previous back surgery to distinguish herniated discs from scar tissue of previous operations; and
3. CT and MRI scan cuts should be no wider than 0.5 cm and should be parallel to the vertebral endplates, and scanner strength should be at least 0.5 Tesla or greater.

Additionally, the AHCPR made the statement that these imaging techniques are generally only used for patients who present with either (1):

1. Back-related leg symptoms and clinically specific, detectable nerve root compromise or a history of neurogenic claudication and other findings suggesting spinal stenosis with symptoms severe enough to consider surgical intervention; or
2. Clinical examination findings or other test results suggesting other serious conditions affecting the spine (such as cauda equina syndrome, spinal fracture, infection, tumor, or other mass lesions or defects).

The authors generally agree with the recommendations set forth by the AHCPR, but will attempt to further elaborate. We also discuss several other situations not addressed by the AHCPR in which these imaging techniques can be useful. Each section also addresses the efficacy studies of these imaging techniques reviewed by the AHCPR and other studies the authors considered useful, but were not reviewed for the guidelines. This section also provides suggestions as to other situations in which these imaging techniques will further assist in patient management.

It is not clear what is meant by "major motor weakness" or "symptoms severe enough to consider surgical intervention," and we cannot therefore directly address the AHCPR recommendations to obtain advanced imaging studies if these features are present. The authors believe that these studies should primarily be reserved for clinical situations in which either:

1. Nonoperative/conservative management will be altered based on the result(s);

2. There is a suspicion of tumor, fracture, or infection undiagnosed by standard radiographs; or
3. When considering an invasive procedure, such as an injection (e.g., epidural or facet) or surgery.

Advanced imaging can aid the clinician in deciding which form of conservative therapy should be provided to the patient. An example would be a case in which an athlete presents with symptoms of low back pain with radiation to the lower extremity. The history and physical exam usually differentiate a disc herniation and an acute spondylolysis with referred pain, but this is not always the case. As the management of this individual will differ significantly, it is important to have a fairly definitive diagnosis before initiating therapy, as treatment for a disc herniation can aggravate symptoms of spondylolysis. When used properly, MRI and other advanced imaging studies can help differentiate between the two diagnoses, and appropriate conservative intervention can be initiated. A similar scenario would be one in which an individual presents with symptoms of back pain exacerbated by extension. This individual could have a spondylolysis or a facet syndrome. Osteopathic manipulation, such as high velocity, low amplitude thrust techniques, would be contraindicated in an individual with a suspected fracture but not in the case of a facet syndrome. Again, advanced imaging would detect the spondylolysis and manipulation would be deferred.

Advanced imaging in cases of suspected tumor, fracture, or infection is clearly indicated when standard radiographs are negative or equivocal. Further discussion is provided in the respective sections concerning which imaging study will best diagnose tumor, infection, or fracture.

Cauda equina syndrome (CES) is a condition in which the nerve routes are bilaterally affected somewhere at or beyond the second lumbar (L2) vertebra. This is the level at which the spinal cord ends and the nerve roots that have not exited the spinal canal travel together for a short distance before leaving the canal at the appropriate spinal level. CES presents with lower motor neuron dysfunction, i.e., either decreased strength, tone, and reflexes or fasciculations of the muscle. A condition similar to CES is the conus medularis syndrome (CMS), a condition in which the last few levels of the spinal cord and the descending roots may be simultaneously affected within the spinal canal. Symptoms and signs of CMS are a mixture of lower motor neuron and upper motor neuron findings. Upper motor neuron findings include increased muscle tone and reflexes, weakness, and spasticity. In both CES and CMS, surgery is recommended to reduce neurologic deficit. In either case, advanced imaging is recommended to view the subject's spine and soft tissue anatomy and detect lesions of either bone or soft tissue that are compressive to the neural elements at either

the cauda or conus level. Advanced imaging studies can also assist in surgical planning for a disc herniation or spinal stenosis, as they will define the anatomy more clearly and can optimize surgical outcome. Similarly, when considering an epidural or facet injection, it is important to ascertain the true diagnosis, as treatment will again differ based on the image findings. An example would be a subject with back pain exacerbated by extension being considered for a facet injection. If the imaging study revealed a spondylolysis at the level in question, the facet injection would not be performed.

The AHCPR guidelines do not address when *not* to use advanced imaging techniques. Herzog and co-workers (44) point out that MRI has been criticized for having too many false-positives leading to unnecessary surgeries. Another concern stems from a recent trend whereby advanced imaging has been used instead of the diagnostic skills of the physician and have been ordered by medical staff who are unclear of the proper use of this imaging tool. While it is true that these techniques may reveal abnormalities not associated with morbidity, it is up to the clinician to use his/her diagnostic skills to determine which of these findings is responsible for disease. Herzog and colleagues further state that [MRI] false-positives are not what result in unwarranted surgeries, but the improper application of the results that is responsible (44). The authors believe that advanced imaging should only be ordered by licensed physicians who clearly understand the purpose of the test and can use it judiciously. Otherwise a consultation should be made to a physician who is capable of making such decisions. This will significantly reduce the cost, as many unnecessary scans will be avoided.

Individuals with acute radiculopathy commonly present with pain radiating from the back or hip into the buttock or leg. Frequently, there is mild neurologic weakness, with strength in affected muscles ranging from 4+/5 to 5–/5, and there may be associated numbness or tingling. There may be decreased reflexes or loss of sensation to pin-prick testing. Initially, conservative management will be guided by the clinical evaluation, making advanced imaging unnecessary. For the small percentage of patients who do not respond to this regimen (45), advanced imaging should be considered only if patient management will be altered by the results.

## MAGNETIC RESONANCE IMAGERY

The magnetic resonance image (MRI) is produced by a technique that uses a powerful magnet, usually on the order of producing a field of 1.0–1.5 Tesla, to pass radio waves in very short pulses through the patient (3). MRI images the proton (H+), which is highly abundant in tissue containing water, proteins, and lipids. When the proton is exposed to a magnetic field, as occurs during an MRI, its minute magnetic field aligns itself with respect to the magnetic field of the MRI. The field of the hydrogen ion can align with or opposite that of the MRI. At certain applied frequencies, the H+ will absorb energy and reverse its direction. The absorbed energy is released when the protons "relax." The rate at which this occurs depends on the relaxation time of the different tissues, and therefore produces signals of varying intensity and contrast (46).

MRI allows imaging of the body in almost any plane desired without the use of ionizing radiation (4), which makes this the imaging method of choice for pregnant women. Additionally, as the quality of magnetic resonance imagery improves, so does the contrasting ability, making MRI the best musculoskeletal imaging method currently available for detecting very minute abnormalities on the order of several millimeters in size. MRI scans are primarily used to examine the neuromusculoskeletal axis in all regions of the body and have gained acceptance as the best noninvasive imaging technique currently available for examining the soft tissue and neural elements of the spine (Figures 5–8 and 5–9). MRI and similar imaging techniques are often reserved for those patients with neurologic deficits or intractable pain that are considered to be amenable to surgery. The major drawbacks to MRI are the cost (around $800–$1,500 per scan), the long time required for scanning (around 30–45 minutes per scan), the small scanner space (which has led to claustrophobia), the patient weight maximum (around 250–300 pounds), the inability to image those patients with ferrometallic implants and the variability of image quality between centers.

The following efficacy studies are those reviewed and used by the AHCPR for inclusion in their guidelines for detecting suspected spinal stenosis and nerve root compression secondary to lumbar disc herniation. Jackson and colleagues (47) compared MRI (1.5 Tesla), CT, myelography, and CT–myelography for detecting lumbar disc herniations as determined at surgery. The study reports no statistically significant differences between methods for rates of accuracy, false-positive tests, sensitivity, or specificity. There was a statistically lower false-negative test rate for MRI and CT–myelography. Masaryk and colleagues (48) prospectively assessed the ability of MRI (0.6 or 1.5 Tesla) and CT–myelography to detect lumbar disc sequestration as determined at surgery. They found 89 percent sensitivity, 82 percent specificity, and 85 percent accuracy for MRI, and 89 percent sensitivity, 45 percent specificity, and 65 percent accuracy for CT–myelography in differentiating disc sequestration from other forms of disc herniation. This study was flawed primarily by its small numbers (n = 20), and no statement is made whether or not the differences are statistically significant between groups.

Szypryt and colleagues (49) prospectively compared the accuracy of MRI (0.15 Tesla) and myelography for

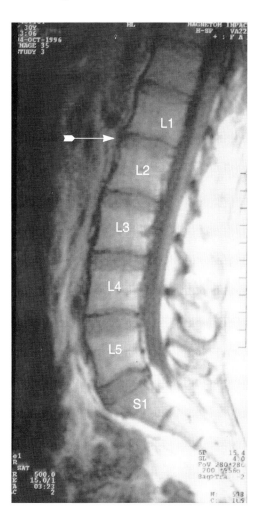

**FIGURE 5–8**

Normal T1–weighted magnetic resonance image in a 30-year-old male. This magnetic resonance image shows normal vertebral body and disc space height and normal disc water content. There is no evidence of disc bulging. There is a small amount of anterior osteophyte presence from the inferior vertebral endplate of L1 *(arrow)*.

diagnosing herniated discs as compared to diagnosis at surgery. Accuracy for MRI and myelography were 88 percent and 75 percent, respectively. This study was primarily flawed by the weak magnetic strength of the MRI.

Bischoff and colleagues (50) compared CT–myelography, MRI (1.5 Tesla), and myelography in 57 patients. Results of the scans were compared to surgical diagnosis. CT–myelogram was the most accurate (76 percent) and most sensitive (78 percent) for detecting a herniated disc, while myelography was the most specific (89 percent). MRI and CT–myelography were equally accurate (85 percent) and sensitive (87 percent) for diagnosing

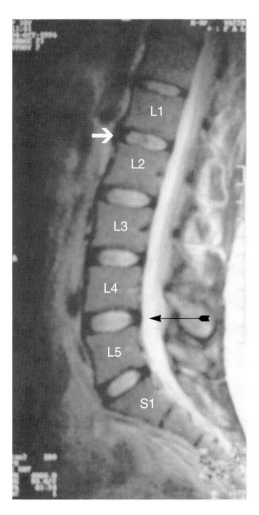

**FIGURE 5–9**

Normal T2–weighted magnetic resonance image in a 30-year-old male. This magnetic resonance image is of the same patient shown in Figure 5–8. Again, there is normal vertebral body and disc space height and normal disc water content. There is no evidence of disc bulging. There is a small amount of anterior osteophyte presence from the inferior vertebral endplate of L1 *(large arrow)*. Several free nerve roots can also be visualized on this scan *(small arrows)*.

spinal stenosis, while myelography was the most specific (89 percent). Sensitivity, specificity, and accuracy values were fairly similar for the MRI, CT–myelogram, and myelogram groups, and no group demonstrated a statistically significant difference over another. No major flaws were identified in this study.

A meta-analysis by Kent and colleagues (51) reviewed the ability of CT, MRI, and myelography to identify lumbar spinal stenosis. They reviewed 116 articles but found only 14 acceptable for review. All 14 were

thought to have significant methodological flaws. The AHCPR used this analysis to formulate recommendations concerning imaging of spinal stenosis. The following studies are those included as part of the meta-analysis where magnetic resonance imaging was concerned. The articles concerning the other imaging techniques are discussed in the appropriate sections.

Modic and colleagues (52) prospectively examined the ability of MRI (0.6 Tesla), CT scan, and myelography to detect herniated disc or spinal stenosis. Patients received MRI and CT and/or myelography. The results were blindly compared to the surgical reports for presence or absence of spinal stenosis or disc herniation. The authors found high agreement between MRI, CT, and myelography, regardless of surgical findings. Compared to surgical findings, there was 82.3 percent, 82 percent, and 71.4 percent agreement with CT, MRI, and myelography, respectively. If MRI and CT were used together, the agreement rate increased to 92.5 percent, whereas combined results of CT and myelogram resulted in 89.4 percent agreement with surgical findings. From the data, it does not appear that any of the imaging techniques resulted in false-positives, e.g., if a scan showed stenosis but a herniation was present at surgery, this was still considered a positive diagnosis in that these patients would have undergone surgery regardless of the ultimate diagnosis. The same rationale was applied if herniation was detected by scanning but stenosis was present at surgery.

Schnebel and colleagues (53) retrospectively reviewed the ability of MRI (1.5 Tesla) scans and CT–myelography to identify spinal stenosis and disc degeneration. Eighteen of the 41 patients in the study had surgical confirmation. The authors found 96.6 percent agreement between MRI and CT–myelogram for detecting these conditions. It is not clear from the data whether MRI or CT–myelogram correctly identified the lesions in those patients undergoing surgery, representing a significant flaw in the reporting of the data from this study.

Epstein and colleagues (54) reviewed data from 60 patients with far lateral lumbar disc herniations who underwent MRI (no strength given), CT, myelogram, and/or CT–myelogram to determine the ability of these tests to identify concomitant lateral recess spinal stenosis. The authors concluded that myelogram and CT–myelogram had the best ability to detect concomitant disc herniation and recess stenosis. The authors also stated that the type of surgery performed in these patients was altered (i.e., had more extensive decompression) by the identification of recess stenosis identified by myelogram and CT–myelogram. It is not clearly stated whether all patients underwent all imaging tests or what criteria were used to determine the ability of a test to detect an abnormality.

Modic and colleagues (55) studied 45 low back pain patients and 20 controls with either a 0.15 Tesla magnet, 0.6 Tesla magnet, or both. It is unclear from the methods how patients were randomized and studied, and it is also unclear how comparisons were made with CT and/or myelogram or surgery/autopsy. The authors concluded that MRI was the most sensitive technique for identifying disc degeneration and disc space infection compared to standard radiographs, CT scans, or myelograms. They also concluded that disc herniation, canal stenosis, and (postsurgical) scarring were equally visualized by all methods. This study was seriously flawed by lack of apparent blinding, randomization, and data presentation. The authors of the meta-analysis concluded that sensitivity for detecting spinal stenosis ranged from 0.80 to 0.97 for MRI, from 0.70 to 1.0 for CT, and from 0.67 to 0.78 for myelography. The studies reviewed in the meta-analysis cannot be used to make any clear statement about the accuracy of MRI for spinal stenosis.

One study not reviewed by the AHCPR was that by Janssen and colleagues (56), who retrospectively compared preoperative MRI (1.5 Tesla), CT–myelography, and myelography in 180 patients suspected of lumbar disc disease (duration of symptoms is not presented). An unspecified number of patients were excluded from the study if they had previous lumbar spine surgery or spinal stenosis. Sixty patients underwent surgery for disc disease at 102 levels. The authors reported accuracy rates of 96 percent (98/102) for MRI, 81 percent (82/102) for myelography, and 57 percent (58/102) for CT–myelography. Sensitivity and specificity were 96 percent and 97 percent, respectively, for MRI, with CT–myelography resulting in 49 percent and 74 percent, respectively. Myelography sensitivity (81 percent) and specificity (79 percent) were intermediate compared to MRI and CT–myelography. The authors concluded that MRI was the imaging technique of choice. The major flaws of this study include the fact that the exclusion criteria are not clearly defined, duration of patient symptoms are not presented, and there is no statement about blinding of the radiologic review of films. As this was a retrospective study, the potential for bias is therefore questioned. The sensitivity and specificity obtained for CT–myelogram is one of the lowest of the studies reviewed by the authors, so the technique used at this facility may need refinement.

Based on the literature reviewed on disc herniation, it appears that CT–myelogram and MRI (Figures 5–10 to 5–12) have slightly better accuracy in detecting herniation than CT (Figure 5–13) or myelogram (Figure 5–14). Even though CT–myelogram and MRI have similar accuracy for diagnosing disc herniation, one should probably consider ordering an MRI as the initial imaging technique, as there is no radiation exposure and no known ill effects. The studies clearly depict MRI as the best technique for visualizing disc degeneration. Accuracy of detection of spinal stenosis by MRI cannot be assessed from the reviewed data. According to the reviewed literature, CT scan and CT–myelography probably have a slight advantage over MRI in detection of spinal stenosis (Figures 5–15 to 5–19). The significant problem with interpreting these data is that MRI magnet strength in several studies was less than 1.0 Tesla and would be considered dramatically inferior to the current imaging capabilities of today's scanners (1.0–1.5 Tesla). These studies also did not consider the advent of three-dimensional reconstructions for computed topography, which are discussed in the section on CT and CT–myelography. In general, when considering an imaging technique, the clear advantage of MRI over other imaging techniques is that it is noninvasive and uses no ionizing radiation or dyes.

The AHCPR recommends an MRI with contrast to evaluate low back pain patients who have had previous surgery, but provide no literature to support their view. Literature on this subject is somewhat scarce, but the results appear to be mixed.

Bernard (57) compared results of enhanced MRI (0.5 Tesla in 29 patients and 1.5 Tesla in 4 others) and CT-discography in low back pain patients who had undergone previous back surgery. The study was designed to compare the ability of these imaging techniques to differentiate between recurrent disc herniation and scar tissue as documented at surgery. Subjects were scanned first with gadolinium-enhanced MRI. If the MRI revealed a mass effect against the neural elements on the symptomatic side at the same level as the previous surgery, the subject underwent CT-discography. Only those subjects with positive discograms (i.e., reproduction of pain character) were referred for surgical confirmation of findings. Enhanced MRI had 72 percent sensitivity, 55 percent specificity, and 67 percent accuracy, whereas CT-discography had 74 percent sensitivity, 60 percent specificity, and 70 percent accuracy for detecting recurrent disc herniations versus scar tissue. This study was primarily flawed by the fact that subjects were removed from further study if no findings were present on the MRI. This raises the possibility of excluding subjects who were falsely determined as negative for scar tissue or recurrent herniation. Additionally, low MRI magnet strength will have decreased resolution, and the eventual outcome of the study.

Tullberg, Grane, Rydberg, and Isacson (58) compared the postoperative changes visible one year after surgery by gadolinium-enhanced MRI (1.0 Tesla) and contrast-enhanced CT scans. The authors found contrast-enhanced CT to demonstrate more extensive scar tissue, but gadolinium-enhanced MRI better delineated the nerve roots and was able to identify root thickening and displacement, not visible by CT. CT and MRI were found to equally identify disc herniations and foraminal stenosis. This study did not compare the findings to surgery, and therefore the conclusions cannot be fully supported.

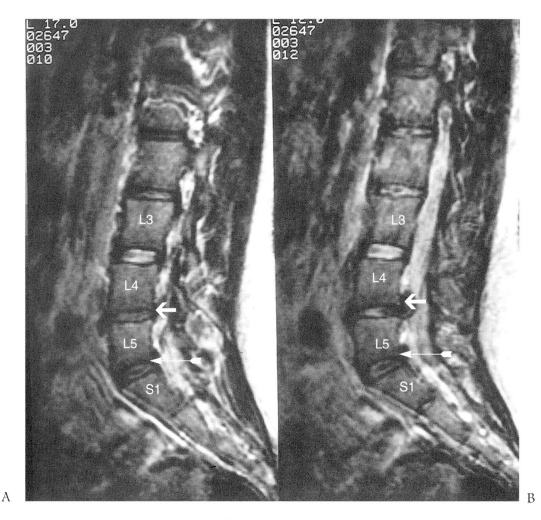

**FIGURES 5–10A, B**

Sagittal T2–weighted magnetic resonance image with large disc herniations. These scans show large disc herniations at the L4–5 *(large arrow)* and L5–S1 *(small arrow)* levels. Figure 5–10A is more left of the midline than is Figure 5–10B, indicating these herniations to be paracentral to the left at both levels. Note the loss of signal intensity from the disc material that has been extruded, signifying a loss of water content and degeneration of the disc material.

Albeck, Wagner, and Knudsen (59) prospectively evaluated contrast-enhanced CT and gadolinium-enhanced MRI (0.3 Tesla) in patients with previous operations for lumbar disc herniation who had recurrent symptoms. Twenty-nine patients were selected based on the clinical signs and symptoms (not specified) and myelography or standard CT scan. All patients underwent CT and MRI imaging with and without contrast material preoperatively. Neuroradiologists unaware of the surgical findings evaluated the studies on two separate occasions. Unenhanced CT and MRI images were evaluated separately, followed by comparison of the contrast-enhanced scans together. Disc pathology and amount of scar tissue were quantified on separate ordinal scales. Disc pathology was defined as definite herniation, probable herniation, possible herniation, probably not a herniation, or definitely not a herniation. Scar tissue was graded as low, moderate, or high amounts. Surgical findings were not classified in a similar manner, only whether or not a herniation was identified intraoperatively. The authors found that the addition of contrast statistically improved the ability of only CT to detect scar tissue. The authors state that there was "enhancement" of scar tissue on enhanced MRI studies as compared to nonenhanced images, but there was not a statistically significant increase in the numbers of scans identified as having increased scar tis-

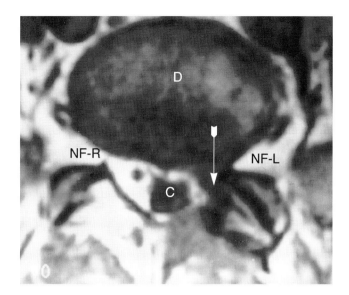

**FIGURE 5–11**

Axial T2–weighted magnetic resonance image with large disc herniation. Magnetic resonance image taken through the disc (D). Note the large left herniation of disc material *(arrow)* into the left neural foramen (NF-L). The right neural foramen is patent (NF-R). There is no evidence of compression of the central canal (C).

sue. The authors report that only the enhanced imaging techniques would have decreased the number of patients being wrongfully operated on. Intraobserver kappa values were 0.53 for enhanced and unenhanced MRI, 0.58 for contrast-enhanced CT, and 0.76 for unenhanced CT images. The authors concluded that gadolinium-enhanced MRI should be used as the primary examination in patients suspected of recurrent disc herniation. This study and its conclusions were flawed by several factors: (1) the intraobserver ratios obtained by the neuroradiologists were well below acceptable; (2) the raw data comparing imaging techniques are not presented; (3) the image find-

ings were not directly compared to the surgical findings; and (4) there are no data presented comparing enhanced MRI and CT scans head-to-head. Based on these errors, the conclusions of this study cannot be supported.

The number and quality of studies comparing post-operative CT-discography or contrast-enhanced CT to gadolinium-enhanced MRI in patients with recurrent back pain remains limited. No clear conclusion can be made from the currently available literature, and more studies in this area are clearly needed. It is the authors' opinion that either contrast-enhanced CT or MRI imaging should be used as opposed to CT-discography for this patient

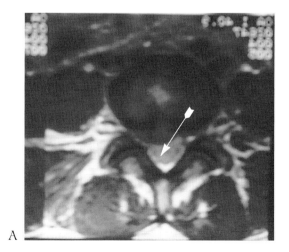

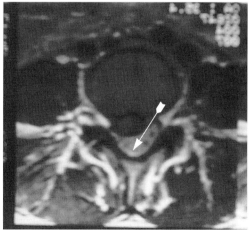

A                                                                                           B

**FIGURES 5–12 A,B**

Axial T2–weighted magnetic resonance image with large disc herniation. Magnetic resonance image is taken through disc and vertebral body in Figure 5–12A. There is clear herniation *(arrow)* compressing the right neural foramen and nerve root. The scan in Figure 5–12B is cut through the disc. There is a large extrusion compressing the central canal *(arrow)*.

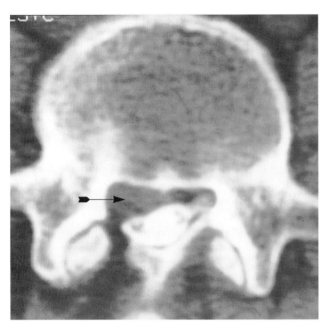

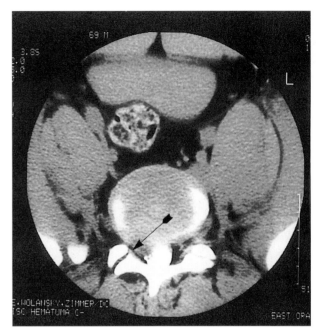

A                           **FIGURES 5–13 A,B**                           B

Computed tomography scans with disc herniations. Both scans reveal right disc herniations. Figure 5–13A shows a large right-sided herniation *(arrow)*. There is also evidence of central canal compression. Figure 5–13B also shows a large right disc herniation, but the scan cannot clearly delineate canal or nerve root compromise. As compared to the magnetic resonance imaging scans in Figures 5–10, 5–11, and 5–12, the computed tomography scans have much lower resolution for disc herniation.

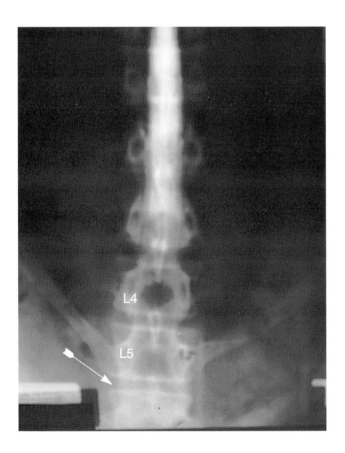

**FIGURE 5–14**

Myelogram with large disc herniation. Myelogram in antero-posterior projection shows complete blockage of contrast at the L5–S1 level, presumably secondary to a large disc herniation at that level *(arrow)*.

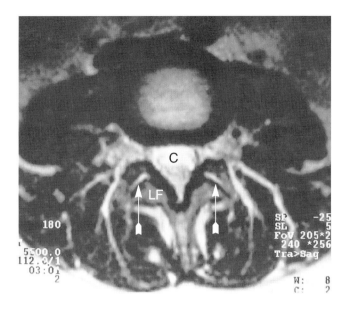

**FIGURE 5–15**

Magnetic resonance image with early degenerative facet changes. This scan displays early thickening of the facets, bilaterally *(small arrows)*, with moderate thickening and buckling of the ligamentum flavum (LF). The central canal (C) caliber is fairly well maintained.

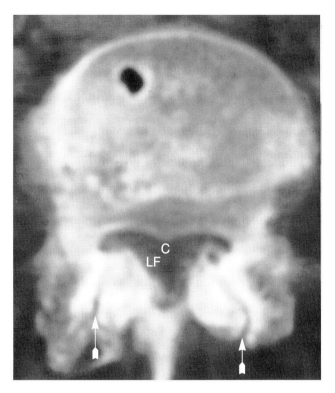

**FIGURE 5–16**

Computed tomography scan of spinal stenosis. This computed tomography scan reveals extensive facet hypertrophy *(small arrows)* and osteophytosis. The caliber of the central canal (C) is reduced by thickening of the ligamentum flavum (LF).

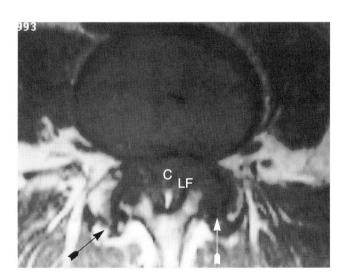

**FIGURE 5–17**

Magnetic resonance image of spinal stenosis. This magnetic resonance scan reveals extensive facet hypertrophy (*small arrows*) and osteophytosis. The caliber of the central canal (C) is reduced by thickening of the ligamentum flavum (LF).

population, because CT-discography is an invasive procedure, and has potentially significant risks. It should be made clear that the history and physical examination will remain the mainstay of diagnosis in this special patient population; imaging studies should be reserved for those situations previously described.

MRI can show minute details once thought to be present only in abnormal populations. It is now known that MRI shows abnormalities in both symptomatic and control populations (60–66), and it is up to the physician to determine when the abnormalities present on imaging are responsible for the patient's symptoms. The physician should be aware of the literature surrounding MRI in asymptomatic subjects, should be able to apply this knowledge to the low back pain patient, and should know when the MRI results are not consistent with the patient's physical exam.

The AHCPR reviewed four articles regarding imaging of asymptomatic patients (65–68), while two others discussed here were not reviewed by the AHCPR (62,63). MRI has shown nonstatistical differences in the number and intensity of changes between low back pain patients

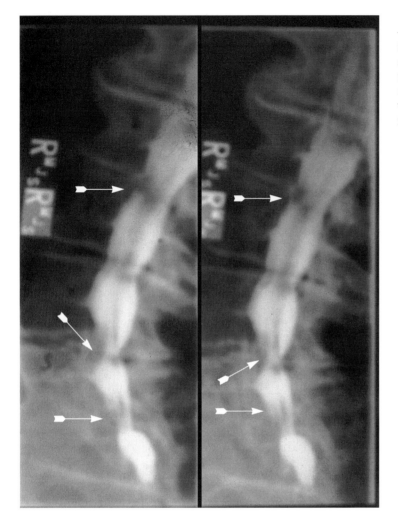

FIGURE 5–18

Standard myelogram with moderately severe spinal stenosis. This figure shows a myelogram taken from the anteroposterior projection. There is evidence of multiple areas of blockage to contrast flow *(arrows)*, with central canal caliber being shown to be very narrow secondary to degenerative changes.

and control groups in the study by Buirski and Silberstein (61) (no strength of MRI scan given), but others have shown that changes are more likely to be associated with low back pain (63,67). Weinreb and colleagues reviewed MRI in asymptomatic nonpregnant and pregnant groups and found nonstatistical differences in the number of bulges and herniations between groups (68). This study used relatively small group sizes (45 and 41, respectively), but yielded a very high p value (0.8). Another flaw of this study was that it did not state what percentage of pregnant women currently had back pain, and therefore did not state which percentage of this subgroup had abnormal scans. Powell and colleagues (66) imaged 302 asymptomatic women, aged 16 to 80 years, 82 pregnant patients, and 56 age-matched nulliparous women for comparison to the pregnant patients with MRI (0.15 Tesla). From the control population, they found an increase in the number of degenerated lumbar discs as the subject's age increased, rising from 6 percent in the group under 20 years to 79 percent in those over age 60 years.

The authors state that over one-third of the controls aged 21 to 40 years had "abnormal discs." They found no increase in the number of bulged or degenerated discs between the pregnant women and their nulliparous controls. Boden and colleagues (65) found 20 percent of asymptomatic controls under the age of 60 years to have a herniated disc and one control had spinal stenosis. Over the age of 60 years, the rate of herniated discs increased to 36 percent and 21 percent had spinal stenosis. Based on these studies, bulging and degenerated discs are common findings in asymptomatic individuals. For this reason, MRI should not be routinely ordered for low back pain, as there is the potential for the patient to unjustly receive a diagnosis of a "herniated disc" when it is merely an incidental finding on imaging.

MRI has been shown to be an accurate and sensitive imaging technique for detecting sequestered lumbar intervertebral disc fragments from other forms of herniations and was slightly better than CT–myelography in this capability (48). The MRI can therefore provide infor-

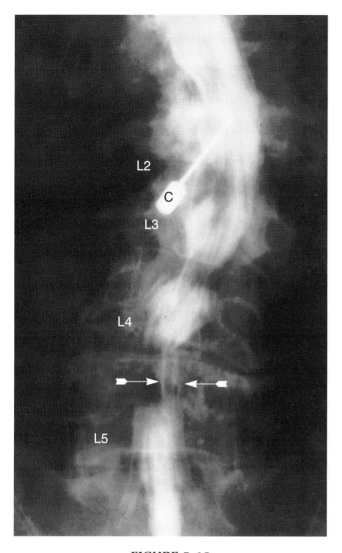

**FIGURE 5–19**

Standard myelogram with severe spinal stenosis. This figure shows a myelogram taken from the anteroposterior projection. The catheter (C) is located at the superior aspect of the L2 vertebra. There is evidence of multiple areas of blockage to contrast flow (*small arrows*), and especially blockage of flow and loss of nerve root filling at the L5 and S1 levels *(dark area—large arrow)*.

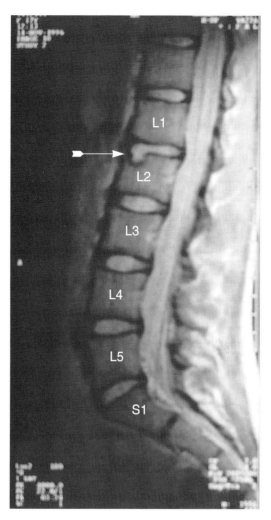

**FIGURE 5–20**

Magnetic resonance image of Schmorl's node. Sagittal magnetic resonance image showing Schmorl's node of superior vertebral end plate of L2 (*arrow*). Note that the vertebral body has no evidence of invasive mass, such as edema or penetration of the anterior vertebral body.

mation on the lumbar spine otherwise unavailable. As sequestered discs are infrequently found in asymptomatic controls and more commonly found in symptomatic low back pain patients (60), the presence of a sequestered disc is more likely to be responsible for producing low back pain. If nonoperative management fails to provide relief in a person with low back pain and subsequent magnetic resonance imaging reveals a sequestered disc, operative intervention would be considered appropriate at that

juncture and should target the affected disc. Additionally, when high-intensity zones (high signal intensity located in the posterior annulus fibrosus distinctly separate from the nucleus pulposus and brighter than the nucleus on T2–weighted images) are present in association with a disc herniation, they are more likely to be associated with symptoms in at least the lumbar (69,70) and cervical spine areas (71). As with sequestered discs, if a herniation has a high-intensity zone and does not respond to nonoperative management, surgical intervention should be considered.

Schmorl's nodes (disc herniation through a vertebral endplate) are common findings in both symptomatic and asymptomatic individuals (19) and may even be more common in those without low back pain (21). MRI findings of inflammation and edema within the vertebral body have been correlated with the presence of symptomatic Schmorl's nodes (61). In contrast to sequestered herniated discs, the presence of a symptomatic Schmorl's node thought to be responsible for low back pain will preclude surgical intervention (Figure 5–20).

Spondylolysis is another condition in which MRI may be useful, as one study has shown MRI to be able to detect changes in the pars interarticularis before both standard radiography and computed tomography (72). Jinkins and colleagues (41) report that foraminal encroachment by spondylolisthesis is easily visualized on MRI, making it useful when radiculopathic symptoms are present in association with posterior element dysfunction.

MRI can also be helpful when searching for tumor or infection. MRI has very high resolution, often allowing small tumors and areas of infection to be easily visualized. Unger (73) reports that MRI is more sensitive (92 percent versus 82 percent) and specific (96 percent versus 65 percent) than bone scintigraphy for detecting acute osteomyelitis.

According to Kraemer (74), certain MRI features have been associated with better nonoperative prognosis for disc herniation, including high signal intensity, supradiscal or infradiscal migration, a wide canal, and a herniation size smaller than one-third of the spinal canal. The authors were unable to find literature to further support or refute this statement. If surgery is being considered for a patient with a disc herniation and several of these findings are present on an MRI at the area of interest, the clinician may consider an aggressive nonoperative approach instead of surgery.

## COMPUTED TOMOGRAPHY

Computed tomography (CT) scans are radiographic images similar to standard radiographs. The difference between CT scans and standard radiographs is that CT scans use multiple projections to view the same area in space to produce an image, whereas radiographs use only one. Tomography is a form of standard radiograph where an image is recorded from one plane (or "slice") of the patient's body. Standard tomograms are produced by using two or more projections of the x-ray beam focused on one object in space. This requires moving the x-ray tube and film to different locations, each time focusing the beam on the desired object of study. Surrounding objects remain superimposed and blurred, while the object of interest becomes more clearly visible. Computed

tomography similarly uses multiple projections in one plane, this time finely focused on a very small area of tissue. The x-ray tube rotates about the patient while electronic detection plates are situated directly opposite the beam collecting information. These plates are comprised of crystal photo-multiplier tubes or contain compressed gases such as Xenon and are much more sensitive to changes than are standard radiograph films. As with standard radiographs, the amount of radiation received by the plates and recorded depends on the density of the object in study; objects with greater density allow less radiation to penetrate, and objects therefore appear white. Less dense objects allow "exposure" of the plates, leading to darker images. As the information is received by the detection plates, it is relayed to a computer, which is able to calculate density measurements for all areas imaged in the two-dimensional arrangement. A composite is formed, and the product is an axial image with high resolution, without the blurring of nearby objects, as is associated with standard tomograms. X-ray dose to the ovaries ranges from 1 to 2 rads and is probably negligible; dose for the testes per slice imaged varies from one to four rads, which is similar to one view of a standard radiograph (3). Resolution is inversely related to the slice thickness imaged and can deteriorate with subject movement. When a metal object is present in or on the patient, it can cast a large shadow across an image and obstruct objects of interest. This "metal artifact" can be a significant problem.

CT scans are most commonly used to evaluate acute intracranial hemorrhage, bony anatomy, the abdomen and pelvis (mostly searching for tumors or lymph node abnormalities), and, until the advent of magnetic resonance imagery, the spine and associated soft tissues. CT remains the method of choice for imaging patients who weigh too much for an MRI scanner and for those who have certain metallic implants.

The following efficacy studies are those reviewed and used by the AHCPR for inclusion in their guidelines for detecting suspected spinal stenosis and nerve root compression secondary to lumbar disc herniation. The AHCPR used the articles reviewed in a meta-analysis by Kent and colleagues (51) to determine the efficacy of CT in diagnosing spinal stenosis and to establish their guidelines (75–80). Schönström and colleagues (80) evaluated 55 patients with suspected spinal stenosis, but only included 24 with central canal stenosis who had "satisfactory CT scans." Each patient had stenosis confirmed by surgery. The authors found a statistically significant difference between 13 controls and 24 stenosis patients with respect to the mean transverse area of the dural sac. Twenty-two of 24 stenotic patients had the narrowest diameter at the level of the facet joints. The authors also found that the ligamentum flavum was a major cause of stenosis in 10 of 24 patients, but they do not state how this was determined (i.e., by surgery or CT scan).

Bolender and colleagues (79) studied 30 normals and 24 spinal stenosis patients (confirmed by surgery) with CT scan to compare dural sac measurements. They also compared CT scans and myelograms in 55 patients with surgically confirmed spinal stenosis. All spinal stenosis patients had dural sac measurements less than 150 mm², while the controls had a mean measurement of 180 mm². They also found that the CT anteroposterior spinal canal measurements from stenosis patients did not correlate with surgical diagnosis or with myelogram findings, which correctly identified stenosis in all but two patients. Dural sac area, however, was more accurate, missing correct diagnosis in only one patient. Both studies concluded that dural sac measurement is the most accurate parameter for diagnosing spinal stenosis by CT scan. Bolender and colleagues concluded that using dural sac measurement is as accurate as myelogram for diagnosing spinal stenosis by CT scan.

Slebus and colleagues (77) obtained CT and myelography on 109 patients with surgery-confirmed spinal stenosis or disc herniation. They found CT to have a specificity of 84 percent and a sensitivity of 88 percent, with myelogram having a specificity of 86 percent and a sensitivity of 81 percent. Stockley and colleagues (75) evaluated the accuracy of CT and myelogram to detect lumbar root encroachment as documented by surgery. The data revealed a correct diagnosis by CT scan in 75 percent (18/24) of patients and a correct diagnosis by myelogram in 56 percent (23/41).

Bell and colleagues (78) compared CT and myelography findings to those determined at surgery for herniated discs and spinal stenosis. Myelography was found to be more accurate than CT scan for both diagnoses (67 percent versus 50 percent for stenosis, and 83 percent versus 72 percent for disc herniation).

Herkowitz and colleagues (76) evaluated the usefulness of CT scanning in 32 patients with blockage on lumbar myelogram. The CT scan demonstrated abnormalities caudad to the level of blockage in 19 patients, but it is unclear from the data presentation what percentage of surgeries were altered based on this information.

The following studies were not reviewed by the meta-analysis of Kent and colleagues but were reviewed by the AHCPR. Jackson and colleagues (81) compared the ability of CT, myelography, CT–myelography, discography, and CT–discography to detect herniated lumbar discs as detected at surgery. CT–discography was the most accurate at 87 percent, with CT–myelography being slightly less accurate at 77 percent. CT–discography was the most sensitive and specific, with the lowest false-positive and false-negative rates of all methods studied. The authors recommended that CT–discography be used

when other tests were nondiagnostic, especially in those with possible foraminal or recurrent herniation (CT–discography was 94 percent accurate for prior surgery and 91 percent for foraminal herniation).

Moufarrij, Hardy, and Weinstein (82) retrospectively compared CT myelography (12.7 cm thick slices) and operative findings in patients suspected of disc herniation. The authors report that CT correctly predicted findings in 48 percent, was partly correct in 24 percent, and was incorrect in 28 percent. Myelogram was accurate in 52 percent, partly correct in 22 percent, and incorrect in 26 percent. These values are significantly lower than most other studies, which leads to questions regarding the study methods, although no flaws are glaringly obvious.

Schipper and colleagues (83) evaluated 461 patients with either CT, myelogram, or both and compared results with the surgical findings. The authors report sensitivities for myelography and CT at 82 percent and 73 percent, respectively, for detecting a herniated disc. Specificity was lower for myelogram (67 percent) than for CT (77 percent). The authors concluded that if CT is used as the first imaging technique after standard radiographs, myelogram usage could be reduced substantially. Fries and colleagues (84) compared CT and myelography in 188 patients with surgically explored low back pain and radiculopathy. Accuracy for detecting a disc herniation was found to be 92 percent for CT and 88 percent for myelography. The authors did find a difference between accuracy for detection at the L5–S1 level, with the CT rate being 92 percent and myelography being 70 percent.

Haughton, Eldevik, Magnaes, and Amundsen (85) evaluated 52 patients who underwent surgical exploration for accuracy of CT versus myelogram. CT was 89 percent accurate, whereas myelogram was 85 percent accurate. There were two false-negative herniations as diagnosed by myelogram and only one by CT scan.

Bosacco and colleagues (86) evaluated 134 patients with suspected disc herniation to compare the ability of CT and myelography to detect herniation as compared to findings at surgery. They excluded patients with previous surgery and spinal stenosis. CT scans with 5 mm cuts per disc space were compared to surgery along with myelograms. Fifty-two of the 134 patients underwent surgery. Myelography was in agreement with surgical findings in 94 percent, while CT agreement was 92 percent. There was an 87 percent agreement between CT and myelography.

Zlatkin and colleagues (87) used CT scan and clinical findings to evaluate the impact of Paget's disease on spinal stenosis in 36 patients. The authors report that 56 percent (20/36) demonstrated spinal stenosis by CT scan, with stenosis being present in 81 percent of symptomatic patients. This study was flawed by the lack of correlation of CT findings to a standard for diagnosis, i.e., there is no confirmation that these patients truly had stenosis.

The following efficacy studies were not reviewed by the AHCPR. Fagerlund and Thelander (88) compared 51 patients for the ability of CT and myelography to detect disc herniation. CT results were divided into normal, slightly bulging, broadly bulging, and herniated discs. Myelography was divided into normal, bulging, and herniated discs The authors report an 89 percent concordance rate between myelography and CT–myelography for normal scans and an 84 percent concordance rate for pathologic changes. Further inspection of the data shows that the CT slightly bulging and normal disc categories were both considered normal for comparison with myelography, yet slightly bulging and broadly bulging discs were considered abnormal when calculating pathologic concordance. It cannot be easily derived from the data presented, but the authors report a 97 percent true positivity rate for CT and 88 percent for myelography based on "findings at surgery and clinical signs." The authors also report that CT imaging of the soft tissues and the intervertebral joints was superior to that of myelography. The authors recommended using CT as the primary examination method (as opposed to myelogram) for imaging the lumbar spine for herniation, unless the level of the lesion is unclear or when complete thoracolumbar junction and lumbar imaging is required. As the findings were not directly correlated to surgical findings in all cases, the conclusions cannot be fully supported. Fagerlund (89) compared CT and CT–myelography in 46 patients suspected of having disc herniation. They found that CT and CT–myelography obtained comparable results in 73 percent, but CT–myelography revealed better imaging in 12 percent and inferior imaging in 15 percent. Based on these results, the authors concluded that CT–myelogram was not indicated when only disc herniation is suspected. It should be noted that the findings of the imaging studies were not confirmed for accuracy. Coste and colleagues (90) reviewed inter- and intraobserver variability in the interpretation of computed tomography of the lumbar spine and found interobserver reliability of 0.7 and intraobserver reliability of 0.9 for herniated discs, but very low interobserver reliability (< 0.2) for facet osteoarthritis and spinal stenosis. The authors therefore recommended only using CT scan for evaluation of herniated discs.

Wiesel and colleagues (91) examined 52 asymptomatic patients aged 21 to 80 years with CT scans. Scans were mixed in with films of patients with surgically proven disease and presented to three blinded neuroradiologists. Not all films were read by all neuroradiologists, as several were considered to be of such poor quality as to be deemed uninterpretable. The neuroradiologists found 16 percent, 31 percent, or 18 percent disc herniations; 9 percent, 4 percent, or 2 percent spinal stenosis; and 4 percent, 16 percent, or 12 percent facet degenerative changes in normal subjects. Scans were abnormal in 20 percent between the ages of 20 and 39 years and increased to 50 percent over the age of 39 years. No false-negatives were reported.

Cervellini and colleagues (92) evaluated 30 asymptomatic postoperative patients and 30 patients with recurrent "sciatic nerve pain" after disc surgery. The authors report that it was not possible to distinguish normal scar from asymptomatic fibrosis. Montaldi and colleagues (93) evaluated 25 patients with successful outcomes post lumbar disc surgery. The subjects underwent CT scan and standard radiographs of the lumbar spine before surgery and at 5–7 days and 6–7 weeks post surgery. The authors found that in 44 percent the operated disc shows changes suggesting a persistence of disc herniation. The authors also found that the outline of the dural sac and the nerve root disappears, and this change persisted from the first to the sixth week postoperatively. The authors concluded that CT scan is not helpful in patients with recurrent or persistent low back symptoms due to the persistent abnormalities present on CT scan postoperatively.

Based on the literature reviewed, CT scanning appears to be as accurate as myelogram for detecting most forms of spinal disease. CT may have a slight advantage over myelogram in its ability to visualize the L5–S1 disc space, can better define anatomy outside of the spinal canal, and can visualize caudal to a level of blockage on myelogram. More advanced CT imaging techniques, such as CT-myelography and CT-discography appear to be slightly more accurate than plain CT or myelography, and are discussed in greater detail earlier in this chapter and elsewhere (Chapter 7). CT appears to be of little value in the postoperative low back patient who has persistent or recurrent symptoms. As stated in the preceding sections, gadolinium-enhanced MRI or contrast-enhanced CT appear to be the imaging methods of choice in this patient population.

Paget's disease of bone is a condition capable of causing low back pain due to lytic, blastic, or a combination of lesions of bone (94). Bone, Cody, and Monsell (95) recommend using CT scan to follow bony changes secondary to Paget's disease, as other imaging techniques are unable to detect changes unless they are of large magnitude and cannot precisely reproduce areas of interest. The authors applied quantitative CT scanning to observe the change in pagetic lesions of the lumbar spine with treatment. The authors found CT to be a valuable tool in observing changes associated with Paget's diseases. CT could potentially be used in patients with Paget's disease who present with new or worsening low back symptoms, to help differentiate between new or progressing lesions and disc herniation or spinal stenosis.

Osteoporosis is another condition for which CT scanning can be useful. Standard radiographs may miss small vertebral compression fractures and require significant bone density loss before displaying osteopenia. A special CT technique known as quantitative computed tomography (QCT) has become one of the most sensitive methods available for measuring vertebral bone density (96). As osteoporotic patients are at risk for low back pain from vertebral compression fractures and can reduce their risk of further fracture through a proper exercise program (97), it is important to identify those at risk as early as possible. Kaplan and colleagues (98) have shown that QCT vertebral bone density measures are strongly inversely correlated with the presence of vertebral compression fractures and could therefore be used to identify patients at risk for further fracture.

Until the advent of MRI, CT and CT–myelography were the imaging techniques of choice for detailing the anatomy of spinal stenosis. Three-dimensional surface reconstructions and multiplanar CT scans became available in the early 1980s, and literature concerning these imaging techniques revealed significant improvements in the ability of CT scans to detect osseous pathology compared to standard CT scanning (99–102). Early scanning technology has been reported to lead to potential false-negatives (100), which have since been improved upon. Three-dimensional CT scanning has not been used as a routine imaging technique, as has MRI, without clear reason why. Three-dimensional CT scanning is currently used in our trauma center to more closely examine the cervical, thoracic, and lumbar spine during cases of severe acute trauma and has proven to be useful in detecting fractures that were missed by standard radiographs or CT scans. Three-dimensional CT scans could potentially be used to better define the anatomy of spinal stenosis prior to planning surgical intervention or to detect fractures or spondylolysis of the lumbar spine. This technique would be especially helpful for patients with ferrometallic implants who cannot be imaged via MRI. To our knowledge, the efficacy of 3D CT has not been directly compared to techniques other than standard CT scans and warrants further research. The AHCPR did not review the use of 3D CT scans, but such scans appear to be helpful under special circumstances for the patient with low back pain, especially under traumatic conditions.

## CT–MYELOGRAPHY

Computed tomography–myelography (CT–myelography) is an imaging technique that utilizes a combination of technologies—computed tomography and myelography—to examine the spine and associated soft tissues. In most cases, the myelogram is performed first and followed up by imaging with CT scan. The potential risks of this technique, therefore, are also additive, combining those associated with myelography and those of CT scanning. Janssen and colleagues (56) report that another problem associated with CT–myelogram is cost; in their study, CT–myelography cost 50 percent more than MRI.

As stated in earlier sections, some believe that CT-myelography is best suited for patients with spinal stenosis or disc herniations concomitantly present with spinal stenosis. This chapter has already presented a number of studies comparing CT-myelography with several other imaging techniques.

The AHCPR reviewed two other studies regarding the efficacy of CT–myelography. Voelker and colleagues (103) reviewed 80 patients with operatively proven spondylosis or disc herniation who had preoperative myelography and CT–myelography. Myelography and CT–myelography results were compared to the diagnosis as described on the operative report. The authors found CT–myelography to correctly diagnose disc herniation in 81 percent, with myelography correctly diagnosing in 79 percent. Both tests combined increased accuracy to 90 percent. CT–myelography accuracy for spondylosis was 83 percent and myelography accuracy was 76 percent, with combined test accuracy of 91 percent. CT–myelography accuracy was not statistically significantly better than myelography for detection of either disc herniation or spondylosis. Both myelography and CT–myelography revealed an accuracy of 70 percent with a combined accuracy rate of 85 percent for detecting recurrent disease associated with low back pain (both disc herniation and/or spondylosis). The combined accuracy rates for detection of spondylosis were statistically significantly improved over myelography alone and combined accuracy for all cases was significantly better than either test alone. The authors concluded that the combination of tests showed better accuracy than each alone and that both myelography and CT–myelography should be simultaneously obtained in patients when a diagnosis remains in question. No mention is made of the role of MRI in management of disc herniation or spondylosis. Ketonen and Gyldensted (104) studied 81 patients with CT–myelography and myelography. The authors compared the results from each imaging method, and 27 patients had surgically confirmed disease. It is unclear from the data presentation how accurate CT–myelography or myelography were for detecting herniations or other pathology in the lumbar spine. The authors claimed that CT–myelography was "superior" to myelography in 68 percent, as CT–myelography was able to demonstrate smaller disc herniations than standard studies. The study does not provide data concerning the surgical confirmation of disease for accuracy or how CT–myelography was deemed "superior." Additionally, it is unclear how significant these "small herniations" were clinically.

The AHCPR did not evaluate the studies by Albeck and Danneskiold-Samsoe (105) or Russell (106), nor did they include the results in their guidelines. Russell (106) states that even with improvements in MRI technology, CT–myelography is considered to be the "gold standard" for demonstrating the soft tissue and bony changes that result in nerve root and spinal cord compression syndromes. Albeck and Danneskiold-Samsoe studied the attitudes of patients to MRI, CT, and myelography (105). They found that myelography was considered the most painful and unpleasant of the three. Many disliked the immobilization of CT scan and the narrow caliber of the MRI scan. Overall, patients reported CT scan as the favored imaging technique.

Based on the literature reviewed in this section, CT–myelography has at least equal capacity to standard myelography. The literature claiming superiority of CT–myelogram over standard myelogram (104) does not present enough data to support this statement. The other studies reviewed in the previous sections provide some evidence that CT–myelography is at least as accurate and probably slightly more so than standard myelography for detection of disc herniation and spinal stenosis. CT–myelography probably has a slight advantage over standard CT scanning in detection of the same disease states.

Summarizing the advanced imaging technique literature, MRI has good to excellent ability to detect disc herniation and spinal stenosis. MRI may be slightly better than CT–myelography for the detection of disc herniation and is probably as good as or better than CT–myelography for the detection of spinal stenosis, especially when using 1.5 Tesla strength MRI magnets. Scanner magnets of strength less than 1.0 Tesla yield less accurate images and may not provide the same accuracy as other imaging techniques. MRI appears to be more accurate than standard CT scans for detection of disc herniation and disc sequestration and is probably at least as accurate as CT scan for spinal stenosis. MRI is probably equal to or slightly better than myelogram for detection of disc herniation. MRI is probably the best method for detecting disc degeneration. In postoperative patients, the following generalizations can be made: (1) contrast-enhanced CT probably shows more extensive scarring than gadolinium-enhanced MRI; (2) enhanced MRI probably displays nerve root thickening and displacement better in this same population; (3) enhanced MRI and CT imaging are probably equally as sensitive in detecting disc herniation and foraminal stenosis; and (4) CT-discography is perhaps equally as sensitive and specific as enhanced MRI for detecting recurrent herniations. CT-myelography is at least as good or slightly better than myelography for detecting disc herniation or spinal stenosis. Standard CT scanning appears to be as accurate as myelogram for detection of either disc herniation or spinal stenosis.

The final recommendations by the AHCPR state that since low back pain is essentially benign (unless other physical or historical findings suggest a medical or surgical emergency), imaging tests such as MRI, CT, CT–myelography, and myelography should be used when surgery is to be considered for specific neurologic loss or for further evaluation of possible serious pathology. As has been stated, imaging can be used for numerous conditions, as needed to provide optimum patient care and comfort. Based on our preceding recommendations, the clinician can comfortably order these more advanced (and more costly) imaging studies when quality of life or activities of daily living function has become impaired and management will be affected or if surgical intervention is being contemplated.

# References

1. U.S. Department of Health and Human Services/Public Health Service Agency for Health Care Policy and Research. Special studies and diagnostic considerations. In: Acute Low Back Problems in Adults, AHCPR Publication No. 95–0642, 1994:59–92.
2. Deyo RA, Bigos SJ, Maravilla KR. Diagnostic imaging procedures for the lumbar spine. *Ann Int Med* 1989; 111(11):865–867.
3. Squire LF, Novelline RA (eds.). *Fundamentals of radiology.* 4th ed. Cambridge: Harvard University Press, 1988:1–31, 312–334.
4. Callaway WJ. Imaging equipment. In: Gurley LT, Callaway WJ (eds.). *Introduction to radiologic technology.* 2nd ed. St. Louis: Multi-Media Publishers, 1986:67–73.
5. Hall FM. Back pain and the radiologist. *Radiology* 1980; 137:861–863.
6. Bejjani FJ. Performing artists' occupational disorders. In: DeLisa JA, Gans BM (eds.). *Rehabilitation medicine: Principles and practice.* 2nd ed. Philadelphia: JB Lippincott, 1993:1165–1190.
7. Stinson JT. Spondylolysis and spondylolisthesis in the athlete. *Clin Sport Med* 1993; 12(3):517–528.
8. Dietrich M, Kurowski P. The importance of mechanical factors in the etiology of spondylolysis. A model analysis of loads and stresses in human lumbar spine. *Spine* 1985; 10(6):532–542.
9. Blanda J, Bethem D, Moats W, Lew M. Defects of pars interarticularis in athletes: a protocol for nonoperative treatment. *J Spinal Disorders* 1993; 6:406–411.
10. Libson E, Bloom RA, Dinari G, Robin GC. Oblique lumbar spine radiographs: importance in young patients. *Radiology* 1984; 151(1):89–90.
11. Daniel JN, Polly DW Jr, Van Dam BE. A study of the efficacy of nonoperative treatment of presumed traumatic spondylolysis in a young patient population. *Mil Med* 1995; 160(11):553–555.
12. Morita T, Ikata T, Katoh S, Miyake R. Lumbar spondylolysis in children and adolescents. *J Bone Joint Surg [Br]* 1995; 77–B:620–625.

13. Schneck CD, Mesgarzadeh M. Imaging techniques relative to rehabilitation. In: DeLisa JA, Gans BM (eds.). *Rehabilitation medicine: Principles and practice.* 2nd ed. Philadelphia: JB Lippincott, 1993:336–377.

14. Troup JDG. The etiology of spondylolysis. *Orthop Clin North Am* 1977; 8(1):57–64.

15. Torgerson WR, Dotter WE. Comparative roentgenographic study of the asymptomatic and symptomatic lumbar spine. *J Bone Joint Surg [Am]* 1976; 58–A(6):850–853.

16. Magora A, Schwartz A. Relation between low back pain and x-ray changes. 4. Lysis and olisthesis. *Scand J Rehabil Med* 1980; 12(2):47–52.

17. Boxall D, Bradford DS, Winter RB, Moe JH. Management of severe spondylolisthesis in children and adolescents. *J Bone Joint Surg [Am]* 1979; 61–A(4):479–495.

18. Biering-Sorensen F, Hansen FR, Schroll M, Runeborg O. The relation of spinal x-ray to low-back pain and physical activity among 60–year-old men and women. *Spine* 1985; 10(5):445–451.

19. Bigos SJ, Hansson T, Castillo RN, Beecher PJ, Wortley MD. The value of preemployment roentgenographs for predicting acute back injury claims and chronic back pain disability. *Clin Orthop Rel Res* 1992; 283:124–129.

20. Leboeuf C, Kimber D, White K. Prevalence of spondylolisthesis, transitional anomalies and low intercrestal line in a chiropractic patient population. *J Manipulative Physiol Ther* 1989; 12(3):200–204.

21. Fullenlove TM, Williams AJ. Comparative roentgen findings in symptomatic and asymptomatic backs. *Radiology* 1957; 68:572–574.

22. Splithoff CA. Lumbosacral junction: roentgenographic comparison of patients with and without backaches. *JAMA* 1953; 152(17):1610–1613.

23. Greenspan A. Spine. In: Greenspan A. (ed.). *Orthopedic radiology: A practical approach.* 2nd ed. Philadelphia: Lippincott-Raven Publishers, 1996:10.3–10.56.

24. Scavone JG, Lathshaw RF, Weidner WA. Anteroposterior and lateral radiographs: an adequate lumbar spine examination. *AJR* 1981; 136:715–717.

25. Steiner ME, Micheli LJ. Treatment of symptomatic spondylolysis and spondylolisthesis with the modified Boston brace. *Spine* 1985; 10(10):937–943.

26. Pavlovcic V. Surgical treatment of spondylolysis and spondylolisthesis with a hook screw. *Int Orthop* 1994; 18(1):6–9.

27. Deyo RA, Diehl AK. Lumbar spine films in primary care: current use and effects of selective ordering criteria. *J Gen Intern Med* 1986; 1(1):20–25.

28. Frazier LM, Carey TS, Khayrallah MA, McGaghie WC. Selective criteria may increase lumbosacral spine roentgenogram use in acute low back pain. *Arch Intern Med* 1989; 149:47–50.

29. Galluccio AC. Spondylolisthesis. Further remarks with emphasis on radiologic aspects. *Radiology* 1946; 46:356–363.

30. Eisenberg RL, Akin JR, Hedgcock MW. Single, well centered lateral view of lumbosacral spine: is coned view necessary? *AJR* 1979; 133:711–713

31. LaRocca H, Macnab I. Value of pre-employment radiographic assessment of the lumbar spine. *Indus Med* 1970; 39(6):253–258.

32. Esdaile JM, Rosenthall L, Turkeltaub R, Kloiber R. Prospective evaluation of sacroiliac scintigraphy in chronic inflammatory back pain. *Arthritis Rheum* 1980; 23(9):998–1003

33. Rosenstein M (ed.). *Organ doses in diagnostic radiology.* Rockville, MD: HEW Publications, 1976.

34. Teters M, Radiation Safety Director, Biomed Associates, Flemington, NJ. Personal communication.

35. Dibos PE, Wagner HN (eds.). *Atlas of nuclear medicine.* Vol. 4. Philadelphia: WB Saunders, 1978.

36. Lowe J, Schachner E, Hirschberg E, Shapiro Y, Libson E. Significance of bone scintigraphy in symptomatic spondylolysis. *Spine* 1984; 9(6):653–655.

37. Miron SD, Khan MA, Wiesen EJ, Kushner I, Bellon EM. The value of quantitative sacroiliac scintigraphy in detection of sacroiliitis. *Clin Rheumatol* 1983; 2(4):407–414.

38. Schütte HE, Park WM. The diagnostic value of bone scintigraphy in patients with low back pain. *Skeletal Radiol* 1983; 10 (1):1–4.

39. Whalen JL, Brown ML McLeod R, Fitzgerald RH Jr. Limitations of indium leukocyte imaging for the diagnosis of spine infections. *Spine* 1991; 16(2):193–197.

40. Deyo RA, Diehl AK. Cancer as a cause of back pain: frequency, clinical presentation, and diagnostic strategies. *J Gen Intern Med* 1988; 3(3):230–238.

41. Jinkins JR, Matthes JC, Sener RN, Venkatappan S, Rauch R. Spondylolysis, spondylolisthesis, and associated nerve root entrapment in the lumbosacral spine: MR evaluation. *AJR* 1992; 159:799–803.

42. Weir MR, Smith S. Stress reaction of the pars interarticularis leading to spondylolysis. A cause of adolescent low back pain. *J Adol Health Care* 1989; 10:573–577.

43. Elliott S, Hutson MA, Wastie ML. Bone scintigraphy in the assessment of spondylolysis in patients attending a sports injury clinic. *Clin Radiol* 1988; 39(3):269–272.

44. Herzog RJ, Guyer RD, Graham-Smith A, Simmons ED Jr. Magnetic resonance imaging. Use in patients with low back or radicular pain. *Spine* 1995; 20(16):1834–1838.

45. Saal JA, Saal JS. Nonoperative treatment of herniated lumbar intervertebral disc with radiculopathy: an outcome study. *Spine* 1989; 14(4):431–437.

46. Edelman RR, Warach S. Magnetic resonance imaging. *NEJM* 1993; 328(10):708–716; 328 (11):785–791.

47. Jackson RP, Cain JE, Jacobs RR, Cooper BR, McManus GE. The neuroradiographic diagnosis of lumbar herniated nucleus pulposus: II. A comparison of computed tomography (CT), myelography, CT–myelography, and magnetic resonance imaging. *Spine* 1989; 14(12):1362–1367.

48. Masaryk TJ, Ross JS, Modic MT, et al. High-resolution MR imaging of sequestered lumbar intervertebral discs. *AJR* 1988; 150:1155–1162.

49. Szypryt EP, Twining P, Wilde GP, Mulholland RC, Worthington BS. Diagnosis of lumbar disc protrusion. A comparison between magnetic resonance imaging and radiculography. *J Bone Joint Surg [Br]* 1988; 70(5):717–722.

50. Bischoff RJ, Rodriguez RP, Gupta K, et al. A comparison of computed tomography-myelography, magnetic resonance imaging, and myelography in the diagnosis of herniated nucleus pulposus and spinal stenosis. *J Spinal Disord* 1993; 6(4):289–295.

51. Kent DL, Haynor DR, Larson EB, Deyo RA. Diagnosis of lumbar spinal stenosis in adults: A metaanalysis of the accuracy of CT, MR, and myelography. *AJR* 1992; 158:1135–1144.

52. Modic MT, Masaryk T, Boumphrey F, Goormastic M, Bell G. Lumbar herniated disk disease and canal stenosis: prospective evaluation by surface coil MR, CT, and myelography. *AJR* 1986; 147(4):757–765.

53. Schnebel B, Kingston S, Watkins R, Dillin W. Comparison of MRI to contrast CT in the diagnosis of spinal stenosis. *Spine* 1989; 14(3):332–337.

54. Epstein NE, Epstein JA, Carras R, Hyman RA. Far lateral lumbar disc herniations and associated structural abnormalities. An evaluation in 60 patients of the comparative value of CT, MRI, and myelo-CT in diagnosis and management. *Spine* 1990; 15(6):534–539.

55. Modic MT, Pavlicek W, Weinstein MA, et al. Magnetic resonance imaging of intervertebral disc disease. *Radiology* 1984; 152(1):103–111.

56. Janssen ME, Bertrand SL, Joe C, Levine MI. Lumbar herniated disc disease: comparison of MRI, myelography, and post-myelographic CT scan with surgical findings. *Orthopedics* 1994; 17(2):121–127.

57. Bernard TN Jr. Using computed tomography/discography and enhanced magnetic resonance imaging to distinguish between scar tissue and recurrent lumbar disc herniation. *Spine* 1994; 19(24):2826–2832.

58. Tullberg T, Grane P, Rydberg J, Isacson J. Comparison of contrast-enhanced computed tomography and gadolinium-enhanced magnetic resonance imaging one year after lumbar discectomy. *Spine* 1994; 19(2):183–188.

59. Albeck MJ, Wagner A, Knudsen LL. Contrast enhanced computed tomography and magnetic resonance imaging in the diagnosis of recurrent disc herniation. *Acta Neurochir* 1996; 138:1256-1260.

60. Jensen MC, Brant-Zawadzki MN, Obuchowski N, et al. Magnetic resonance imaging of the lumbar spine in people without back pain. *N Engl J Med* 1994; 331:69–73.

61. Takahashi K, Miyyazaki T, Ohnari H, Takino T, Tomita K. Schmorl's nodes and low-back pain. Analysis of magnetic resonance imaging findings in symptomatic and asymptomatic individuals. *Eur Spine J* 1995; 4(1):56–59.

62. Buirski G, Silberstein M. The symptomatic lumbar disc in patients with low-back pain: magnetic resonance imaging appearances in both a symptomatic and control population. *Spine* 1993; 18(13):1808–1811.

63. Erkintalo MO, Salminen JJ, Alanen AM, Paajanen HE, Kormano MJ. Development of degenerative changes in the lumbar intervertebral disk: results of a prospective MR imaging study in adolescents with and without low-back pain. *Radiology* 1995; 196(2):529–533.

64. Boos N, Rieder R, Schade V, Spratt KF, Semmer N, Aebi M. The diagnostic accuracy of magnetic resonance imaging, work perception, and psychosocial factors in identifying symptomatic disc herniations. *Spine* 1995; 20: 2613–2625.

65. Boden SD, Davis DO, Dina TS, Patronas NJ, Wiesel SW. Abnormal magnetic-resonance scans of the lumbar spine in asymptomatic subjects. *J Bone Joint Surg [Am]* 1990; 72(3):403–408.

66. Powell MC, Wilson M, Szypryt P, Symonds EM, Worthington BS. Prevalence of lumbar disc degeneration observed by magnetic resonance in symptomless women. *Lancet* 1986; 2(8520):1366–1367.

67. Paajanen H, Erkintalo M, Dahlström S et al. Disc degeneration and lumbar instability. Magnetic resonance examination of 16 patients. *Acta Orthop Scand* 1989; 60(4):375–378.

68. Weinreb JC, Wolbarsht LB, Cohen JM, Brown CE, Maravilla KR. Prevalence of lumbar intervertebral disk abnormalities on MR images in pregnant and asymptomatic nonpregnant women. *Radiology* 1989: 170(1): 125–128.

69. Aprill C, Bogduk N. High-intensity zone: A diagnostic sign of painful lumbar disc on magnetic resonance imaging. *Br J Radiol* 1992; 65(773):361–369.

70. Schellhas KP, Pollei SR, Gundry CR, Heithoff KB. Lumbar disc high-intensity zone: correlation of magnetic resonance imaging and discography. *Spine* 1996; 21(1):79–86.

71. Schellhas KP, Smith MD, Gundry CR, Pollei SR. Cervical discogenic pain: prospective correlation of magnetic resonance imaging and discography in asymptomatic subjects and pain sufferers. *Spine* 1996; 21(3):300–312.

72. Yamane T, Yoshida T, Mimatsu K. Early diagnosis of spondylolysis by MRI. *J Bone Joint Surg [Br]* 1993; 75(5): 764–768.

73. Unger E, Moldofsky P, Gatenby R, Hartz W, Broder G. Diagnosis of osteomyelitis by MR imaging. *AJR* 1988; 150:605–610.

74. Kraemer J. Presidential address: natural course and prognosis of intervertebral disc diseases. *Spine* 1995; 20(6): 635–639.

75. Stockley I, Getty CJM, Dixon AK, et al. Lumbar lateral canal entrapment: clinical, radiculographic and computed tomographic findings. *Clin Radiol* 1988; 39: 144–149.

76. Herkowitz HN, Gaffin SR, Bell GR, Bumphrey F, Rothman RH. The use of computerized tomography in evaluating non-visualized vertebral levels caudad to a complete block on a lumbar myelogram. *J Bone Joint Surg [Am]* 1987; 69–A(2):218–24.

77. Slebus FG, Braakman R, Schipper J, van Dongen KJ, Westendorp-de Serière M. Non-corresponding radiological and surgical diagnoses in patients operated for sciatica. *Acta Neurochir* 1989; 94:137–43.

78. Bell GR, Rothman RH, Booth RE, et al. A study of computer-assisted tomography. II. Comparison of metrizamide myelography and computed tomography in the diagnosis of herniated lumbar disc and spinal stenosis. *Spine* 1984; 9(6):552–556.

79. Bolender NF, Schönström NSR, Spengler DM. Role of computed tomography and myelography in the diagnosis of central spinal stenosis. *J Bone Joint Surg [Am]* 1985; 67–A:240–246.

80. Schönström NSR, Bolender NF, Spengler DM. The pathomorphology of spinal stenosis as seen on CT scans of the lumbar spine. *Spine* 1985; 10(9):806–811.

81. Jackson RP, Cain JE, Jacobs RR, Cooper BR, McManus GE. The neuroradiographic diagnosis of lumbar herniated nucleus pulposus: I. A comparison of computed tomography (CT), myelography, CT–myelography, discography and CT–discography. *Spine* 1989; 14(12): 1356–1360.

82. Moufarrij NA, Hardy RW, Weinstein MA. Computed tomographic, myelographic, and operative findings in patients with suspected herniated lumbar discs. *Neurosurgery* 1983; 12(2):184–188.

83. Schipper J, Kardaun JW, Braakman R, van Dongen KJ, Blauuw G. Lumbar disk herniation: diagnosis with CT or myelography. *Radiology* 1987; 165(1):227–231.

84. Fries JW, Abodeely DA, Vijungco JG, Yeager VL, Gaffey WR. Computer tomography of herniated and extruded nucleus pulposus. *J Comput Assist Tomogr* 1982: 6(5): 874–887.

85. Haughton VM, Eldevik OP, Magnaes B, Amundsen P. A prospective comparison of computed tomography and myelography in the diagnosis of herniated lumbar disks. *Neuroradiology* 1982; 142(1):103–110.

86. Bosacco SJ, Berman AT, Gabarino JL, Teplick JG, Peyster R. A comparison of CT scanning and myelography in the diagnosis of lumbar disc herniation. *Clin Orthop Rel Res* 1984; 190:124–128.

87. Zlatkin MB, Lander PH, Hadjipavlou AG, Levine JS. Paget disease of the spine: CT with clinical correlation. *Radiology* 1986; 160(1):155–159.

88. Fagerlund MK, Thelander UE. Comparison of myelography and computed tomography in establishing lumbar disc herniation. *Acta Radiol* 1989; 30(3):241–246.

89. Fagerlund MK. Computed tomography in low back pain before and after myelography. A qualitative comparison. *Acta Radiol* 1988; 29(3):353–356.

90. Coste J, Judet O, Barre O, et al. Inter- and intraobserver variability in the interpretation of computed tomography of the lumbar spine. *J Clin Epidemiol* 1994;47(4): 375–381.

91. Wiesel SW, Tsourmas N, Feffer HL, Citrin CM, Patronas N. A study of computer-assisted tomography. I. The incidence of positive CAT scans in an asymptomatic group of patients. *Spine* 1984; 9(6):549–551.

92. Cervellini P, Curri D, Volpin L, Bernardi L, et al. Computed tomography of epidural fibrosis after discectomy: a comparison between symptomatic and asymptomatic patients. *Neurosurgery* 1988; 23(6):710–713.

93. Montaldi S, Fankhauser H, Schnyder P, de Tribolet N. Computed tomography of the postoperative intervertebral disc and lumbar spinal canal: investigation of twenty-five patients after successful operation for lumbar disc herniation. *Neurosurgery* 1988; 22:1014–1022.

94. Cotran RS, Kumar V, Robbins SL. The musculoskeletal system: the skeletal system. In: Cotran RS, Kumar V, Robbins SL (eds.). *Robbins pathologic basis of disease.* 4th ed. Phiadelphia: WB Saunders, 1989:1315–1345.

95. Bone HG, Cody DD, Monsell EM. Application of quantitative computed tomography to Paget's disease of bone. *Semin Arthritis Rheum* 1994; 23(4):244–247.

96. Yu W, Gluer CC, Grampp S, et al. Spinal bone mineral assessment in postmenopausal women: a comparison between dual X-ray absorptiometry and quantitative computed tomography. *Osteoporos Int* 1995; 5(6):433–439.

97. Sinaki M, Mikkelsen BA. Postmenopausal spinal osteoporosis: flexion versus extension exercises. *Arch Phys Med Rehabil* 1984; 65:593–596.

98. Kaplan FS, Dalinka M, Karp JS, Fallon MD, et al. Quantitative computed tomography reflects vertebral fracture morbidity in osteopenic patients. *Orthopedics* 1989; 12(7):949–955.

99. Hadley MN, Sonntag VK, Hodak JA, Lopez LJ. Three-dimensional computed tomography in the diagnosis of vertebral column pathological conditions. *Neurosurgery* 1987; 21(2):186–192.

100. Wood GW, Koltai PJ, Meagher DJ et al. Three-dimensional interactive analysis of craniofacial and spinal computed tomography. *Acta Radiol Suppl (Stockholm)* 1986; 369:703–705.

101. Jurik AG, Albrechtsen J. The use of computed tomography with two- and three-dimensional reconstructions in the diagnosis of three- and four-part fractures of the proximal humerus. *Clin Radiol* 1994; 49(11):800–804.

102. Sundberg SB, Clark B, Foster BK. Three-dimensional reformation of skeletal abnormalities using computed tomography. *J Pediatr Orthop* 1986; 6(4):416–420.

103. Voelker JL, Mealey J, Eskridge JM, Gilmor RL. Metrizamide-enhanced computed tomography as an adjunct to metrizamide myelography in the evaluation of lumbar disc herniation and spondylosis. *Neurosurgery* 1987; 20:379–384.

104. Ketonen L, Gyldensted C. Lumbar disc disease evaluated by myelography and postmyelography spinal computed tomography. *Neuroradiology* 1986; 28:144–149.

105. Albeck MJ, Danneskiold-Samsoe B. Patient attitudes to myelography, computed tomography and magnetic resonance imaging when examined for suspected lumbar disc herniation. *Acta Neurochir* 1995:133(1–2):3–6.

106. Russell EJ. Computed topography and myelography in the evaluation of cervical degenerative disease. *Neuroimaging Clin N Am* 1995; 5(3):329–348.

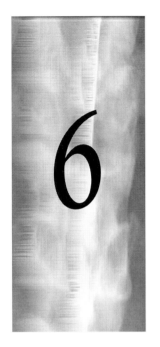

# 6 Physiologic Assessment: Electromyography and Nerve Conduction

*Joel M. Press, M.D., and Jeffrey L. Young, M.D.*

E
lectrodiagnostic studies, electromyography, and nerve conduction velocities (EMG/NCV) are an extension of the clinical examination and should be guided by pertinent information gathered from the history, physical examination, and anatomic or radiologic data. Electrophysiologic information needs to be interpreted in light of this clinical picture. It is important to keep in mind that the electrodiagnostic examination evaluates the physiology of the nerves and muscles studied *at that time*. Some abnormalities might not yet have appeared; others may have resolved, leaving no detectable residual deficit. The electrodiagnostic impression must be based on the entire clinical picture. A lack of electrophysiologic abnormality does not necessarily mean that there is or has not been nerve damage. Conversely, lack of nerve damage does not mean that the patient is free of pathology.

This chapter describes the chronology of electrophysiologic events that occur with nerve injuries, the usefulness and limitations of various aspects of electrophysiologic testing, and the sensitivity and specificity of these tests, as well as reviews and critiques the conclusions of the Agency for Health Care Policy Research (AHCPR) as to the relative value of EMG/NCV for patients with acute low back disorders.

## ANATOMY

The spinal nerves are composed of dorsal and ventral roots (Figure 6–1). The axons of the ventral root originate primarily from cells in the anterior and lateral gray columns of the cord, whereas those of the dorsal roots originate in the dorsal root ganglia. The dorsal root ganglia are usually situated within the entrance of the bony intervertebral foramina (1,2). The ganglia are situated along the distal portion of the dorsal root near the area where the dorsal and ventral roots join to form the spinal nerves. The spinal nerve is formed at about the level of the intervertebral foramina. Disruption of the nerve root by a herniated disc occurs prior to the exit at the intervertebral foramina and, therefore, proximal to the dorsal root ganglia (3). As a result, the sensory fibers distal from the ganglia to the periphery are not affected. However, the afferent fibers from the dorsal root ganglia to the spinal cord can be affected, explaining why hypesthesia can be present despite normal sensory studies. Almost all muscles are innervated by more than one root level. The only exception to this may be the rhomboids, which are felt to be exclusively C5 in origin (4). Needle electromyography is based entirely on finding abnormalities in myotomal distributions. There is controversy regarding some muscles and their specific nerve root supply, which is complicated and fueled by the natural variability in muscle innervation (4). For this reason, when

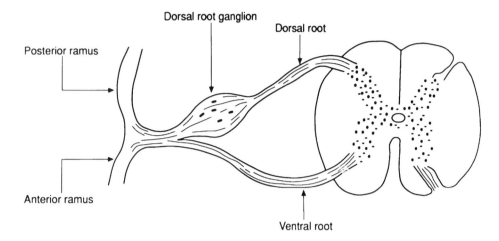

**FIGURE 6–1.**

Spinal nerve root anatomy. Note that the spinal nerves terminate by dividing into anterior and posterior rami.

electromyographic studies are performed, a number of muscles with overlapping innervations need to be studied to get the clearest picture of which nerve root is the most likely one affected. Sensory dermatomes overlap to a great extent. Due to the extensive sensory overlap, as well as myofascial pain syndromes and nonneural causes simulating radicular pain, it is difficult to assess sensory symptoms well with standard nerve conduction studies (3,5).

## CHRONOLOGY/PATHOPHYSIOLOGY

In order to use electrophysiological studies efficiently and effectively in patients with spine problems, an understanding of the chronology and pathophysiology of changes that occur with nerve injury, and in particular radiculopathy, is essential (Table 6–1). Compression of the nerve tissues may induce structural damage to the nerve fibers, impairment of intraneural blood flow, and formation of intraneural edema as well as axonal transport block (6). Some electrodiagnostic changes occur from the onset of irritation or damage to a nerve. If the initial injury to the nerve fibers is mild, a focal conduction slowing or block occurs, which can be very transient (neurapraxia) or when more persistent, with focal demyelination (7,8,9,10). With this type of injury the sensory or motor deficit may last only hours to days. Electromyographic changes of spontaneous single muscle fiber discharges, e.g., positive waves and fibrillation potentials, or changes in the parameters of the motor unit action potential (MUAPs) never occur since there has not been any axonal loss. Weakness that is apparent clinically may be recognized electrophysiologically as a reduced recruitment pattern on maximal contraction (11). However, if weakness is minimal, the recruitment pattern may not be identified as reduced. Then, with minimal con-

traction, a reduced recruitment interval can be seen. The reduced recruitment interval occurs because there are fewer motor units available and the first unit will fire more rapidly at the moment the second unit is recruited.

Other electrodiagnostic changes that can be detected from the onset of nerve injury are changes in the H-reflex latency and amplitude of the compound muscle action potential (CMAP). The H-reflex latency is prolonged in S1 radiculopathies from the onset (3). Opinions regarding what constitutes a significant difference in H-reflex latency from side to side in unilateral radiculopathies varies from 1.0 to 2.0 msec (11,12,13,14). The reduc-

| TABLE 6–1 *Chronology of findings in acute radiculopathy* | |
|---|---|
| **TIME FROM ONSET** | **FINDINGS** |
| 0–4 days | Reduced recruitment, prolonged H-reflex, decreased number of F waves |
| 7 days | Positive waves in the paraspinal muscles |
| 12–14 days | Positive waves in the proximal limb muscles, fibrillations in the paraspinals |
| 18–21 days | All electrodiagnostic abnormalities present |
| 5–6 weeks | Innervation of motor unit potentials present |
| 6 mos–1 yr | Increased amplitude or reinnervated motor unit potential |

tion in the amplitude of the CMAP, especially as compared to the normal side, over the appropriate muscle group can also be seen early after nerve injury (11).

With more severe injuries, axonal loss occurs. If a mixed nerve is involved, typically sensory abnormalities are prominent, muscle stretch reflexes are reduced or lost, and denervation occurs in the muscles of that myotome (3). The electrophysiologic hallmark of findings of axonal degeneration are the spontaneous single muscle fiber discharges called positive sharp waves and fibrillation potentials. Positive sharp waves are first noticeable in paraspinal muscles (posterior primary ramus distribution) within 7 to 10 days following loss of axon function (11). By 14–18 days, positive sharp waves can appear in the limb muscles, beginning proximally and quickly becoming evident throughout the involved myotome. Soon the positive waves are accompanied by fibrillation potentials (11,15,16). By 18–21 days, all muscles in the involved myotome have abnormalities including positive sharp waves and fibrillation potentials. Positive sharp waves start out as large amplitude waves of approximately 200 microvolts that gradually drop in amplitude over many weeks to approximately 100–150 microvolts (17,18). Fibrillation potentials follow a similar course. With time, if reinnervation of muscle fibers remains incomplete, both positive sharp waves and fibrillation potentials decrease in amplitude to values between 20 and 50 microvolts. As the nerve root pathology resolves, paraspinal muscles, which are the first muscles to show abnormalities on EMG, are also the first muscles to reinnervate and cease fibrillating. Proximal limb muscles follow suit, followed by the more distal muscles. Most radiculopathies do not show the presence of positive waves and fibrillations within the first 3 weeks of symptoms, so electrodiagnostic studies are not pursued early in the course. However, if the patient has had previous episodes of radicular symptoms or prior spinal surgery, it may be useful both diagnostically and from a medical–legal standpoint to perform initial electrodiagnostic studies as soon as possible after the appearance of new symptoms (19). If positive waves are seen within the first week or two, they can be assumed to have been present prior to the onset of new neuropathology. New electromyographic abnormalities seen 4 to 6 weeks later can be assumed to represent new pathology if none were present at first.

In chronic radiculopathies, fibrillation potentials are typically seen only in distal muscles. If the radiculopathy resolves (does not become chronic), the spontaneous single muscle fiber discharges (positive sharp waves and fibrillation potentials) begin to diminish in 5 to 6 weeks and disappear in 6 months or less unless the root lesion was severe (16). Evidence of reinnervation (long duration, large amplitude polyphasic MUPs) may be found after several weeks following onset of symptoms, but this does not become readily apparent unless the radiculopathy has been quite severe (16). Absence of positive waves (i.e., absence of denervation) even though weakness is present portends a good prognosis, assuming there has been sufficient time since onset of nerve compromise for them to develop (16).

## Specific Electrodiagnostic Studies

There are many specific steps that comprise a comprehensive electrodiagnostic evaluation. Each of these is discussed separately to delineate their usefulness and limitations in evaluating patients with back pain. Specific procedural details of each of these studies are not discussed in this chapter as they are explained fully in standard electrodiagnostic texts (20,21).

### Nerve Conduction Studies

Distal peripheral motor and sensory nerve conduction studies are often normal in a single level radiculopathy. They may be useful though to evaluate the possibility of nerve entrapment or peripheral neuropathy, which may mimic symptoms of radiculopathy. In radiculopathy, if the root lesion is purely demyelinative, there will be no change in the compound muscle action potential (CMAP) amplitude following stimulation distal to the lesion. If axonal degeneration occurs at one root level, the CMAP amplitude may still be relatively preserved, either through reinnervation of the muscles by fibers from the other uninvolved roots, or if the relative contribution of the injured root to that muscle is small compared to the uninvolved levels. Root compromise is nearly always incomplete and rarely do the majority of motor fibers degenerate. When considerable axon degeneration does occur, the CMAP amplitude may be reduced. Maximum reduction is reached 7 days post injury, and is easily recognized in the peroneal muscle groups in L5 radiculopathy and in the tibial groups when S1 is involved (4). A reduction of the CMAP of a specific muscle of more than 50 percent compared to the uninvolved side is probably significant. In general, the CMAPs are likely to be significantly reduced only in situations where considerable axonal degeneration has occurred, or especially when multiple nerve roots are acutely involved. In clinical situations where the muscle is very weak yet the CMAP is large, prognosis for recovery is good. Chronic nerve root compression, such as occurs with central lumbar stenosis, tends not to cause axonal degeneration until late in the course of progression.

Sensory nerve action potentials and conduction velocities are often normal in radiculopathies. Since the lesion in a herniated disc is almost always proximal to the dorsal root ganglion, degeneration of peripheral sensory fibers does not occur (4,22,23). However, in a far lateral lumbar disc herniation, particularly at the L5–S1 level, the dorsal root ganglion may be injured and cause abnormal sensory studies.

### H-Reflex

The H-reflex is the electrophysiologic analogue to the ankle muscle stretch reflex. It measures afferent and efferent conduction mainly along the S1 nerve root and is used in localizing nerve root compromise at that level (12,13,24,25,26,27). Investigators disagree as to which component, the latency or the amplitude of the response, is the most important in determining S1 root pathology. Comparing side-to-side latency differences is even more critical in tall patients with long limbs (and therefore longer nerves) as absolute latencies may be prolonged on the sole basis of nerve length. A side-to-side latency difference of at least 1.0–2.0 msec is significant. H-reflex latency shows a high correlation with S1 nerve root pain production, as demonstrated by selective nerve root blocks (18). Amplitude differences of $< 25–50$ percent compared to the uninvolved side or $< 1$ mV are also significant (4,7,28). Since the amplitude of this reflex is sensitive to contraction of the plantar flexor muscles, caution is recommended about accepting a significant finding based solely on amplitude changes.

There are a number of advantages in performing H-reflex studies in patients with spine problems as part of the electrodiagnostic evaluation. H-reflex parameters can become abnormal as soon as root injury occurs and therefore are detectable much earlier than standard electromyography (29). Because the H-reflex is able to look at both afferent and efferent pathways, it can give information about the status of sensory fibers which is not available with standard EMG that evaluates only motor nerve fibers. H-reflexes are also helpful in distinguishing S1 from L5 radiculopathies. Because these two levels are involved in over 90 percent of lumbar radiculopathies, H-reflex studies may help put together a clinical picture that is not otherwise clear. If surgery is contemplated, H-reflexes may assist in localizing the involved level and help guide the surgical approach. As with the physiologically similar phasic myotactic reflexes, however, it is important to recognize that symmetrically absent H-reflexes are not necessarily abnormal and that the percentage of absent responses increases in the elderly (30).

Certain limitations need to be understood in performing H-reflex studies (25). They provide direct information only about the segmental level being studied, i.e., S1, although by inference they also provide information about L5 (14,29). The H-reflex is sometimes normal in people with proven S1 radiculopathies, presumably because of incomplete root involvement with sparing of the fibers over which the reflex is mediated (28). H-reflex studies give no information about chronic vs. acute radiculopathies, nor do they correlate with the severity of the radiculopathy. H-reflex studies, once unelicitable, may remain so indefinitely (28). H-reflex studies reveal nothing about etiology of the S1 root pathology and, in fact, do not even specifically localize the lesion to the root because they can be abnormal in peripheral neuropathies (often bilaterally), tibial or sciatic nerve injuries, lumbosacral plexus, spinal cord injury, and even CNS disorders. Evaluation of other peripheral nerves via standard nerve conduction studies may be helpful if the clinical situation warrants. Furthermore, patient relaxation is important because mild muscle contraction of the antagonist muscles inhibits the H-reflex (15,29).

In conclusion, the H-reflex may be part of an electrodiagnostic study in patients with low back and leg complaints when considering a possible S1 nerve injury. When EMG abnormalities on needle exam are limited to the paraspinal muscles, a prolonged H-reflex suggests an S1 radiculopathy. H-reflex studies are especially important when EMG abnormalities are inconclusive. They may be helpful in making a diagnosis early in the course of nerve irritation in a patient with radicular symptoms before needle EMG findings are present.

### F Wave

The F wave is a late muscle potential that results from the backfiring of antidromically and supramaximally activated anterior horn cells (18,25,31,32). F wave studies have been shown by some to be useful in the diagnosis of lumbar nerve root lesions when the side-to-side minimal latency difference is $> 2.0$ msec (27,33). Like H-reflexes, F wave abnormalities occur immediately after injury to a nerve root. In one study, F wave abnormalities were found to be the only abnormality in up to 15 percent of patients with radiculopathy (7). Other studies have found that the F waves are most often abnormal when other abnormalities are also present and are rarely the only abnormality noted (4,27). Unlike the H-reflex, the F wave can be elicited at many spinal levels and from any muscle.

There are a number of limitations of the F wave in evaluating patients with spine problems. First, F wave studies, like needle EMG, assess only motor fibers, not sensory fibers (29). Second, only a small population of all the fibers of a nerve are evaluated with each stimulus, and if these are not involved the study will be normal. Third, F wave studies, like the H-reflex, look at the entire pathway of the nerve and small focal abnormalities tend to be obscured by the longer segments. Fourth, because the F wave is elicited by stimulating the nerve of the muscle studied, and all muscles receive more than one nerve root innervation, it is not specific for a given nerve root level. Fifth, like the H-reflex, the F wave cannot distinguish between acute and chronic changes. Sixth, because there is a range of latencies, 10 to 20 stimuli are required for each nerve studied to determine the shortest and longest latencies. Finally, as with H-reflexes, a variety of conditions can injure the nerve pathways at sites other that the nerve root and result in abnormal F waves. In conclusion, although there are many limitations, F wave studies may be useful in evaluating radiculopathies and should be utilized as clinical indications dictate.

### Needle Examination

The chronology of electrophysiologic changes that occur with nerve injury has been discussed. The steps in performing a proper needle examination study are well documented (11). Needle electromyography is probably the single most useful electrodiagnostic study in evaluating patients with low back pain for evidence of nerve injury. In spite of the fact that EMG only evaluates motor fibers, the diagnostic yield is considerably higher than with other techniques (4,28,34). Although the needle examination is an excellent way to evaluate limb symptoms associated with back pain, the studies are not always abnormal even though true nerve injury exists. There are a few explanations based on electrophysiologic grounds. First, there can be weakness in the presence of a normal needle examination owing to neurapraxia or conduction block (e.g., the nerve is not conducting normally but no axonal injury occurred). Second, if only a few axons degenerate, the lesion could be missed by random sampling of the muscles (4). Third, the timing of the needle exam is also important. If the examination is performed more than 4 to 6 months after symptoms have occurred, reinnervation by collateral sprouting has probably halted the occurrence of spontaneous single muscle fiber discharges (positive waves and fibrillations). If performed less than 2 to 3 weeks following onset, spontaneous single muscle fiber discharges have not yet appeared. Therefore, the needle examination done "too early," i.e., less than 2 to 3 weeks, or "too late," i.e., more than 4 to 6 months, does not reveal the abnormalities that may be prominent between these time limits.

The needle study is particularly useful in localizing a nerve injury to a specific root level. It is important to sample a variety of muscles in a multisegmental distribution that are innervated by different peripheral nerves. Then, if the abnormalities are confined within a single myotome but fall outside the distribution of a single peripheral nerve, the evidence is strongly in favor of a radiculopathy. However, individual variations in muscle innervation occur, sometimes making exact localization less precise (32). Clinical experience has shown that certain muscles have higher yields for positive needle exam findings in specific nerve root injuries (16) (Table 6–2).

The needle examination can help differentiate acute from chronic denervation. In an acute radiculopathy, pos-

itive waves, fibrillation potentials, and fasiculations are usually present in the affected muscle at rest. Chronic radiculopathy without significant ongoing denervation will show large or giant motor unit potentials with polyphasia and often very small fibrillation potentials or positive waves.

Needle examination of paraspinal muscles in suspected radiculopathies or nerve injury is essential. Paraspinal fibrillation potentials indicate that the lesion is proximal to the posterior primary ramus, eliminating the concern of a possible plexopathy (4,15,35). Chronologically, paraspinal muscles are also the first muscles to show fibrillation following onset of radiculopathies in patients with low back or neck pain. They are the first to stop showing fibrillations as the patient recovers (18). Of all patients with positive EMG findings 3 weeks or greater after onset of symptoms, about 70 percent will have abnormalities in the distribution of the posterior primary rami (paraspinal muscles) and 90 percent in the anterior rami distribution (16). Ten to 30 percent of all cases of lumbar radiculopathy have EMG abnormalities only in the distribution of the posterior primary rami (11,16). Evaluating the paraspinal muscles as part of the needle examination is thus quite important.

There are limitations to the needle examination of the paraspinal muscles. First, fibrillation potentials have been shown to be present in the paraspinal muscles for up to 3 days after lumbar myelography (36). Similar findings have been noted in the paraspinal muscles after lumbar epidural injections, as well as lumbar selective nerve root blocks in which abnormalities may last for as long as 4 weeks (18). Second, as paraspinals are the first muscles to reinnervate, needle EMG findings may not be noted because reinnervation has already occurred at the time of the examination. Furthermore, there may be incomplete root involvement that does not affect the posterior ramus (4). Like other aspects of electrodiagnostic abnormalities, positive sharp

| TABLE 6–2 |
| :---: |
| *Common electrodiagnostic study findings in lumbar radiculopathy* |

| | |
| --- | --- |
| L3 | Adductors, iliopsoas |
| L4 | Anterior tibialis, quadriceps. Decreased saphenous SNAP |
| L5 | Anterior tibialis, hamstrings, hip abductors, tensor fascia lata, medial gastrocnemius. Peroneal F wave may be abnormal |
| S1 | Gluteus maximus, medial hamstrings, lateral gastrocnemius. +/− sural SNAP |

waves and fibrillation potentials in paraspinal muscles are only indicative of very proximal nerve or muscle pathology, not diagnostic of radiculopathy. Other causes for these changes include metastatic disease affecting the proximal nerve roots, anterior horn cell disease, inflammatory myopathies (e.g., polymyositis), and particularly diabetes mellitus, which can cause widespread fibrillation potentials throughout the paraspinal muscles (28). Because of overlapping innervation, questions have been raised about the localizing value of paraspinal EMG findings. The specificity of this information is probably enhanced if care is taken to examine the main muscles of the deeper group of intrinsic back muscles, the multifidi (33). Anatomic data indicate relatively localized innervation by dorsal rami in this muscle (37). It is most prudent to try to correlate findings in peripheral muscles with paraspinal muscle findings for precise localization of nerve root injuries. Complete relaxation of the patient can be difficult in the paraspinals, causing misinterpretation of distant motor units as positive waves. Nonreproducible trains or bursts of positive waves in the paraspinals are usually normal and are generated by the needle passing through an endplate zone (38).

The significance of positive sharp waves and fibrillation potentials in the paraspinal muscles in patients who have undergone spinal surgery is controversial (39,40). Recurrent herniation of a lumbar disk, for instance, is not common, but when it does occur, it usually occurs at the same level and side as it did originally. After reviewing 77 EMGs in 60 patients, Johnson and colleagues concluded that EMG abnormalities present at one level at least 3 cm lateral to the scar are probably not related to trauma from surgery but rather are active radiculopathy (40). They also claimed that inserting needle electrodes 2 to 3 cm from the midline and deeper than 3 cm in the muscle is likely to be at the level of the vertebral body spine of the root innervating that particular muscle (15). However, See and Kraft showed that in 20 patients who had undergone laminectomy for root compression, EMG changes in the paraspinal for periods of up to 41 months postoperatively can occur, even without recurrent radiculopathy (41). These findings were usually present at both 1 and 3 cm lateral from the midline and at multiple vertebral levels. Absence of spontaneous single muscle fiber discharges on needle examination of the paraspinal muscles at the site of the surgical scar decreases the possibility that a new radiculopathy is present. In conclusion, positive waves and fibrillations in the paraspinal muscles of patients who have undergone lumbar surgery or other invasive procedures, e.g., recent injections, or even recent electrodiagnostic studies, should be correlated with the clinical history, physical findings, and anatomic studies and should never be used alone to diagnose radiculopathies.

Although the presence of positive waves and fibrillation potentials confined to a specific myotome is the most reliable EMG evidence of acute radiculopathy, analysis of motor unit potentials and their recruitment patterns plays a role in evaluating patients with subacute, chronic, and old resolved radicular syndromes. Abnormal motor unit recruitment occurs almost immediately after the onset of any nerve injury in which interrupted conduction of nerve impulses occur (11,21,23). Evaluating radiculopathy by abnormal recruitment intervals or frequencies has been described and felt possibly to be of particular benefit early in the course of the nerve injury before positive sharp waves and fibrillation potentials occur (23). Johnson suggested in early and mild L5 radiculopathy a recruitment interval of 70–90 msec in the extensor digitorum longus as compared to the normal interval of 100–120 msec was significant (40,42). However, motor unit recruitment abnormalities are unlikely to be recognized unless muscle weakness is easily detectable clinically. Mild weakness is accompanied by only minimal alterations in recruitment intervals, which can be difficult to detect, even for an experienced electromyographer. Although the recruitment pattern at maximal contraction is thought to be indicative of the number of active motor unit potentials, Johnson and colleagues showed this parameter to be a less sensitive finding in patients with radiculopathy than positive sharp waves and fibrillations (20).

Changes in motor unit size and configuration are seen in patients following the acute phase of radiculopathy. They are due to reinnervation of denervated muscle fibers and include polyphasic potentials, often of long duration and sometimes of large amplitude, but such changes by themselves cannot be considered evidence of ongoing, active nerve degeneration. In radiculopathy, reinnervation occurs by intramuscular collateral sprouting from the distal portions of the remaining viable nerves. There are always many viable nerves supplying any given muscle in monoradiculopathy because muscles are innervated by more than one nerve root. As viable nerves sprout, they begin to reinnervate the denervated muscle fibers. Then, when the nerve discharges, it activates not only its own muscle fibers but also some of those belonging to an adjacent denervated nerve fiber. The recorded motor unit potential under such conditions is larger and wider than normal and may be polyphasic. Polyphasicity has long been recognized as one of the electrophysiologic abnormalities found in radiculopathy (18,28,43,44). It should be noted that when a muscle fiber is reinnervated, it stops fibrillating. Therefore, persistent fibrillations indicate ongoing nerve degeneration, a reflection of chronic radiculopathy. Although it is not uncommon for pain to persist chronically following acute radiculopathy, it is relatively uncommon to find evidence of progressive nerve degeneration. Such findings are more often seen in the chronic, progressive narrow spinal canal syndromes (16).

In conclusion, the needle examination appears to be the most reliable aspect of the electrodiagnostic examination in patients with low back complaints and provides the highest yield of abnormalities in radiculopathy (3,34,45). Nerve conduction studies and late responses also yield useful information, which, when taken within the entire context of the patient's complaints, physical findings, and anatomic studies, aids in diagnosing nerve injuries in the back and upper and lower extremities.

## Accuracy of Electrodiagnostic Studies

For decades, clinical investigators have been comparing EMG results, which reveal the electrophysiologic properties of nerve and muscle, with imaging studies, which delineate anatomic configuration of the tissues (46,47,48). Comparisons between surgically "proven" nerve root compromise and EMG findings have also been made (26,48,49). This concept is based on fallacious reasoning. The misconception that the two can be compared to one another with accuracy comes from the observed high coincidence of nerve root pathology at the site of, and often caused by, disk protrusion and other anatomic distortions. While it is true that distorted spinal architecture can damage a nerve root, it is also well known that nerve root pathology can be demonstrated in the absence of macroanatomic abnormality (50,51). Furthermore, disk protrusion can be seen at postmortem examination in the spine of almost all patients over the age of 40 years, the majority of whom were asymptomatic for radiculopathy (52). The EMG reveals the presence and to some degree the extent of motor nerve degeneration. This information is provided neither by imaging studies nor by direct observation of the tissues during surgery. In radiculopathy, during the acute or subacute phase of muscle fiber denervation, the observation of fibrillation, i.e., the sensitivity of the test, approaches 100 percent accuracy; i.e., either there has been nerve degeneration (fibrillation is present) or there has not. By the time muscle fibers have been reinnervated, EMG must rely on findings that are sometimes less obvious than fibrillation potentials, but the presence of such findings indicates that nerve degeneration has led to reinnervation of muscle fibers. The specificity for radiculopathy, based on the findings of positive waves and fibrillation potentials is not known; however, it greatly increases when the distribution of the abnormalities is clearly segmental (53). The EMG also allows recognition of the segmental level involved as long as the abnormality is distributed to at least three or four muscles distributed within a single myotome. Detection of anatomic abnormality at another level does not alter the location of nerve root pathology. Some studies have attempted to compare findings on physical examination with those on EMG (47,54). This is also improper. The EMG is an extension of the physical examination; one does not supplant the other. The presence or absence of EMG abnormalities always adds information. At times the EMG reveals abnormality when no neurologic deficits can be found on physical examination. This is particularly true in chronic radiculopathy such as with spinal stenosis (54,55,56).

## CLINICAL AND ELECTROPHYSIOLOGIC PRESENTATIONS OF RADICULOPATHIES

The most common referral to an electrophysiology laboratory for leg pain or back pain is to evaluate for potential radiculopathy. Patients often present with symptoms of numbness, tingling, dysesthesias, or weakness in various distributions. Although radiculopathy is most commonly due to a herniated disc or degenerative foraminal stenosis, electrophysiologic studies reveal only the presence of nerve root irritation, not the cause of the radiculopathy. Table 6–3 shows some common signs, symptoms, and clinical points to consider when evaluating patients for potential radiculopathy. Included in this table are common entrapment neuropathies and other common clinical conditions that may be seen in patients that mimic spine problems. Details of all the potential peripheral nerve entrapments that can mimic radiculopathy is beyond the scope of this text, but are well documented (20,21,57,58,59,60). It is important to note that some peripheral nerve entrapments may present with symptoms very similar to radiculopathy (Table 6–3). All patients presenting with numbness, tingling, or pain in an extremity must not be assumed to only have radiculopathy. Although not common, examples of concomitant cervical radiculopathy and rotator cuff tear, or plantar fasciitis and an S1 radiculopathy occur in clinical practice. Furthermore, the "double crush" syndrome is well documented where a nerve can be injured in more than one place, possibly due to the first injury making the nerve more susceptible to injury in a second location (61). An example is tarsal tunnel syndrome with a L5 radiculopathy. Understanding the anatomy of peripheral nerves and their dermatomal distributions can lead to more effective electrophysiologic evaluation of patients with suspected spinal problems.

## AHCPR GUIDELINES

The AHCPR guidelines provided only three major conclusions with respect to electrodiagnostic studies.

1. EMG/NCV studies, including H-reflexes, may be appropriate in the lower limbs if there is a question of nerve root dysfunction with leg symptoms lasting greater than 4 weeks.

**TABLE 6–3**
*Signs, symptoms, and differential diagnosis of lumbar radiculopathy*

| NERVE ROOT | CLINICAL FINDINGS | DIFFERENTIAL DIAGNOSIS |
|---|---|---|
| L3 | P/D in groin, medial thigh. Weak hip flexion | Psoas and adductor strain |
| L4 | P/D in hip to groin and anterior thigh to medial leg and foot. Decreased knee MSR. Weak knee extensors, ankle dorsiflexors | Saphenous nerve entrapment, anterior compartment syndrome |
| L5 | P/D in back of thigh and anterior tibial region to first web space on dorsum of foot; weak ankle dorsiflexion, great toe extension; diminished medial hamstring MSR; SLR positive | Peroneal neuropathy at the fibular head, or anterior compartment syndrome |
| S1 | P/D from hip to posterior thigh and calf to lateral aspect of foot; weak plantar flexors and ankle eversion; diminished ankle MSR; SLR positive | Deep posterior compartment syndrome, ACL injury with posterior tibial translation, plantar fasciitis, "chronic" hamstrings strain; persistent "tennis leg" |

P/D = paresthesias and/or dysesthesias, MSR= muscle stretch reflex, SLR = straight leg raise, SNAP = sensory nerve action potential, ACL = anterior cruciate ligament.

2. No physiologic testing is necessary if the diagnosis is obvious on clinical examination.
3. Surface EMG and F wave tests are not recommended for assessing patients with acute low back pain symptoms.

The guidelines reviewed 52 articles, of which eight met their reviewers criteria for adequate evidence of efficacy. In general, these recommendations are adequate for a patient with acute low back pain. In most of these cases with low back pain less than 4 weeks there is rarely need for any electrophysiologic testing except in situations stated below. The AHCPR guidelines, although only barely touching the surface of the overall uses of electrodiagnostic studies, provide accurate information regarding the evaluation of acute back pain. The limitations of the studies they reviewed will be discussed.

The diagnostic accuracy ("true positives" and "true negatives") of the four studies discussed in the guidelines of the needle examination (electromyography or EMG) were based on surgical and CT scan findings (12,46,62,63). The panel acknowledged that these studies have poor clinical descriptions, faulty cohort assembly, and biased test interpretation. Furthermore, to com-

pare the true accuracy of a physiologic test on anatomic abnormalities alone (either imaging studies or at surgery) is suspect. Many anatomic "abnormalities" on radiologic imaging exist in asymptomatic patients (64). Similarly, electrophysiologic abnormalities can exist in patients with "normal" imaging studies.

The accuracy of precisely detecting and localizing nerve root compromise with EMG was also evaluated by the panel, which looked at three studies. Aeillo showed that needle EMG was abnormal in all 24 patients who had positive findings at surgery. However, the exact root level was noted only in 9 percent (62). They claimed one false positive EMG where the EMG was positive with no evidence of herniation found at surgery. In fact, there are no "false positives" with EMG. Either the exam reveals membrane instability or positive sharp waves and/or fibrillations or it does not. Positive EMG findings, such as positive sharp waves and/or fibrillation potentials, indicate that some irritation of the nerve has occurred. Correlation with symptoms and or anatomy is not always clear. Chemical factors have been implicated as a causative factor in radiculopathy and can explain the positive EMG with negative anatomic corroboration (50,51). In a related study, Aeillo showed that the true positive rate, as defined by positive EMG along with positive surgical findings, varied from 71 percent to 100 percent and the true negative rate, as defined by negative EMG and negative surgical findings, was from 38 percent to 88 percent (63). Again, all of these studies compared the presence or absence of EMG findings (physiologic parameters) with the results of surgical exploration (anatomic parameters). In a study of 100 patients with clinical evidence of L5 or S1 radiculopathy, Young showed that the needle EMG predicted the correct level in 84 percent of 95 patients with positive surgical findings (48)

In another attempt to explore the usefulness of electrodiagnostic studies, the study by Khatri looked at the outcome of patients treated surgically and nonsurgically for radicular pain who had positive EMGs and positive imaging studies (CT scans). They showed that 81 percent (13 of 16) of the surgically treated patients were better, and 47 percent (9 of 19) of the nonsurgically treated patients were better at 1-year follow-up. However, 67 percent (16 of 24) of the patients with negative EMGs and negative imaging studies were better (46). One could surmise that patients with radicular symptoms with positive EMGs and positive imaging studies may respond better to surgical treatment. However, longer term follow-up studies (e.g., 4 and 10 years of follow-up) have shown that patients fare equally well whether they receive surgical or nonsurgical care (65). The prognostic usefulness, or lack thereof, of electrodiagnostic studies is still undetermined. Other types of studies, such as the H-reflex and the F wave, which were discussed in detail previously, were reviewed briefly by the panel. They thought that H-reflexes which evaluate the S1 nerve root may have some role if low back symptoms persist for a number of weeks and radiculopathy is suspected (13,62,63). However, as previously stated, a number of studies have shown some limitations of H-reflexes that render them not clinically very meaningful in and of themselves (4,29). They may, however, add some useful information to the rest of the electrodiagnostic examination.

The two studies of surface EMG reviewed have also shown significant problems with these techniques which limit their usefulness in the clinical management of radiculopathy and low back pain (66,67). In the study by Arena, only the upper trapezius was studied, not a specific low back muscle. A review of surface EMG by Haig and colleagues, endorsed by the American Board of Electrodiagnostic Medicine in 1995, stated, "there is no clinical indication for the use of surface electromyography in the diagnosis and treatment of disorders of nerve or muscle" (68). No discussion was presented in that review about the usefulness of surface EMG in low back pain. DeLuca looked at the fatigue patterns exhibited by low back muscles in patients with and without low back pain. He found that the pattern of fatigue exhibited by the six

median frequency curves can be used to distinguish individuals who have low back pain from those who do not with an accuracy of at least 84 percent (69). Jalovarra looked at surface EMG activity in the paraspinal muscles of patients with different degrees of low back and leg pain. Patients with only local low back pain had significantly higher EMG activities than those with unilateral radiating pain without verified disc herniation, those with verified disk herniation, and controls (70). They concluded that surface EMG may be a valid tool for indirectly assessing pain in low back pain patients but not for classification into different diagnostic groups.

No discussion was presented in the AHCPR guidelines with respect to the role of nerve conduction studies in the diagnosis of patients with acute low back pain. These patients can have a normal EMG, although nerve injury exists. EMG findings may not become apparent for 2 to 3 weeks after a nerve injury has occurred, when positive sharp waves and fibrillations become apparent. A nerve conduction block, or neurapraxia, can occur almost immediately after a nerve is compressed and cause slowing of the nerve conduction across a segment of nerve such as in a herniated nucleus pulposus. True neurogenic weakness can occur without EMG findings. Wilbourne has shown that there is a reduction of the compound muscle action potential amplitude 7 days post injury in the peroneal muscles in L5 radiculopathy and the tibial muscles in S1 radiculopathy (4). These findings may or may not be of significant clinical value in managing patients with low back pain.

Sensory nerve studies, which evaluate the sensory fibers from the dorsal root ganglion, can potentially be useful in the evaluation of patients with low back pain and radiculopathy. An absent or delayed sensory nerve action potential may suggest the presence of a far lateral disk herniation because the nerve injury has occurred distal to the dorsal root ganglion, which in the lumbar spine is located at about the level of the intervertebral foramen.

### Indications for Electrophysiologic Testing in Patients with Back Pain

The utility of electrodiagnostic testing in a given patient may be estimated following a thorough history and physical examination, a review of supplemental information (i.e., imaging studies), and through an appreciation for the chronology of electrophysiologic changes that occur following nerve injury. Some helpful guide as to the indications and limitations of electrodiagnostic studies are worthy of review:

1. *To establish and/or confirm a clinical diagnosis.* Pain in the lower extremities and back is often referred from pain-sensitive structures other than nerve tissue. This pain may even appear to follow a dermatomal pattern. If

there is no electrophysiologic abnormality, the studies give the physician confidence that this is the case, which may help in patient management and reassurance. With nerve injury, however, a properly timed EMG can show evidence of the nature, location, and severity of the injury. A thorough electrophysiologic exam may alert the examiner to the possibility of unsuspected pathological condition, i.e., concomitant peripheral neuropathy with radiculopathy, an active common peroneal nerve entrapment superimposed on a chronic L5 radiculopathy. In a small percentage of patients, the diagnosis of radiculopathy is established by EMG when the diagnosis on clinical grounds seems unlikely (16). In medicolegal situations, an electrodiagnostic study done early in the course of the injury, i.e., the first few days, if positive waves and fibrillation potentials are present, may indicate that some pre-existing injury is present. If the examination is initially negative and later positive, this indicates a new injury.

2. *To localize nerve lesions.* Signs or symptoms of nerve injuries in the extremities can be from a number of causes, including root lesions (radiculopathy), lumbosacral plexus or root lesions (i.e., metastasis, retroperitoneal hematoma), or peripheral nerve injuries (i.e., meralgia paresthetica, saphenous nerve entrapment, tarsal tunnel syndrome). Various conduction studies and EMG can evaluate many of these nerve segments to specifically localize the lesion. Occasionally, what may appear clinically as a single level radiculopathy may in fact be multilevel or, in the case of spinal stenosis, bilateral. Frequently, clinical assessment only predicts a uniradicular lesion, but EMG may reveal involvement of two roots. This has importance in planning an operative approach (48).

3. *To determine the extent of nerve injury.* A properly timed EMG can differentiate between a neurapraxic injury (conduction block) and active axonal degeneration. It can also semiquantitatively assess the degree of reversible motor axon damage and the severity of the neuronal deficit. This information may have significant impact on the aggressiveness of treatment for a lumbar radiculopathy. The acuteness or chronicity of the lesion may also be obtained.

4. *To correlate findings on anatomic studies.* The existence of nerve root dysfunction cannot be determined or even assumed from diagnostic procedures that determine structural pathology (29). EMG can show if physiologic nerve injury has occurred or is ongoing and if these findings correlate with the symptoms and radiologic studies. This information may have significant importance as to what type of treatment is instituted (surgical vs. nonsurgical). Furthermore, in presurgical candidates it is useful to know what nerve root levels are most involved in order to plan the most appropriate approach and level. Selective nerve blocks can complement EMG studies in localization of pathology.

5. *To assist in prognosis.* The paucity of positive sharp waves and fibrillation potentials in acute radiculopathy with proper timing of the exam may portend an excellent prognosis for return of muscle strength (16). Comparing the compound muscle action potential of a very weak muscle to that of the same muscle on the asymptomatic side gives an idea of the extent of neurapraxia and potential recovery. A side-to-side amplitude difference of greater than 50 percent is probably significant (16). Recovery is prolonged and less complete when more than one root is involved, which may be determined at times only by EMG (22,48). Normal electrophysiologic findings have correlated with poor postoperative results (71).

## Limitations of Electrophysiologic Tests

The EMG is not a perfect test and should not be done in every patient referred for evaluation of low back pain. Some of the limitations of electrophysiologic testing and situations in which it may not be necessary to obtain them are described here.

1. *In the first 2 to 4 weeks after onset of symptoms.* In most cases if the clinical situation and examination are strongly suggestive of radiculopathy, treatment can be instituted without an EMG. Many findings may not be seen if the exam is done too early. If the patient has progressive neurologic deficits, the results of the EMG will not be important because the patient will require emergent care. If a patient is not improving to the extent that is anticipated for that level of care, an EMG may be useful, but not in the very acute situation.

2. *In unequivocal radiculopathy.* When the clinical history and the motor, sensory, and reflex changes are consistent, EMG adds little information and generally is not necessary. It may be required if the patient is not improving with treatment, and may still pick up coexisting pathologies.

3. *When the history and examination are highly inconsistent with acute radiculopathy.* If the clinical situation is not clear, some important points must be considered. When a patient with back or neck pain is being evaluated, acute radiculopathy is unlikely if the pain is confined to the axial skeleton, if it involves both lower limbs, or if it occurs intermittently. Additionally, if there is no detectable neurologic deficit on physical examination, acute radiculopathy is highly improbable and electrodiagnostic studies may not be needed.

4. *When there has been no change in clinical situation in previously studied patients.* Many patients have had multiple EMGs in an attempt to determine an etiology for nonsegmental, nondermatomal complaints. When multiple studies have been done, and they have been of high

quality, with no change in the clinical signs or symptoms, very little information will be gained with further studies.

5. *The results will not change medical or surgical management.* For whatever reasons (e.g., extreme illness, patient refusing surgery), if the results of the studies will in no way change the treatment plan, EMG should probably be avoided.

6. *Barriers to acquiring sufficient information are present.* If a patient cannot be moved from prone to supine (or vice versa) or if dressings, casts, or stabilizing devices cannot be repositioned or temporarily removed, the information from performing the electrodiagnostic studies may be limited.

## The EMG Evaluation and Report

A thorough, comprehensive electrophysiologic medical consultation is an essential component in the overall approach to the evaluation and management of patients with spine problems. The evaluation must include a thorough history and physical examination preceding the appropriate electrodiagnostic studies. The electrophysiologic report should include a number of important pieces of data for the referring physician. First, the electrophysiologic findings should be correlated with any physical findings noted or discrepancies identified. Inconsistencies may have as much importance in the clinical management of the patient as consistent results, if not more. Second, the degree of certainty or "hardness" of the finding needs to be conveyed to the referring physician. A diagnosis of an S1 radiculopathy by H-reflex changes only will carry different weight compared to abundant spontaneous discharges in an S1 myotomal distribution. Third, the diagnoses that have been excluded can be as important as those confirmed. Fourth, information should be noted about potential diagnoses that are suggested by the clinical examination but not supported by the electrophysiologic study. Fifth, significant concomitant pathology noted, e.g., tarsal tunnel syndrome superimposed on a lumbar radiculopathy, should be mentioned. Sixth, any change from previous studies may be useful information. Seventh, the degree of acuteness or chronicity of the lesions identified need to be stated. Finally, prognosis, when possible, is critical information for managing patients. This is particularly important when the EMG shows only neurapraxic changes in contrast to significant axonal degeneration.

## Cost and Harm

The cost-effectiveness of a given electrodiagnostic study is difficult to determine. No other available test is able to give the level of dynamic physiologic information that electrodiagnostic studies can provide. In general, the examination can be completed in less than 1 hour. The cost may vary from $200 to $1,000 depending on the number of nerves and muscles studied. Patient comfort is variable and often dependent on the skill of the examiner in accurately and gently placing the electromyography electrodes.

Needle precautions are required with electromyographic studies, as they are whenever a needle is used and the potential for the examiner to be exposed to blood or blood products exists. There are no common complications. Pneumothorax from over-zealous needle examination of intercostal muscles has been anecdotally described to the authors. Bleeding complications are a potential problem in patients on anticoagulants or with bleeding diatheses. In general, EMG/NCV are a very safe procedure to perform in adequately trained practitioners.

## FUTURE RESEARCH

Much research needs to be done to evaluate the usefulness of electrodiagnostic studies for low back pain. Specifically, it needs to be determined if there is any prognostic value of EMG/NCV in low back pain. Does a patient with 2+ positive waves and fibrillations clinically do as well or as poorly as a patient with 4+ findings. Do EMG/NCV findings correlate at all with outcome in patients treated surgically or nonsurgically? What effect, if any, do epidural corticosteroids and selective nerve root injections have on EMG/NCV findings? Many of these answers will require serial electrodiagnostic studies in randomly controlled groups of patients with similar presentations and clinical findings.

*S*ummary

The effectiveness and reliability of the electrodiagnostic examination in detecting pathology in patients with spine problems is high but must always be understood in light of its capabilities and limitations. Indiscriminate use of this or any testing procedure should be avoided. Electrodiagnostic studies are examiner-dependent and, when possible, should be performed by a physician who is a specialist in electrodiagnostic medicine. Ideally, this physician is involved in the diagnosis and management of the patient studied. Electrodiagnostic studies evaluate nerve physiology in a certain chronological sequence but do not measure pain. Suggested guidelines have been given for possible situations where an EMG may or may not be helpful in treating patients with spine problems, which in turn leads to better care.

# References

1. Glantz RH, Haldeman S. Other diagnostic studies: electrodiagnosis. In: Frymoyer JW (ed.). *The adult spine: principles and practice.* New York: Raven Press, 1991:541–548.
2. Goss CM (ed.). *Gray's anatomy of the human body.* 29th ed (American). Philadelphia: Lea & Febiger, 1973:1466.
3. Weichers DO. Radiculopathies. *Phys Med Rehab—State Art Rev* 1989; 3:713–724.
4. Wilbourne AJ, Aminoff MJ. The electrophysiologic examination in patients with radiculopathies and nerve. *Muscle Nerve* 1988; 11:1099–1114.
5. Travell JG, Simons DG. *Myofascial pain and dysfunction: the trigger point manual.* Baltimore: Williams & Wilkins, 1983.
6. Rydevik B, Braun MD, Lundborg G. Pathoanatomy and pathophysiology of nerve root compression. *Spine* 1984; 9:7–15.
7. Fowler T, Danta G, Gilliatt R. Recovery of nerve conduction after a pneumatic tourniquet: Observations on the hind limb of the baboon. *J Neurol Neurosurg Psychiatry* 1972; 35:638–647.
8. Gilliatt R. Acute compression block. In: Sumner AJ (ed.). *The pathophysiology of peripheral nerve disease.* Philadelphia: WB Saunders, 1980:287–315.
9. Gilliatt RW. Chronic nerve compression and entrapment. In: Summer AJ (ed.). *The physiology of peripheral nerve disease.* Philadelphia: WB Saunders, 1980:316–339
10. Gilliatt R. Recent advances in the pathophysiology of nerve conduction. In: Desmedt J (ed.). *Developments in electromyography and clinical* neurophysiology. Vol. 2. Basel: Karger, 1983:2–18
11. Johnson EW. Electrodiagnosis of radiculopathy. Advanced concepts in evaluation of focal neuropathy. Inst. course of American Association Electromyography and Electrodiagnosis, Las Vegas, 1985
12. Baylan SP, Yu J, Grant AE. H-reflex latency in relation to ankle jerk, electromyographic, myelographic, and surgical findings in back pain patients. *Electromyogr Clin Neurophysiol* 1981; 21:201–206.
13. Braddom RL, Johnson EW. Standardization of H-reflex and diagnostic use in S1 radiculopathy. *Arch Phys Med Rehabil* 1974; 55:161–166.
14. Schuchmann JA. H-reflex latency in radiculopathy. *Arch Phys Med Rehabil* 1978; 59:185–187.
15. Johnson EW, Melvin JL. Value of electromyography in lumbar radiculopathy. *Arch Phys Med Rehabil* 1971; 52:239–243.
16. MacLean IC. Acute radiculopathy. Presented at EMG and Neurophysiology: A High Intensity Review. Chicago, April 6, 1989.
17. Johnson EW. The EMG examination. In: Johnson EW (ed.): *Practical electromyography.* Baltimore: Williams & Wilkins, 1988:1–21
18. Saal JA. Electrophysiologic evaluation of lumbar pain. Establishing the rationale for therapeutic management. *Spine—State Art Rev* 1986; 1:21–46.
19. Spindler, HA, Felsenthal, G. Electrodiagnostic evaluation of acute and chronic radiculopathy. *Phys Med Rehabil Clin North Am* 1990; 1:53.
20. Johnson EW. Electrodiagnosis of radiculopathy. In: Johnson EW (ed.). *Practical electromyography.* Baltimore: Williams & Wilkins, 1988:229–245
21. Kimura J. *Electrodiagnosis in diseases of muscle and nerve.* Philadelphia: FA Davis, 1985.
22. Benecke R, Conrad B. The distal sensory nerve action potential as a diagnostic tool for the differentiation of lesions in dorsal roots and peripheral nerves. *J Neurol* 1989; 223:231–239.
23. Eisen A. Electrodiagnosis of radiculopathy. In: Aminoff MJ (ed.). Symposium on electrodiagnosis. *Neurol Clin* 1985; 3:495–510.
24. Aeillo I, Rosati G, Serra G, et al. The diagnostic valve of H-index in S1 root compression. *J Neurol Neurosurg Psychiatry* 1981; 44:171–172.
25. Fisher, MA. AAEM Minimonograph #13: H reflexes and F waves physiology and clinical indications. *Muscle Nerve* 1992; 15:1223–1233.
26. Leyshon A, Kirwan EOG, Wynn PCG. Electrical studies in the diagnosis of compression at the lumbar root. *J Bone Joint Surg* 1981; 63B:71–75.
27. Tonzola RF, Ackil AA, Shahani BT, Young RR. Usefulness of electrophysiological studies in the diagnosis of lumbosacral root disease. *Ann Neurol* 1981; 9:305–308.
28. Wilbourne AJ. The value and limitations of electromyographic examination in the diagnosis of lumbosacral radiculopathy. In: Hary RW (ed.). *Lumbar disc disease.* New York: Raven Press, 1982:65–109.
29. Haldeman S. The electrodiagnostic evaluation at nerve root function. *Spine* 1984; 9(1):42–45.
30. Weintraub JR, Madalin K, Wong M, Wilbourn AJ, Mahdad M. Achilles tendon reflex and the H response. *Muscle Nerve* 1988; 11:972.
31. Marshall TM. Nerve pinch injuries in football. *J Kentucky Med Assoc* 1970; VOL:648–649.
32. Young RR, Shahani BJ. Clinical value and limitation of F-nerve determination. *Muscle Nerve* 1978; 13:248–249.
33. Fisher MA, Shivde AJ, Teixera C, et al. The F-response: A clinically useful physiological parameter for the evaluation of radicular injury. *Electromyogr Clin Neurophysiol* 1979; 19:65–75.
34. Aminoff MJ, Goodin DS, Parry GJ, et al. Electrophysiologic evaluation of lumbosacral radiculopathies: Electromyography, late responses, and somatosensory evoked potentials. *Neurology* 1985; 35:1514–1518.
35. Eisen A, Schamer D, Melmed C. An electrophysiological method for examining lumbosacral root compression. *Can J Neurol Sci* 1977; 2:117–123.
36. Weber RJ, Weingarden SI. EMG abnormalities following myelography. *Arch Neurol* 1979; 36:588.
37. Jonsson B. Morphology, innervation, and electromyographic study of the erector spinae. *Arch Phys Med Rehabil* 1969; 50:638–641.
38. Weichers DO. Electromyographic insertional activity in normal limb muscles. *Arch Phys Med Rehabil* 1979; 60:359.
39. Fisher MA, Kaur D, Houchins J. Electrodiagnostic examination, back pain and entrapment of posterior rami. *Electromyogr Clin Neurophysiol* 1985; 25:183–189.
40. Johnson EW, Burkhart JA, Earl WC. Electromyography in postlaminectomy patients. *Arch Phys Med Rehabil* 1972; 53:407–409.
41. See DH, Kraft GH. Electromyography in paraspinal muscles following surgery for root compression. *Arch Phys Med Rehabil* 1975; 56:80–83.

42. Johnson EW, Stocklin R, LaBan MM. Use of electrodiagnostic examination in a university hospital. *Arch Phys Med Rehabil* 1965; 46:573–578.

43. Hoover BB, Caldwell JW, Krusen EM, et al. Value of polyphasic potentials in diagnosis of lumbar root lesions. *Arch Phys Med Rehabil* 1970; 51:546–548.

44. Lajoie WJ. Nerve root compression: correlation of electromyographic, myelographic and surgical findings. *Arch Phys Med Rehabil* 1972; 53:390–392.

45. Rodriguez AA, Kanis L, Rodriguez AA, et al. Somatosensory evoked potentials from dermatomal stimulation as an indicator of L5 and S1 radiculopathy. *Arch Phys Med Rehabil* 1987; 68:366–368.

46. Khatri BO, Barvah J, McQuillen MP. Correlation of electromyography with computed tomography in evaluation of lower back pain. *Arch Neurol* 1984; 41:594–597.

47. Lane ME, Tamhankar MN, Demopoulos JJ. Discogenic radiculopathy: use of electromyography in multidisciplinary management. *N Y State J Med* 1978; VOL:32–34.

48. Young A et al. Variations in the pattern of muscle innervation by the L5 and S1 nerve roots. *Spine* 1983; 8:616–624.

49. Fisher MA, Shivde AJ, Teixera C, et al. Clinical and electrophysiological appraisal of the significance of radicular injury in back pain. *J Neurol Neurosurg Psychiatry* 1978; 41:303–306.

50. Marshall LL, Trethewie ER, Curtain CC. Chemical radiculitis: A clinical, physiological and immunological study. *Clin Orthop Rel Res* 1987; 129:61–67.

51. Saal JS. The role of inflammation in lumbar pain. *Phys Med Rehabil: State Art Rev* 1990; (4)2:191–199.

52. McCrae, DL. Asymptomatic intervertebral disc protrusions. *Acta Radiol* 1956; 46:9–27.

53. American Association of Electrodiagnostic Medicine. Guidelines in electrodiagnostic medicine. *Muscle Nerve* 1992; 15:229–253.

54. Hall S, Bartlesen JD, Onotrio BM, et al. Clinical features, diagnostic procedures and results of surgical treatment in 68 patients. *Ann Intern Med* 1985; 103:271–275.

55. Seppalainen AM, Alaranta H, Solni J. Electromyography in the diagnosis of lumbar spinal stenosis. *Electromyogr Clin Neurophysiol* 1981; 21:55–66.

56. Jacobson RE. Lumbar stenosis: An electromyographic evaluation. *Clin Orthop Rel Res* 1976; 115:68–71.

57. Herring SA, Weinstein SM. Electrodiagnosis in sports medicine. *Phys Med and Rehabil: State Art Rev* 1989; 3(4):809–822.

58. Hirasawa Y, Sakakida K. Sports and peripheral nerve injury. *Am J Sports Med* 1983; 11:420–426.

59. Pease WS. Entrapment neuropathies. *Phys Med Rehabil: State Art Rev* 1989; 3(4):741–756.

60. Takazawa H, Sudo N, et al. Statistical observation of nerve injuries in athletes. *Brain Nerve Injuries* 1971; 3:11–17.

61. Thomas JE, Lambert EH, Csevz KA. Electrodiagnostic aspects of the carpal tunnel syndrome. *Arch Neurol* 1967; 16:635–641.

62. Aeillo I, Serra G, Migliore A. Tugnoli V, Roccella P, Cristofori MC, Manca M. Diagnostic uses of H-reflex from vastus medialis muscle. *Electromyogr Clin Neurophysiol* 1983; 23; 159–166.

63. Aeillo I, Serra G, Tugnoli V, Cristofori MC, Migliore A, Roccella P, Rosati G. Electrophysiological findings in patients with lumbar disc prolapse. *Electromyogr Clin Neurophysiol* 1984 May; 24(4):313–320.

64. Boden SD, Davis Do, Dina TS, Patronas NJ, Wiesel SW. Abnormal magnetic resonance scans of the lumbar spine in asymptomatic subjects. *JBJS* 72–A 1990; (3):403–408.

65. Weber H. Lumbar disc herniation: A controlled prospective study with ten years of observation. *Spine* 1983; 8(2):131–140.

66. Arena JG, Sherman RA, Bruno GM, Young TR. Electromyographic recordings of low back pain subjects and non-pain controls in six different positions: Effects of pain levels. *Pain* 1991 Apr; 45(1):23–28.

67. Sihoven T, Partanen J, Hanninen O, Soimakallio S. Electric behavior of low back muscles during lumbar pelvic rhythm in low back pain patients and healthy controls. *Arch Phys Med Rehabil* 1991 Dec; 72:1080–1087.

68. Haig AJ, Gelblum JB, Rechtien JJ, Gitter, AJ. Technology assessment: The use of surface EMG in the diagnosis and treatment of nerve and muscle disorders. *Muscle Nerve* 1996; 19(3):392–395.

69. DeLuca CJ. Use of the surface EMG signal for performance evaluation of back muscles. *Muscle Nerve* 1993; 16(2):210–216.

70. Jalovaara P, Niinimaki T, Vanharanta H. Pocket-size, portable surface EMG device in the differentiation of low back pain patients. *European Spine Journal* 1995; 4(4):210–212.

71. Tulberg T, Svanborg E, Isacsson J, Grane P. A preoperative and postoperative study of the accuracy and value of electrodiagnosis in patients with lumbosacral disc herniation. *Spine* 1993; 18(7):837–842.

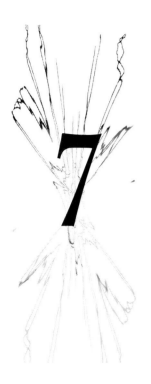

# 7 Physiologic Assessment: Somatosensory Evoked Potentials

*Jerrold N. Rosenberg, M.D., and Erwin G. Gonzalez, M.D.*

Almost every American will experience disabling back pain at some point in his or her adult life. The direct costs of physician visits, diagnostic evaluations, and therapy compose a major portion of the health care dollar. When one also considers the indirect costs of time lost from work, disability benefits, litigation, and lost productivity, it becomes a significant percentage of our entire gross national product (1). The Agency for Health Care Policy Research (AHCPR) recently convened a 23-member multidisciplinary panel of experts and published a Clinical Practice Guideline (Number 14) on Acute Low Back Pain Problems in Adults (2). As part of this review, they considered somatosensory evoked potential (SEP) diagnostic evaluations. They concluded that SEPs "may be useful in assessing suspected spinal stenosis and spinal cord myelopathy" (2). This review, however, was quite limited and failed to identify the clinical usefulness of SEP evaluation in acute low back pain.

## HISTORY

Somatosensory evoked potentials (SEPs) are the electrical manifestations generated by the nervous system in response to a repetitive external stimulus. This stimulus excites the large myelinated fibers in peripheral nerves and results in afferent volleys that ascend through the spinal cord to the somatosensory cerebral cortex. These stimuli may be physiological or electrical. They were first described by Caton in 1875, but it was not until 1947 that Dawson (3) was able to record them in the laboratory. Since then SEPs have been applied in both research and clinical medicine, helping in the diagnosis and prognosis of clinical syndromes.

## TECHNIQUE

A detailed description of the equipment and techniques of obtaining SEP recordings is beyond the scope of this review. However, a brief understanding of the application principles and nomenclature is necessary to appreciate the clinical advantages of SEP evaluation.

The somatosensory evoked response can be elicited by stimulation of either a mixed nerve, a dermatome, or a cutaneous nerve. The stimulus excites the largest myelinated fast conducting Group Ia muscle or II cutaneous afferent nerve fiber and travels to the dorsal root ganglion. It then ascends ipsilaterally in the posterior column to synapse in the dorsal column nuclei of the nucleus cuneatus or nucleus gracilis. The potential crosses in the medial lemniscus to the ventral posterior lateral nucleus of the thalamus where there is a second synapse and then travels directly to the sensory cortex. The central nervous system has a built in "amplifier effect" increasing the signal at each synapse as it proceeds rostrally. SEP abnormalities are most commonly associated with disorders of touch, vibration, and conscious proprioception (4). Coincidentally, these are also the fibers responsible for the most common symptoms associated with low back syndromes.

Actual recording techniques vary from laboratory to laboratory. The afferent volleys may be recorded over the peripheral nerve, spinal cord, or scalp with various surface and/or needle electrodes. The arrangement of the recording electrodes is referred to as a "montage" or recording location. When using surface electrodes, the skin and scalp under the electrode must be prepared with an abrasive paste to reduce skin impedance. Since the SEP is of low amplitude—0.1 to 3μV—signal averaging is required, usually 250–1,000 sweeps. Monopolar (referential) recordings are in general of larger amplitude, more consistent, and easier to obtain. However, they may be more susceptible to contamination from muscle artifact and electromagnetic interference. Bipolar (differential) recordings have not been shown to represent valid anatomic physiological correlates (5).

Short latency SEPs refer to the portion of the wave form that typically occurs within 25 ms after stimulation in the upper extremity and 50 ms in the lower extremity. A mid-latency SEP usually occurs within 100 ms while a long latency SEP refers to a time greater than 100 ms. Near field potentials are those potentials where both recording electrodes are close to one another and the biological source of the potential. For example, Cz'-Fz' are both cephalic sites. Far field potentials are those potentials where the biological origin is located at a distance from the recording electrode. This most commonly involves montages where the recording electrode is cephalic and the reference is noncephalic, placed on the arm or leg. Any combination of the above may be attempted in making recordings. In our laboratory, we have found monopolar, cephalic, short latency recordings to be the most clinically useful.

Multichannel recordings are usually required to increase the yield of any study. Spinal recordings are described by the level of the recording. For example, a recording electrode may be inserted into the T12 intervertebral space and referenced to the T11 intervertebral space. This is referred to as a "T11/T12 spinal recording montage." When making scalp recordings, the international 10–20 EEG system is utilized (Figure 7–1A). This

system divides the scalp into equidistant sections 10–20 percent between the nasion and inion in the sagittal plane and between the right and left preauricular points in the coronal plane. For example, Cz-Fz describes the active recording electrode being placed at Cz and referenced to Fz. Many investigators have found that 1–2 cm posterior to these standard EEG locations is more advantageous for recording SEPs and refer to these locations as "prime" (Figure 7–1B). This is depicted as Cz'-Fz'. Figure 7–2 demonstrates different wave form recordings from different cortical recording sites.

One source of confusion when discussing SEPs involves the use of recording nomenclature. The problem is that there is no universally accepted nomenclature for reporting wave forms. Initially, they were described by the latency at which they typically appeared. A P40 wave, for example, denotes a positive wave form at 40 ms. Figure 7–3 depicts a P38 wave form. Note that it is a down-going wave form electrically described as positive. This is a typical recording when stimulating the tibial nerve at the ankle of an adult. It will, however, vary from laboratory to laboratory and from patient to patient depending on their height and so forth. Some laboratories report the wave forms in terms of their arrival. For example, P1 occurred at 38 ms.

To date, the most reliable recording parameter is peak latency. The patient's height, however, is a variable that must be considered when establishing normal values (6). Amplitude measurements are somewhat variable, although side to side differences of greater than 50 percent are usually considered significant. Interpeak differences, duration measurements, and wave form analysis have yet to be proved as significant. Refinement in analytical techniques remains an ongoing area of research.

One simple method of stimulation is segmental cutaneous nerve activation (CSEP) (7,8). Eisen and co-workers (9,10) were able to demonstrate that abnormal SEPs occurred most frequently when sensory deficits predominated and that there was a good correlation between physiological, myelographic, and operative findings with this technique. They utilized amplitude reduction, abnormal morphology, and latency prolongation as their criteria for evaluation. Table 7–1 summarizes the different cutaneous nerve stimulation sites, segments, and the normal latencies following segmental sensory stimulation

Mixed nerve stimulation involves the direct repetitive stimulation of a mixed nerve, usually the tibial or peroneal in the lower extremity. This may take place at either the ankle or the knee. This form of stimulation is most often used because it yields the most consistent wave forms (11). Mixed nerve stimulation, however, may elicit multiroot stimulation and therefore can not localize single nerve root lesions (9–12). Its greatest clinical usefulness thus far has been limited to investigations of spinal cord pathology and intraoperative monitoring tech-

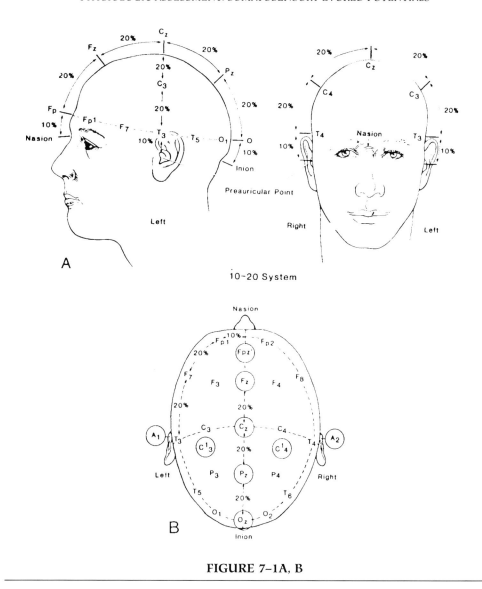

**FIGURE 7–1A, B**

*A:* International 10–20 System of Electrode Placement based on four anatomic landmarks of the nasion, inion, and bilateral preauricular points. *B:* The most common electrode sites for recording SEPs are circled. From *Practical Electromyography,* 2nd ed, edited by E. Johnson. Baltimore: Williams & Wilkins, 1988.

niques. Figure 7–4 depicts a mixed nerve stimulation technique with both spinal and cortical recordings.

Dermatomal evoked potentials offer the most promise with regard to segmental specificity and is the main focus of this chapter. This technique requires the use of large stimulation electrode strips over "signature areas" and increased stimulation intensity. Figure 7–5 depicts the standard signature areas of the lower extremity. The wave forms are smaller and more dispersed than either mixed nerve or cutaneous evoked responses. They have, however, been demonstrated to be an accurate and reproducible tool (13–15).

There is little required in terms of patient preparation. Myogenic silence, however, is mandatory as motor activity can obliterate the SEP recording. To account for this, one reduces the stimulus until the slightest muscle contraction is physically observed. In our laboratory we promote silence in the testing room by dimming the lights and reminding the patient not to speak during the examination. Patients may be either seated or supine and supported by pillows for comfort. It is unusual to sedate a patient. When necessary, chloral hydrate is recommended. Valium may also be used but it may reduce the amplitude of the wave form (16).

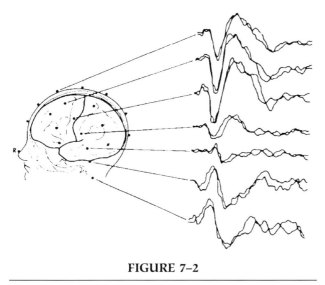

**FIGURE 7–2**

A set of normal evoked potential recordings from multiple locations on the cortex. From *Evoked Potential Primer,* Rianer Spehlmann, MS Butterworth Publishers, Boston, MA, 1985.

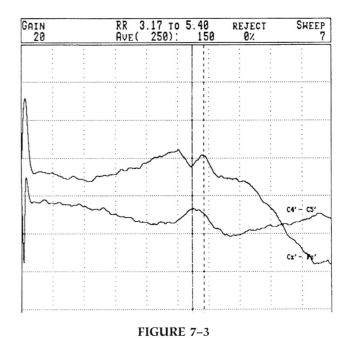

**FIGURE 7–3**

Normal mixed nerve stimulation SEP recording. *Upper line* represents Cz'/Fz' recording site while *lower line* represents C3'/C4' montage. P1 is 38.3 ms.

**TABLE 7–1**
*Results of segmental sensory stimulation*

| CUTANEOUS NERVE | STIMULATION SITE | SEGMENT | LATENCY TO N20 OR P40 (MEAN, SD) |
|---|---|---|---|
| Musculocutaneous | Forearm | C5 | 17.4 (1.2) |
| Median | Thumb | C6 | 22.5 (1.1) |
| Median | Adjoining surfaces of index and middle fingers | C7 | 21.2 (1.2) |
| Ulnar | Little finger | C8 | 22.5 (1.1) |
| Lateral femoral cutaneous | Thigh | L2 | 31.8 (1.8) |
| Saphenous | Knee | L3 | 37.6 (2.0) |
| Saphenous | Ankle | L4 | 43.4 (2.2) |
| Superficial peroneal | Above ankle | L5 | 39.9 (1.8) |
| Sural | Ankle | S1 | 42.1 (1.4) |

From Eisen AA: The somatosensory evoked potential. Minimonograph 19, Rochester, MN, AAEE, 1982.

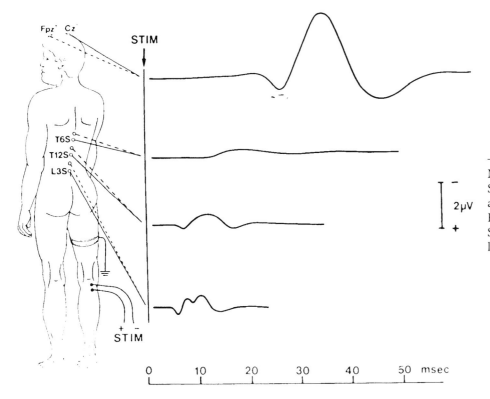

## FIGURE 7–4

Normal mixed nerve stimulation SEP recording at several locations along the neurophysiological tract. From *Evoked Potential Primer,* Rianer Spehlmann, MS Butterworth Publishers, Boston, MA, 1985.

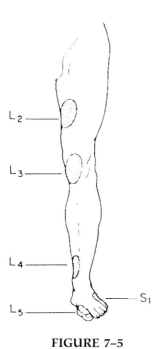

## FIGURE 7–5

Dermatological stimulation signature areas. Redrawn from Katifi HA, Sedgwixk EM. Evaluation of dermatomal SEP in diagnosis of lumbral sacral root compression. *J Neurol Neurosurg Psych* 1987; 50:1204–1210.

## AHCPR REVIEW

As noted previously, the AHCPR reviewers limited the usefulness of SEPs to spinal stenosis and spinal cord myelopathy. Their literature search, however, reviewed only one article on SEPs, a report by Dr. Walter Stolov and Dr. Jefferson Slimp entitled "Dermatomal Somatosensory Evoked Potentials in Lumbar Spinal Stenosis," published in 1988 (17).

In this report, the authors restricted their evaluation to patients with lumbar spinal stenosis. This included only two pathologic conditions, central stenosis and lateral recess stenosis. Sixty-eight patients referred for symptoms of spinal stenosis were reviewed. Of those 68 patients, 38 percent (26 patients) met all criteria for the diagnosis of spinal stenosis, including CT and/or myelography confirmation. Of the 26 stenotic patients, 25 (96 percent) had bilateral multilevel dermatomal SEP abnormalities while only 59 percent had bilateral EMG abnormalities. It is interesting to note that of the original 68 patients, 49 demonstrated abnormal SEPs. Ten percent of these were considered false-positive as reflected by negative myelography. Of the 14 patients with normal SEPs, EMGs were positive in six but only one had structural changes on myelography or less than 1 percent false-negative.

They concluded that dermatomal SEPs were more likely than EMG to detect root compromise in lumbar central and lateral recess stenosis.

## CRITIQUE OF LITERATURE
## REVIEWED BY AHCPR

Obviously, a literature review of one article is inadequate. It is impossible to determine the efficacy of a technique if the literature search is limited to only two specific diagnostic entities. Additionally, this particular article was not a review of the topic under consideration—acute low back pain. In fact, this study failed to even discuss the length of symptomatology in the patients evaluated. Patients with classic radicular findings (low back pain) were not included and mixed nerve/cutaneous SEP stimulation techniques were not addressed. It also used myelography as the basis for confirming the pathologic condition. This is certainly open to criticism. While it does confirm the value of dermatomal SEPs in the diagnosis of lumbar spinal stenosis, it does not rule out the usefulness of SEPs in radiculopathy.

## RATIONALE FOR USE

Acute low back symptoms are most frequently sensory in nature, including pain and radiating paresthesias. Motor weakness is often a late finding (18). There can be many neurologic and musculoskeletal etiologies. Of primary concern is a nerve root injury resulting from a posterior lateral disc protrusion or rupture. Other potential injuries that may mimic the clinical symptoms of a nerve root injury include peripheral nerve injury distal to the root such as a lumbar plexopathy, carcinomatous root invasion, diabetic radiculopathy, and so forth. Musculoskeletal etiologies, including facet joint inflammation, sacroiliac joint inflammation, piriformis syndrome, and simple muscle spasms, further complicate the diagnosis.

Routine electrodiagnostics traditionally include NCVs and electromyographic studies. There are significant limitations in utilizing routine studies in the evaluation of acute back syndromes. The details are discussed in Chapter 6. In an attempt to address these shortcomings, F wave (19) and H reflex techniques (20,21) were developed. The value of H reflexes or F waves in radiculopathy has been somewhat successful, as confirmed by the AHCPR (2). F wave techniques, however, require maximal stimulation and may result in multiroot activation, thereby missing a single root lesion. H reflex studies are limited to S1 root lesions. These factors contribute to the limited sensitivity of routine EMG/NCV examinations (22) and provide a significant rationale for the use of SEPs in radiculopathy.

Similarly, electromyographic evidence is limited in acute situations. EMG changes from radiculopathy, including fibrillations and positive sharp waves, will only be present if motor nerve function is disrupted and Wallerian degeneration has developed. This process takes several days even at the paraspinal level. Recent attempts to evaluate recruitment patterns immediately after injury remain somewhat subjective.

SEP evaluations offer several theoretical advantages over routine neurodiagnostic techniques. First, SEP conduction, in contrast to routine neurodiagnostics and F wave and H reflexes, are a true conduction across the nerve root site. Type Ia and type II fibers are directly stimulated (10). Coincidentally, these are also the very fibers predominantly responsible for the majority of sensory symptoms in patients with low back pain.

Second, SEPs are helpful in ruling out other peripheral nerve etiologies for acute low back pain. For example, SEPs have been demonstrated to be helpful in the evaluation of plexopathies (23). To ensure that the abnormal SEP is not the result of a central nervous system injury, a central conduction time needs to be determined (10). This can be accomplished by subtracting the cortical SEP latencies from the cervical or lumbar potential. It should not exceed 7.5 ms in the arm or 22.5 ms in the leg. The SEP again has the advantage of being abnormal in plexopathies soon after injury while routine EMG studies are not.

Third, SEPs may have significant prognostic value. For example, SEPs have been demonstrated to have prognostic value when studying a plexopathy. The preservation of SEPs in the presence of denervation and absent motor responses is regarded with a favorable prognosis in plexopathies (24,25). In addition to its prognostic value in plexus injuries, SEP has been established to have prognostic value in several other clinical syndromes including coma (26), head injury (27), and cerebrovascular accidents (28,29). Narayan (27) studied 133 severely head injured patients and found that "multimodality" evoked potentials were the most accurate single prognostic indicator, with a 91 percent accuracy when compared to clinical examination, CT scan, and intracranial pressure. La Joie and colleagues (29) reported that of 42 patients with right hemiplegia and absent SEPs, only one had functional improvement on the involved side. Those patients with preserved SEPs had significantly more functional improvement following rehabilitation. Feinsod and associates (30) described 76 patients with myelographically proven herniated discs and compared their SEPs to those of 65 healthy subjects. Of particular interest was the finding that postoperative SEP changes correlated well with improvement or worsening of the patient's condition. Gepstein and co-workers (31) also looked at the predictive value of SEPs. In their study, they looked at 41 consecutive surgeries for herniated intervertebral disc (27 patients) and spinal stenosis (14 patients) intraoperatively and correlated their results with 3 months and 1 year postsurgical follow-up. Postoperatively, patients evaluated their pain on a scale of 0 to 100, and success of surgery was determined using standard review criteria. In most cases, there was an immediate reduction in latency following adequate decompression of the nerve roots. The degree of normalization at time of surgery correlated with symptomatic relief after surgery, suggesting that SEPs are valuable in determining the adequacy of lumbar nerve decompression and for prediction of the successful relief of symptoms. While there is limited scientific support to document the prognostic value of SEPs in radiculopathy, one suspects that it may serve this function as well.

## OTHER LITERATURE

Specific literature regarding the use of SEPs in acute radiculopathy is limited but growing. In particular, the use of SEPs in radiculopathy has been hampered by technical difficulties. After cutaneous stimulation, the only spinal SEP parameter that can be monitored with any consistency is latency. This, however, may be absent in 50 percent of normal patients (29). Seyal and colleagues (32) reported an increased yield of 41 percent when cortical and spinal SEPs were utilized. They studied 21 patients with lumbosacral radiculopathies and made both spine and scalp recordings from multiple mixed nerves. Spinal SEPs were abnormal in 10 patients, three of whom had normal EMGs. Eisen and co-workers (33) reported a 57 percent yield using cortical SEPs and cutaneous nerve stimulation when using the criteria of a latency prolongation of three standard deviations and a 50 percent decrease in amplitude. Walk and colleagues (34) also found SEPs useful in the electrodiagnostic evaluation of lumbosacral radiculopathy, particularly when EMG is nondiagnostic. They performed SEP studies in 59 patients with clinical radiculopathy and compared them with the results of myelography, CT scan, MRI, and EMG. Of 38 patients with abnormal myelogram/CT, 32 (84 percent) had abnormal SEPs while 11 (29 percent) demonstrated EMG abnormalities. All 21 patients with normal myelograms had normal SEPs. They went on to define a subset of patients with radiculopathy and weakness or reflex changes and found SEPs to be more sensitive than EMG. Perlik and associates (18) demonstrated a high yield of abnormal SEPs in patients with compressive root lesions, often in the absence of focal clinical signs and normal EMG. Specifically, they reported cortical SEPs to be helpful in diagnosing radiculopathy in 21 of 27 (78 percent) patients with CT and myelogram confirmed evidence for root injuries when using a scalp recording technique.

They, however, confirmed the clinical difficulty of making these recordings. Thus, depending on the laboratory, the abnormal criteria, and/or patient population, CSEP has a diagnostic yield of 40–85 percent when compared to myelography.

Mixed nerve SEPs have been shown to be easier to perform and more effective in localizing the injury site in cases of myelopathy due to spondylosis (33–36). Additionally, mixed nerve SEPs have been demonstrated as helpful in various lesions of the cauda equina and the conus medullaris (37). Noterman and Velk (38) found that tibial and deep peroneal along with saphenous and sural nerve SEPs correlated well with surgical findings in 66 percent of cases. Knutsson and associates (39) reported a restitution of the SEP after autotraction in four of five patients with low or abolished SEP. Keim and co-workers (40) found tibial nerve SEPs as a useful screen in patients with spinal stenosis. Cassvan and Sook Park (41) reported a 71 percent diagnostic yield using peroneal nerve. They clinically evaluated 49 patients suffering from L5 radiculopathy. Twenty-eight had identifiable SEPs and 20 of those had identifiable abnormalities, a diagnostic yield of 71 percent compared to EMG with 64 percent. The combined positive yield of EMG and SEPs was 85 percent, assuming that the clinical diagnosis was correct. Seyal and associates (42) reported increased specificity in spinal recordings of mixed tibial nerve SEPs in comparison to scalp recordings. SEPs were recorded from 22 nerves in 12 normal adults, aged 18 to 42. Spinal and scalp recording montages were employed. They concluded that SEP potentials were reproducible and useful. Notermans and colleagues (43) reported over a 60 percent correlation of SEPs with EMG and imaging. This study was interesting because 50 percent of the subjects had surgical correction confirming their pathology. Twenty normals underwent routine mixed nerve SEP evaluations. The same test was then performed on 20 patients with clinical evidence of lumbosacral disc prolapse. All patients with previous history of surgery were excluded from the study. In 71 percent of all patients, the findings of SEPs showed a good correlation with those of the radiological examinations. Of the patients who underwent surgery, 66 percent showed abnormal SEP results. However, the difficulty with mixed nerve stimulation in radiculopathy involves the physiologic multisegmental composition of the mixed nerve, making it unlikely to show significant changes when a single nerve root is compressed. For the same reason, mixed nerve SEPs appear particularly helpful in diagnosing multiroot disease, spinal stenosis, and so forth.

Some investigators have also questioned the use of dermatomal SEPs (DSEPs) in radiculopathy. Aminoff and colleagues (44), for example, found that dermatomal SEPs correctly identified lesions in only 5 of 19 patients while providing misleading information in 10 patients. They also performed peroneal mixed nerve SEPs on all patients and found them normal in all patients. In this work, all patients had clinical features of unilateral L5 and/or S1 radiculopathies. Patients with bilateral symptoms were excluded but two with radiologic evidence of spinal stenosis were included. Each patient's nonsymptomatic side served as the control. For the DSEPs, a latency difference of three standard deviations or an amplitude decrease of 75 percent was considered abnormal. Of the five patients in whom the DSEP correctly identified the lesion, one patient was of particular interest. Here the clinical and radiological findings suggested an L5 radiculopathy while the DSEP suggested an S1 root, which was confirmed at surgery. They concluded that mixed nerve SEPs were of no value and DSEPs were of limited value. They concede that their use of a latency difference of three standard deviations rather than an absolute side to side differences of 2–3 ms is an explanation for the limited sensitivity of DSEPs in their study.

In another study, Aminoff and colleagues (45) compared the diagnostic utility of EMG, F wave, H reflex studies, and peroneal dermatomal SEPs in evaluating 28 patients with clinically unequivocal L5 or S1 compressive root lesions. Twenty-seven had radicular pain and 24 had motor or sensory segmental signs on examination. Thirty-two controls were used with similar heights. A greater than three standard deviation in latency or 75 percent amplitude decline was again considered abnormal. DSEPs confirmed the diagnosis in only 7 of the 28 patients in contrast to EMGs, which confirmed the diagnosis in 21 patients. Late responses confirmed the diagnosis in only 5 of 28. They conclude that EMG is more valuable than DSEPs, but it is unclear how they confirmed the diagnosis.

Rodriquez and co-workers (46) compared the results of dermatomal SEPs (DSEPs) to electromyography in 50 patients referred for evaluation and to imaging studies in 31 of these patients. They report that side to side amplitude variations were too variable to be of use. Sixty-five percent of abnormal DSEPs were based on side to side latency changes, whereas 35 percent were based on an absent unilateral response. In this report a greater than three standard deviations was chosen as the method to determine a side to side latency abnormality while an absent unilateral response was also considered an abnormal DSEP. Imaging techniques included myelopathy or CT and were considered abnormal if "impingement" was present. The criteria for an abnormal EMG were not reported. They found that 60 percent had EMG abnormalities, 52 percent had DSEP abnormalities, and 60 percent had imaging irregularities. DSEP sensitivity was approximately 70 percent when compared to either EMG and imaging, whereas the specificity was 90 percent in comparison to imaging and 70 percent versus EMG. They

concluded that DSEPs added little to the diagnosis of radiculopathy. Although this is an interesting report, it is difficult to draw many conclusions. The patient populations were not clearly identified nor were the diagnostic criteria. It is unclear if the referred patients had acute or chronic symptoms, the degree of symptomatology (subjective pain or loss of reflexes), what the EMG findings were, and how the "impingement" was determined. While this report suggests that DSEPs are not better than EMG and imaging techniques, it suggests that they are comparable in sensitivity and specificity.

In one of the most comprehensive articles to date, Dumitru and Dreyfuss (47) concluded that neither segmental nor dermatomal SEPs could accurately diagnose those persons with well-defined unilateral/unisegmental radicular lesions at values approaching a sensitivity of 90 percent or better while maintaining a specificity also exceeding 90 percent. In this study, clearly defined inclusion criteria were established, including historical and physical data, anatomic imaging, and electrodiagnostic results, to identify a patient population with unquestionable radicular disease. Standard techniques for SEP stimulation were then employed, including bilateral lower extremity stimulation. Regression equations evaluating for age and height were then applied. In isolated L5 radicular insults, segmental and dermatomal SEP studies were found to maintain a 93 percent specificity but sensitivity was reduced to 70 percent and 60 percent, respectively. With isolated S1 lesions, sensitivity was reduced to 30 percent and 20 percent, respectively. A significant number of false-positives were also identified. Almost 20 percent of patients with an isolated L5 lesion demonstrated abnormal S1 SEPs while 10 percent of patients with an S1 lesion had abnormal L5 SEPs. The authors expanded their analysis to evaluate both latency and amplitude changes at 2.0, 2.5, and 3 standard deviations without a significant change in their conclusions.

In total, 20 test patients met their inclusion criteria while a control group of 43 subjects were tested. Of the 20 patients, 10 had L5 lesions while the remaining 10 patients had S1 lesions. This study does identify and address many of the concerns of previous studies. The strict inclusion criteria clearly document the existence of isolated nerve root pathology in the test group. It does not rely on a single abnormality but a combination of history, physical examination, and imaging findings. It also addresses the two most significant biological variables in SEP recordings, age and height. It suggests that there is a high degree of biological variation in patients, reducing the sensitivity in SEP analysis. It also suggests that even in dermatomal pathways, there may be significant neural fiber splitting and multiroot entry. Another explanation for the low yield of DSEP would be that only few radicular lesions are complete and some SEP transmission may be unimpeded and thus yield relatively normal conductions, thereby reducing its sensitivity. Furthermore, it suggests that at the time of evaluation, demyelination may not be a significant component of the pathologic condition. Remyelination of the radicular lesion may have also occurred, reducing the sensitivity of the technique. This would not be true in cases of spinal stenosis and in fact may explain the reports of persistent abnormal SEPs in this patient population (48,49). Finally, the existence of "central amplification" may further limit the sensitivity.

While this work raises multiple questions regarding the use of SEPs to identify unilateral radicular lesions, some questions are still left unanswered. First, one should always be careful what conclusions to draw from a study with a small patient population of only 10 patients in each group. It is also unclear why they chose a bilateral stimulation technique to evaluate a unilateral lesion. Finally, as the authors point out, in long-standing pathology, remyelination repair may have already begun, limiting the sensitivity of DSEP. This, however, does not preclude the usefulness of SEPs in acute radiculopathy. A logical follow-up would be to increase the patient population and look at the variations in the results correlated with clinical acuteness.

Despite these concerns, many investigators have reported the value of dermatomal SEPs in radiculopathy (50–53). Dermatomal SEPs should be more root-specific than either cutaneous or mixed nerve SEPs. Drs. Slimp, Stolov, and associates (54), the co-authors of the one AHCPR article reference, were among the first to document the reproducibility of DSEPs in clinical practice. They recorded scalp DSEPs from C4, C5, C6, C7, C8, T2, T4, T6, T8, T12, L2, L3, L4, L5, and S1 from 25 normal subjects. Latency responses were correlated to height and/or vertebral column length and were found to be reproducible. Liguori and colleagues (55) were also among the first to report the reproducibility of dermatomal SEP values and suggest the role dermatomal SEPs may play in diagnosing lumbar radiculopathy.

In another paper, Saal and co-workers (56) demonstrated that abnormalities in DSEP correlated well with CT scans, discograms, and MRI. In particular, they focused on upper lumbar root lesions, an area difficult to evaluate with routine EMG. In this report 100 consecutive patients who presented with upper lumbar radicular complaints were evaluated with a control of 20 normals. Abnormalities were defined as greater than 2.5 ms difference between latencies of each leg. They found a 100 percent correlation with anatomical abnormalities at L2 and L4 with an 80 percent correlation at L3. Their conclusion was that there is a high correlation between DSEPs and imaging techniques.

Green and colleagues (57,58) have also demonstrated the role of dermatomal SEPs in radiculopathy and

confirmed pathology in 90 percent of patients. In this report they studied 129 subjects ranging in age from 21 to 82 years with both cervical and lumbar symptoms. Side to side comparisons for DSEPs were utilized as the criteria for determining abnormality. They concluded that lower extremity DSEPs were more sensitive but do not detail how the diagnosis was confirmed. One is left to assume that the comparison was only to symptomatic complaints and imaging techniques. They used two standard deviations as their abnormal criteria.

Yasuaki, Tokuhashi, and associates (59) presented an interesting report on 94 cases of lumbosacral radiculopathy. Of those patents, 52 patients had pathology confirmed by operation and 42 had radiographic confirmation. The main purpose of this report, however, was to compare DSEPs to the Semmes-Weinstein esthesiometer. Their conclusion was that DSEPs were more sensitive. Nevertheless, they identified a sensitivity rate of 54 percent with operative findings. It is unclear if this number represents abnormal DSEPs in only those patients with radiculopathy or if it includes patients with stenosis, spondylolisthesis, and/or spondylolysis, all of which were identified at surgery and/or on imaging studies.

Scarff and associates (60,61) stimulated the medial aspect of the first toe and found DSEP abnormalities in 93 percent of their cases. This was directly contrasted to EMGs where only 50 percent and myelography where 81 percent had abnormalities confirmed at surgery. In this report, they evaluated over 300 patients over 3 years on the neurosurgical and orthopedic services. Thirty-eight consecutive patients with technically adequate DSEPs underwent myelography and operation. They considered an absent unilateral response, a latency delay of greater than 3 ms between sides, and/or a 75 percent decrease in side to side amplitude as significant. Thirty-five of the 38 had positive DSEPs for the root involved and confirmed in surgery. Two with bulging discs had normal DSEPs and a third had abnormal studies for the contralateral side. There were no false-positives. Myelograms were normal in five patients with confirmed pathology. They concluded that DSEPs were even more sensitive than myelography (the gold standard) in identifying radicular pathology.

The design of this study is impressive in that over 300 studies were performed, and all of the 38 reported patients underwent surgical correlation of their pathology. It is unclear what the exclusion criteria were and what became of the other 262 patients. It is also of note that few other investigators have been able to confirm the reliability of using a 75 percent side to side amplitude decrease as a diagnostic criterion for DSEPs.

Needless to say, these results are quite different from those reported by Aminoff (44). The differences may be explained in several ways. Scarff and Aminoff studied different patients. Aminoff selected patients who had clinical indications of unilateral radicular dysfunction at the L5–S1 level. Scarff examined patients with local radicular herniated disc prolapses established by surgery. Furthermore, Scarff's criteria for establishing abnormality were less strict. He used 1.5 times the standard deviation and found 90 percent abnormalities, whereas Aminoff used 3 times the standard deviation and found only 30 percent abnormalities. Interestingly, Notermans used 2 times the standard deviation and found abnormality in 60 percent of the cases.

Masafumi, Machida, and colleagues (62) reported recording the DSEP on the scalp of 50 healthy patients and 40 patients who later underwent exploratory surgery. They found that DSEPs correctly and accurately predicted the level and degree of pathology in all but six patients (85 percent). Of the 40 patients who underwent surgery, 13 had L5 root compression, 20 had S1 root compression, one had S2 root compression, and six had no compression. In the 33 patients with root compression, all had abnormal DSEPs. A normal DSEP was found in one patient who had a central herniation but normal sensation clinically. When compared to myelography, six patients demonstrated abnormalities not present at surgery while two herniations identified at surgery were not present on myelography, for a total of eight misleading interpretations. Their technique for stimulation is carefully described and is considered a good standard for dermatomal stimulation. It is also interesting to note that the authors did include patients with acute low back pain syndromes. This is one of the only articles reviewed that addressed the duration of symptoms in their patient populations. Their conclusions were that DSEP is a valuable noninvasive tool for the evaluation of herniated lumbosacral disc.

There may be several explanations for the false-negatives and false-positives of myelography. Certainly anatomical variations may not correlate with true neurophysiological abnormalities. A laterally prolapsed disc may be difficult to identify. Minor bone changes, needle artifacts, thickening of the ligamentum flavum, or arachnoid adhesions may be misinterpreted as nerve root compression. It is unclear if there was a difference between the results of acute or chronic patients. One of the most impressive aspects of this study is that the majority of patients had surgical confirmation of the presumed pathology by exploratory surgery. The large number of subjects, as well as the high degree of sensitivity and specificity of the results, is a strong indication of the role that DSEPs may play in the evaluation of acute low back pain.

Other techniques have been investigated with various results. These include attempted stimulation using magnetic pulses (63), paraspinal muscle stimulation (64), and needle stimulation of motor points. These techniques are early in their development and remain unsubstantiated.

## FURTHER STUDY

While current scientific knowledge is not yet sufficient to suggest that SEPs be utilized in the routine evaluation of all patients with radicular symptoms, there are strong indications that it may become a valuable tool. Just as the sensitivity and specificity of electrodiagnosis (EMG/NCV) has improved with the additional techniques of conducting across specific peripheral compression sites of nerve lesions, so too may SEP. It is clear that further investigation should be carried out to better determine indications, techniques, and the ideal abnormal parameters. Prospective as well as additional retrospective studies need to be developed looking at patient acuteness and confirmed diagnosis. Larger populations of normal and abnormal patients need to be evaluated. Special emphasis should be placed on the prognostic value of SEPs. These studies could be coordinated with rehabilitation efforts and long-term follow-up needs to be addressed. Outcome comparisons might be monitored when using SEPs in place of imaging techniques to make treatment decisions.

## COST ANALYSIS

In this day and age of health care reform, no report on diagnostic testing can be complete without some comment on cost-effectiveness. Most laboratories charge several hundred dollars for an SEP test. Medicare reimbursement varies from state to state but averages $100–$200. In contrast, EMGs, CT scans, MRIs, and myelograms cost several times this amount. There can be little argument that the best method to control costs is to identify which tests yield the most accurate data and affect clinical decision making. In reviewing the literature, it appears that SEPs cannot yet stand alone as a diagnostic test but must be utilized in combination with clinical examination, EMG, and imaging when indicated. It does appear from the literature that SEPs are as sensitive as most imaging studies and offers the theoretic advantage of being a physiologic study. Furthermore, there are no known complications from a properly performed SEP examination. It is a safe, noninvasive procedure with little or no discomfort to the patient. Therefore, it may be considered before these more expensive tests in the physician's diagnostic tree. When used in combination with other routine neurodiagnostic testing, it also more effectively rules out other diagnostic considerations and may provide valuable insight into prognosis. This information may ultimately lead a particular patient either directly to rehabilitation or to surgery, thereby curtailing prolonged ineffective rehabilitation efforts and/or unnecessary surgery.

# Summary

While new imaging techniques are gaining popularity in the diagnosis of acute lumbar syndromes, they remain limited in their correlation to clinical situations. CT and MRI reveal anatomic abnormalities but do not provide insight into the physiological function or prognosis. The degree of false-positive readings is also of concern. Many persons with "significant" degenerative disc disease on MRI are in fact nonsymptomatic. Others with acute back pain are in fact primarily disabled by the musculoskeletal components of their injury and their disc pathology, while present, may not be clinically significant. In contrast, SEPs are a direct physiological evaluation tool. They provide objective, reproducible, sensitive, and noninvasive information about patients whose clinical signs and symptoms may be equivocal.

The literature on the value of SEPs in low back pain has varied from enthusiastic to poor. As with most procedures, it is clear that patient selection and technique are critical. There is little doubt that the SEP does measure a physiologic function. The observation of SEP improvement during surgical decompression of the involved nerve root intraoperatively is unequivocal. The major criticism of the technique revolves around the ability or inability to identify a specific unilateral isolated nerve root lesion. In some experienced laboratories, the sensitivity and specificity is greater than in others. What is critical is identifying whether there is neurologic dysfunction and to what degree so that treatment decisions can be made.

The AHCPR panel only considered one resource with two diagnostic categories in a small patient population. Many more studies are currently available describing both the benefits and the limitations of SEPs in low back pain. Clearly, many questions regarding the use of SEP in acute low back pain remain to be answered.

# References

1. Holbrook et al. The frequency of occurrence, impact, and cost of selected musculoskeletal conditions in the United States, Amer Acad Ortho Surg 1984.
2. Clinical Practice Guidelines #14, Acute Low Back Problems in Adults U.S. Dept. of Health and Human Services, AHCPR Pub;1994; No. 95–0642.
3. Dawson GD. Investigations in a patient subject to myoclonic seizures after sensory stimulation. *J Neuro Neurosurg Psychiatry* 1947; 10:141–162.
4. Chiappa K. *Evoked potentials in clinical medicine.* New York: Raven Press, 1983.
5. DeLisa J, Mackenzie K, Baran E. *Manual of nerve conduction velocity and somatosensory evoked potentials.* 2nd ed. New York: Raven Press, 1987:151–159.
6. Alonso JA, Hajdu M, Gonzales E, et al. Cortical somatosensory evoked potentials: Effects of positional change. *Arch Phys Med Rehabil* 1989; 70:194–98.
7. Eisen A, Hoirch M, Moll A. Evaluation of radiculopathies by segmental stimulation and somatosensory evoked potentials. *Can J Neurol Sci* 1983; 10:178–82.
8. Gonzalez E, Hajdu M. Disparate involvement of short and long latency somatosensory evoked potentials in nerve root decompression. *Arch Phys Med Rehabil* 1983; 64:494.
9. Eisen A, Elleker G. Sensory nerve stimulation and evoked cerebral potentials. *Neurology* 1983; 30:1097–1105.
10. Eisen A, Aminoff M, Somatosensory evoked potentials In: Aminoff M (ed.). *Electrodiagnosis in clinical neurology.* 2nd ed. New York: Churchill Livingstone, 1986:532–573.
11. Simpson RK, Blackburn JG, Martin HS, et al. Peripheral nerve fiber and spinal cord pathway contributions to the somatosensory evoked potentials. *Exp Neurol* 1981; 73:700.
12. Watanabe J, Tanaka H. Identification of alpha-motor nerve fiber potentials in lumbar epidural space and its clinical significance. *Spine* 1990; 15(11):1131–1137.
13. Green J, Gildenmeister R, Hazelwood C. Dermatomally stimulated somatosensory cerebral evoked potentials in the clinical diagnosis of lumbar disc disease. *Clin Electroencephalogr* 1983; 14:152–160.
14. Katifi HA, Segwich EM. Evaluation of the dermatomal somatosensory evoked potential in the diagnosis of lumbo-sacral root compression. *J Neurol Neurosurg Psychiatry* 1987; 50:1204–1210.
15. Katifi HA, Sedgwick EM. Somatosensory evoked potentials from posterior tibial nerve and lumbo-sacral dermatomes. *Electroencephalogr Clin Neurophysiol* 1986; 65(4):249–259.
16. Prevec TS, et al. Effect of valium on evoked cerebral cortex activity. Neurologija 1997; 25(1–2): 77–80.
17. Stolov, WC, Slimp JC, Dermatomal somatosensory evoked potentials in lumbar spinal stenosis. Am Assoc Electromyography and Electrodiagnosis, Electroencephalography Soc Joint Symp, 1988:17–22.
18. Perlik S, Fisher MA, Patel DV, et al. On the usefulness of somatosensory evoked responses for the evaluation of lower back pain. *Arch Neurol* 1986; 43:907–913.
19. Kimura J. F-wave velocity in central segment of the median and ulnar nerves. A study of normal subjects in patients with Charcot-Marie-Tooth disease. *Neurology* 1974; 24:539–546.
20. Braddom RL, Johnson EW. Standardization of H reflex and diagnostic use in S1 radiculopathy. *Arch Phys Med Rehabil* 1966; 55:161–166.
21. Lane ME. Recent developments in the electrodiagnosis of radiculopathies. *Bull Hosp Jt Dis Orthop Inst* 1984; 44(1):56–64.
22. Aminoff MJ, Goodin DS, Parry GJ, et al. Electrophysiological evaluation of lumbosacral radiculopathies: Electromyography, late responses, and somatosensory evoked potentials. *Neurology* 1985; 35:1514–1518.
23. Synek VM. Validity of median nerve somatosensory evoked potentials in the diagnosis of supraclavicular

brachial plexus lesions. *Electroencephalogr Clin Neurophysiol* 1986; 65(1):27–35.

24. Jones SI, Winn Parry CB, Landi A. Diagnosis of brachial plexus traction by sensory nerve action potentials and somatosensory evoked potentials. *Injury* 1981; 12:376–382.

25. Synek VM. Somatosensory evoked potentials from musculocutaneous nerve in the diagnosis of brachial plexus injury. *J Neurol Sci* 1983; 61:443–452.

26. Zentner J, Ebner A. Prognostic value of somatosensory and motor evoked potentials in patients with non-traumatic coma. *Eur Arch Psych Neurol Sci* 1988; 237:184–187.

27. Narayan RK, Greenberg RP, Miller JD. Improved confidence of outcome prediction in severe head injury. *J Neurosurg* 1981; 54:751–762.

28. Robinson RL, Richey ET, Kase CS. Somatosensory evoked potentials in pure sensory stroke and related conditions. *Stroke* 1985 16:818–823.

29. La Joie, WJ, Reddy NM, Melvin JL. Somatosensory evoked potentials: Their predictive value in right hemiplegia. *Arch Phys Med Rehabil* 1982; 63:223–226.

30. Feinsod M, Blau D, Findler G, et al. SEP to peroneal nerve stimulation in patients with herniated lumbar discs. *Neurosurg* 1982; 11(4):506–511.

31. Gepstein R, Brown M. SEP in lumbar nerve root decompression. *Clin Orthop Related Res* 1989; 69–71.

32. Seyal M, Sandhu LS, Mack YP. Spinal segments somatosensory evoked potentials in lumbosacral radiculopathies. *Neurology* 1989; 39:801–805.

33. Eisen A, Hoirch M. Electrodiagnostic evaluation of radiculopathies and plexopathies using somatosensory evoked potentials. *Electroencephalogr Clin Neurophysiol* 1982; 36(Suppl):349–357.

34. Walk D, Fisher M, et al. SEP in the evaluation of lumbosacral radiculopathy. *Neurology* 1992; 42:1197–1202.

35. Ganes T. Somatosensory conduction times and peripheral cervical and cortical evoked potentials in patients with cervical spondylosis. *J Neurol Neurosurg Psychiatry* 1980; 43:683–689.

36. Perlik SJ, Fisher MA. Somatosensory evoked response evaluation of cervical spondylitic myelopathy. *Muscle Nerve* 1987; 10(6):481–489.

37. Ertekin C, Mutlu R, Sarica, Y. Electrophysiological evaluation of the afferent spinal roots and nerves in patients with a conus medullaris and cauda equina lesions. *J Neurol Sci* 1980; 48:419–433.

38. Noterman SLH, Velk NMT. Cortical and spinal somatosensory evoked potentials in patients suffering from lumbosacral disc prolapse. *Electromyogr Clin Neurophysiol* 1988; 28:33–37.

39. Knutsson E, Skoglund CR, Natchev E. Changes in voluntary muscle strength, somatosensory transmission and skin temperature concomitant with pain relief during autotraction in patients with lumbar and sacral root lesion. *Pain* 1988 33:173.

40. Keim H, Hajdu M, Gonzalez EG. Somatosensory evoked potentials as a diagnostic aid in the diagnosis and intraoperative management of spinal stenosis. *Spine* 1985; 10:338–344.

41. Cassavan A, Sook Park Y. Cortical somatosensory evoked potentials following peroneal nerve stimulation in lumbosacral radiculopathies. *Electromyogr Clin Neurophysiol* 1983; 23:393–402.

42. Seyal M, Sandhu LS, Mack YP. Spinal segmental somatosensory evoked potentials in lumbar radiculopathies. *Neurology* 1989; 39(6):801–805.

43. Notermans S, Velk N. Cortical and spinals SEP in patients suffering from lumbosacral disc prolapse. *Electromyogr Clin Neurophysiol* 1988; 28:33–37.

44. Aminoff MJ, Goodin DS, Barbaro NM. Dermatomal somatosensory evoked potentials in unilateral lumbosacral radiculopathy. *Ann Neurol* 1985; 17(2):171–176.

45. Aminoff M, Goodin D, et al. Electrophysiologic evaluation of lumbosacral radiculopathies. *Neurology* 1985; 35:1514–1518.

46. Rodriquez A, Kanis L, et al. Somatosensory evoked potentials from dermatomal stimulation as an indicator of L5 and S1 radiculopathy. *Arch Phys Med Rehabil* 1987; 68:366–368.

47. Dumitru D, Dreyfuss P. Dermatomal/segments somatosensory evoked potential evaluation of L5/S1 unilateral/unilevel radiculopathies. *Muscle Nerve* 1996; 19:442–449.

48. Herroir LD, Trippi AC, Gonyeau M. Intraoperative use of dermatomal SEP in lumbar stenosis surgery. *Spine* 1987; 12:379–383.

49. Snowden ML, Haselkorn JK, Kraft GH, et al. Dermatomal SEP in the diagnosis of lumbosacral spinal stenosis comparison with imaging studies. *Muscle Nerve* 1992; 15:1036–1044.

50. Eisen A. Electrodiagnosis of radiculopathies. *Neurol Clin* 1985; 3(3):495–510.

51. White A. *Lumbar spine surgury: Techniques and complications.* 2nd ed. St. Louis: Mosby, 1987:204–218.

52. Gonzalez EG, Hajdu M, Bruno R, et al. Lumbar spinal stenosis: Analysis of pre and postoperative somatosensory evoked potentials. *Arch Phys Med Rehabil* 1985; 66:11–15.

53. Downey JA, Myers SJ, Gonzalez EG. *The physiological basis of rehabilitation medicine.* 2nd ed. Boston: Butterworth-Heinemann, 1994.

54. Slimp J, Rubner D, Snowden M, Stolov W. Dermatomal SEP: Cervical, thoracic, and lumbosacral levels. *Encephalogr Clin Neurophysiol* 1982; (84) 55–70.

55. Liguori R, Taher G, Trojaborg W. Somatosensory evoked potentials from cervical and lumbosacral dermatomes. *Acta Neurol Scand* 1991; 84(2):161–166.

56. Saal JA, Firtch W, Assl JS, et al. The value of somatosensory evoked potentials testing for upper lumbar radiculopathy: A correlation of electrophysiologic and anatomic data. *Spine* 1992; 17(6):133–137.

57. Green J, Hamm S, Benfante P, et al. Clinical effectiveness of dermatomal evoked cerebrally recorded somatosensory responses. *Clin Electroencepalogr* 1988; 19(1);14–15.

58. Green J, Gildenmeister R, Hazelwood C. Dermatomally stimulated somatosensory cerebral evoked potentials in clinical diagnosis of lumbar disc disease. *Clin Electroencephalogr* 1983; 14:152–160.

59. Tokuhashi Y, Satoh K, et al. A quantitative evaluation of sensory dysfunction in lumbosacral radiculopathy spine. 6(11):1321–1328.

60. Scarff TB, Dallmann DE, Bunch WH, Dermatomal somatosensory evoked potentials in the diagnosis of lumbar root entrapment. *Surg Forum* 1981; 32:489–491.

61. Scarff T, Dallmann P, et al. Herniated lumbosacral discs. *Lancet* 1980; 81:85–93.

62. Machida M, Asai T, Sato K, et al. New approach for diagnosis in herniated lumbosacral disc dermatomal SEPs. *Spine* 1986; 11(4):380–384.

63. Tsuji S, Murai Y, Yarita M. Somatosensory potentials evoked by magnetic stimulation of the lumbar cauda equina and leg nerves. *Ann Neurol* 1988; 24(4):568–573.

64. Zhu Y, Haldeman S, et al. Paraspinal muscle evoked cerebral potentials in patients with unilateral low back pain. *Spine* 1993; 8:1096–1102.

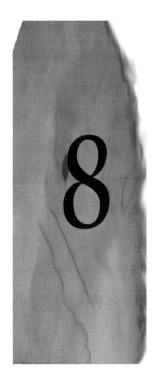

# 8 Physiologic Assessment: Thermography

*Robert G. Schwartz, M.D.*

Thermography involves measuring temperature and recording the findings with color images. Liquid crystal systems utilize small inflated pillows with rubberized surfaces embedded with cholesteric liquid crystals. The pillows must be manually placed on the skin, one side at a time, and left in place for a sufficient duration of time to achieve full color expression of the measured temperature.

Infrared systems are easier to use and less operator-dependent; they also provide greater resolution and mapping clarity over liquid crystal. With electronic systems, no contact with the body surface is required, and entire regions of the body can be assessed at one time. Infrared systems are able to measure temperature changes of at least 1° C, with a resolution of 1 mm square, up to a depth of 6 mm (1).

Both liquid crystal and electronic infrared thermography are harmless to the patient. Costs of the study are generally less then those of CT scanning or electromyography with nerve conduction velocities.

## BASIS FOR THERMOGRAPHY

The regulation of skin temperature is dependent on the rate of blood flow from the cutaneous vasculature, which is under sympathetic control. In order for thermography to be a useful test for pain, there must be concurrent change in skin temperature.

Sympathetic nerve fibers arise from the sympathetic ganglion, join the peripheral nerves via the rami communicans (distal to the nerve root), and terminate upon tissue of mesodermal or ectodermal origin. These nerve fibers endings do not terminate with sensory nerve fibers, but rather with the microvasculature (Figure 8–1).

Since the sensory nerve fibers and microvasculature to the skin do not exactly correlate in their distribution, sympathetic changes cannot be expected to follow dermatomal distributions.

A given region of the body surface ordinarily differs by < 0.5° C from the homologous region on the contralateral side (2). When performed according to the Wexler protocol (three separate sets of measurements, done in 15-minute intervals, with the subject equilibrating in a cooled, temperature controlled environment) abnormal findings present as an interside difference of ≥1° C (2,3).

Thermography is a physiologic test that, *like all physiologic tests,* does not provide specific causal information. There is no structural imaging system that can be

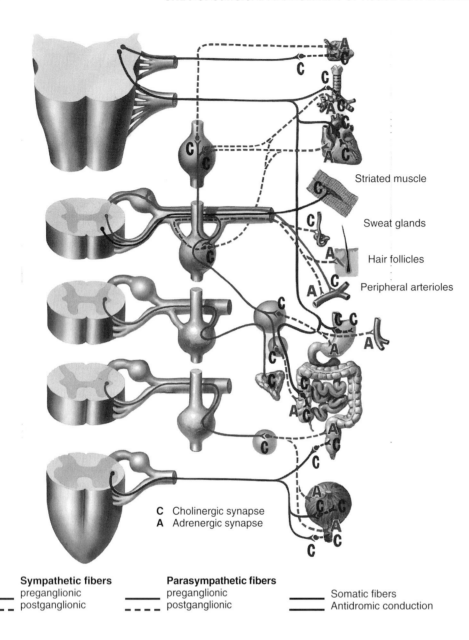

Striated muscle

Sweat glands

Hair follicles

Peripheral arterioles

**C** Cholinergic synapse
**A** Adrenergic synapse

**Sympathetic fibers**
——— preganglionic
– – – postganglionic

**Parasympathetic fibers**
——— preganglionic
– – – postganglionic

——— Somatic fibers
——— Antidromic conduction

**FIGURE 8–1**

Autonomic innervation of the somatic and visceral system. Reprinted with permission from Netter F. *Atlas of Human Anatomy.* West Caldwell, NJ: Ciba-Geigy, 1992.

used as a correlate to thermography. Electrophysiologic assessment of sympathetic function with skin galvanic impedance studies have demonstrated excellent correlation with thermography (4).

## THE AHCPR'S GUIDELINE ON ACUTE LOW BACK PAIN (5)

The AHCPR panel determined that thermography is not useful in the evaluation of acute low back pain due to radiculopathy. The conclusions in the guideline are correct, but the studies from which the conclusion is derived are inappropriate.

There are numerous articles on thermography. The panel, however, notes that it only reviewed 17 articles, of which only one satisfied their review criteria (6). The panel then notes that it reviewed an additional four articles. No explanation is given as to why the additional four articles that were used were chosen over others that covered the same material.

## EVIDENCE OF EFFICACY

In the study by Mills (6), which met the AHCPR criteria, the panel wrote, "all the asymptomatic subjects had temperature differences on thermography of less than

1.9° C in the feet and less than 1° C in other parts of the lower limbs."

The same study is used to quote, "of the 19 patients who went on to have surgery, only 53 percent had results on the preoperative thermography in agreement with surgical findings."

It is curious to note that the reference quoted for these statements (1) used liquid crystal, not infrared recording equipment; (2) specifically stated that they intentionally chose not to follow the Wexler protocol; and (3) described a method of measurement that had never been used before, nor replicated since.

The panel goes on to say that it reviewed 81 citations for meta-analysis reliability and found only one to be usable (6). The quoted reference ". . . found no discriminant value for thermography in diagnosing lumbar radiculopathy. True positive and true negative rates were both 48 percent."

Upon reviewing the quoted citation, one finds out that it was (a) written by one of the principal investigators awarded the contract by the AHCPR, (b) specifically in reference to liquid crystal thermography and (c) the criteria utilized for inclusion into the meta-analysis were overly restrictive.

Criteria for assessment of this physiologically oriented test included (1) anatomic findings of nerve root compression at surgery; (2) correlation to anatomic imaging reference tests that do not image the sympathetic system; (3) the referring diagnosis was not known prior to the test being performed; (4) the test result was not used to assist in making a diagnosis upon its completion; and (5) the use of cohort methods whereby patients who were known not to have sciatica, but had the appropriate symptoms, were studied and compared to those who did have sciatica.

The first two criteria applied assume that the diagnosis of radiculopathy can only exist in an anatomically imaged or surgically remediable basis and disregard known human anatomy with respect to the sympathetic system. The third and fourth criteria are transparently unrealistic.

The last criterion is a study feature that is idealistic. It is, however, rarely part of any study. Including this criterion with the first four essentially assures that no study could ever survive such a screen. In fact the one acceptable article was not a clinical study at all, but a meta-analysis itself.

The panel further concludes, "Chafetz, Wexler and Kaiser (8), evaluating 15 asymptomatic subjects with no current back pain and no history of back surgery or disability from back pain, found that 40 percent had abnormal thermograms."

The study cited, however, notes a 100 percent sensitivity and 60 percent specificity of patients who had demonstrated CT changes. It further explains, "the only discrepancies were three asymptomatic volunteers whose thermograms were interpreted as normal by the more experienced of the two interpreters but as abnormal by the other interpreter."

The reference continues, "for the purposes of this study these three asymptomatic volunteers were regarded as having positive thermograms, thereby maximizing the number of false positives and lowering the specificity from a possible 80 percent to the reported 60 percent."

The panel also writes, "Harper, Low, Fealy, et al. (9) evaluated thermography in 37 asymptomatic subjects (carefully screened for no history of back pain, back surgery, or disease or injury affecting the lower extremities). . . . " "The different readers interpreted thermograms as probably or definitely abnormal in 56–81 percent of the asymptomatic controls." Upon reading the reference, the authors conclude, "the sensitivity of thermography ranged from 78 percent to 94 percent compared with 81 percent to 92 percent for imaging studies and 77 percent for EMG. The specificity of thermography ranged from 20 percent to 44 percent. Thermography predicted the level of radiculopathy correctly in less than 50 percent of cases." The reference notes that the authors had attended only a single thermography course prior to commencing their study of the procedure.

The panel uses an article by Perelman, Adler, and Humpreys (10) to report, ". . . in 16 asymptomatic subjects with no low back complaints (. . .) 25 percent were found to have abnormal thermograms." The panel notes, ". . . temperature differences were not measured."

The panel then cites Aminoff and Onley (11) to report that "abnormal thermograms, defined as temperature differences between sides greater than three standard deviations from the mean for all asymptomatic subjects, were found in 7 percent of the asymptomatic subjects."

Perelman's (10) article does note that ". . . 75 percent of (the control group) had normal thermograms." The panel does not explain why they chose to quote the articles 25 percent false positive rate when the same authors found that in symptomatic patients who underwent thermography and CT scanning ". . . there was complete agreement in 99 patients, or 85 percent."

Interestingly, Aminoff's article (11) concludes, "in patients with clinically unequivocal radiculopathy, thermography and electrophysiologic study were similar in diagnostic sensitivity, and the two methods agreed on the presence or absence of abnormality in 71 percent of cases." "However, the thermographic findings had limited localizing value. . . . Moreover, thermographic abnormalities appeared not to follow a dermatomal distribution." Despite the fact that sensory nerves and arterioles to the skin do not have to correlate in their anatomic distribution, the authors note that with a 2.5 standard of deviation level, the false positive rate is 15 percent.

## AHCPR CONCLUSION

The panel concludes, "the one study meeting review criteria found that thermography did not accurately predict either the presence or absence of lumbar nerve root compression found at surgery. In addition, several studies have shown thermography of the lower limbs as abnormal in a substantial proportion of asymptomatic subjects without back problems."

In as much as the sympathetic nerve fibers arise from the sympathetic ganglion and join the peripheral nerves via the rami communicans (distal to the nerve root), it is easy to understand why one would conclude that thermography is not the test of choice for nerve root compression. Despite reaching the correct conclusion, however, the panel has demonstrated little insight into normal anatomy and physiology of the human sympathetic nervous system.

The panel has selected to comment on only portions of some articles and has limited its citations to other articles such that questions concerning the validity of the methods used are raised. It is easy to find current, well-respected publications that report thermography is a useful tool to evaluate the functional integrity of autonomic nerve fibers (12,13,14,15,16,17,18). Despite this, there is little favorable reference to the appropriate use of thermography mentioned in the report.

## Summary

Research on thermography in low back pain should address patients who are felt to have sympathetic pain—not only in helping diagnosis and plan intervention for those patients, but also in evaluating the effectiveness of treatment.

Study methods should be consistent with accepted thermographic performance and interpretive standards. Medical specialists in sympathetic pain should play an integral role in any research that evaluates this procedure.

The role of thermography in the evaluation and treatment of low back pain should be limited to only those cases in which there is an index of suspicion for sympathetic dysfunction.

Specialists who have interest in sympathetic dysfunction have successfully utilized thermography to advance both the understanding of this syndrome as well as its diagnosis and treatment. An example of this is Ochoa's work (19), whereby subsets of sympathetic pain syndromes have been described. Two such subsets include the "CCC" and "ABC" syndromes. In the "CCC" syndrome, afflicted patients complain of cold hypesthesia, cold hyperalgesia, and regionalized hypothermia. In the "ABC" syndrome, symptoms include warm hyperalgesia, erythalgia, and regionalized hyperthermia.

Thermography has been instrumental in the identification of sympathetic pain subsets and has been utilized to follow the results of treatment. It offers an objective measurement of autonomic physiology. Without such measurements, diagnosis of this condition may be entirely dependent on subjective patient responses to treatment. If it is assumed that all sympathetic pain syndromes are by their very nature responsive to sympathetic block, then treatment would remain a speculative endeavor.

## References

1.  Hubbard J. Thermography: Toss the bathwater, not the baby. *APS Bulletin*, 1993; Jan:7.
2.  Uematsu S. Quantification of thermal asymmetry. Part 1: Normal values and reproducibility. *J Neurosurg* 1988; 69:525–555.
3.  Abernathy M. *Medical thermology*. Washington, DC: American Academy of Thermology, 1986.
4.  Koor I. *The collected papers of Irvin M. Koor*. Newark: American Academy of Osteopathy, 1988
5.  Bigos S, Bowyer O, Braen G, et al. Acute Low Back Problems in Adults. Clinical Practice Guidelines No. 14, AHCPR Publication No 95–0642, Rockville, Agency Of Health Care Policy & Research, Public Health Service, U.S. Department of Health and Human Services, 1994.
6.  Mills GH, The evaluation of liquid crystal thermography in the investigation of nerve root compression due to lumbosacral lateral spinal stenosis. *Spine* 1986; 1:427.
7.  Hoffman Richard, Diagnostic accuracy and clinical utility of thermography for lumbar radiculopathy. *Spine* 1991; 6:623.
8.  Chafetz N, Neuromuscular thermography of the lumbar spine with CT correlation. *Spine* 1988; 13:922.
9.  Harper CM. Utility of thermography in the diagnosis of lumbosacral radiculopathy. *Neurology* 1991; 41:1010.
10. Perelman R. Electronic infrared thermography. *J Neurol Orthop Med Surg* 1985; 6:7.
11. Aminoff M. The role of thermography in the evaluation of lumbosacral radiculopathy. *Neurology* 1989; 39:1154.
12. Hooshmand H. *Chronic pain*. Boca Raton: CRC Press, 1993.
13. Stanton-Hicks M. *Reflex sympathetic dystrophy*. Boston: Kluwer Academic Publishers, 1990.
14. Bonica J. *The management of pain*, 2nd ed. Philadelphia: Lea & Febiger, 1990.
15. Klippel J. *Practical rheumatology*. Baltimore: Mosby, 1995.
16. Teasell R (ed.). *The autonomic nervous system*. Philadelphia: Hanley & Belfus, 1996.
17. Tollison D (ed.). *Sympathetic pain syndromes: Reflex sympathetic dystrophy and causalgia*. Philadelphia, Hanley & Belfus, 1996.
18. Raj P. *Pain medicine*. St. Louis: Mosby, 1996.
19. Ochoa J. The human sensory unit and pain: New concepts, syndromes and tests. *Muscle Nerve* 1993; 10:1009.

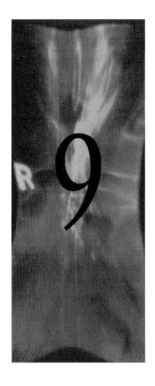

# 9 Epidural Steroid Injection

*Robert E. Windsor, M.D., and Krystal W. Chambers, M.D.*

ow back pain is the leading cause of disability in people under 45 years of age and the third leading cause in people over this age. In industrialized societies 3–4 percent of the working population has a temporarily disabling low back injury and more than 1 percent are considered permanently disabled as a result of low back injury (1). Low back pain and its associated cost have become a serious problem for industrialized societies. The medical cost of treating this condition is over $16 billion per year. If legal costs and lost productivity are accounted for, this figure increases dramatically to $50 billion per year (2). Lumbar epidural steroid injection (L-ESI) for the treatment of low back pain with radicular symptoms has been in use for over 40 years. There have been numerous studies examining the efficacy of injecting cortisone into the epidural space.

No general agreement on selection criteria, route of epidural administration, number of injections, or medications used has been reached. Despite controversy in the medical literature, L-ESI has remained an accepted means of treating low back pain with radicular symptoms (3,4).

In an effort to determine which treatments are effective and cost-efficient for low back pain, the Agency for Health Care Policy and Research (AHCPR) panel examined the medical literature regarding lumbar epidural injections. Based on their review, they concluded that lumbar epidural injections are of no therapeutic benefit in the treatment of acute low back pain without radiculopathy. They further concluded that epidural injections are invasive and pose rare but serious potential risks. It was the opinion of the panel that epidural steroid injections may be useful as an attempt to avoid surgery.

## HISTORY

Report of the first epidural injections for the treatment of low back pain was in 1901 (5,6). Cathelin, Pasquier, and Leri in two separate studies reported on the injection of cocaine into the epidural space. In 1925, Viner injected 20 cc of 1% procaine and 50–100 cc of Ringer's lactate solution, normal saline, or petrolatum into the sacral epidural space (7). The epidural injection of cortisone for the treatment of lumbar radiculopathy was first reported by Robechhi in 1952 (8).

In 1953, Livre and colleagues reported their experience with the injection of hydrocortisone and contrast into the epidural space of 46 patients with sciatica (9). They thought that 23 patients had good or very good results and 8 had mediocre results; the rest were considered failures.

In 1960, Brown and Goebert and colleagues in two separate studies were first to report the use of epidural steroid injections in the United States (10,11). Brown injected 40–100 cc of normal saline followed by 80 mg of methylprednisolone into the caudal epidural space of four patients suffering from sciatica for 6 months to 2 years. He reported complete relief of pain in all subjects for at least 2 months. Goebert and colleagues injected 30 cc of 1% procaine hydrochloride and 125 mg of hydrocortisone acetate into the caudal epidural space of 239 patients three times on consecutive or alternating days. He reported that 58 percent had good relief, 8 percent had fair relief, and 34 percent had poor results.

In 1970, Swerdlow and Sayle-Creer reported on their experience after injecting 550 patients with saline, 0.3–0.4% lidocaine, or 80 mg of methylprednisolone and lidocaine over the previous 12 years (12). They divided their patients into acute, chronic, and recurrent groups. In the chronic group, they found that there was no difference between the saline and local anesthetic groups alone (20 percent improved) and that the steroid group performed significantly better (45 percent) than the nonsteroid groups. In the acute and recurrent groups, there was no statistical difference between the groups.

There have been numerous reports on the use of epidural steroid injections for the treatment of lumbosacral radiculopathy since 1970 (9,10,13–34). A few reports have evaluated the effects of the epidural injection of steroids and other substances on low back pain without radiculopathy (30,35). The medical literature regarding epidural injections for lower back problems is fraught with difficulty. Most studies were poorly designed with no control groups, adequate outcome criteria, or follow-up protocols. Additionally, many of these studies varied on route and timing of injection, volume of injectant, number of injections, positioning of the patient, and use of fluoroscopic guidance.

Despite these differences, most studies have indicated a favorable outcome for the use of epidural steroid injection for lumbosacral radiculopathy (4). Controversies continue to exist regarding the use of fluoroscopic guidance (20,21,22,36), number of injections (31,32,37), site and route of injection (14,17,18,19,27,28,29,30,31,37,38,39), and volume and type of injectant (17,31,37). The procedure is illustrated by Figures 9-1 through 9-9.

## AHCPR REVIEW

The panel screened 74 articles to evaluate the efficacy of epidural injection of various substances for the treatment

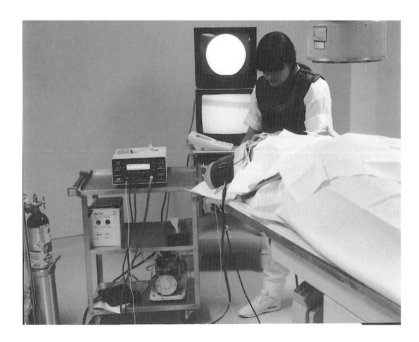

**FIGURE 9–1.**

A procedure room for invasive spinal procedures should have the following items: crash cart, cardiac monitoring/defibrillation unit, IV access, and pulse oximetry.

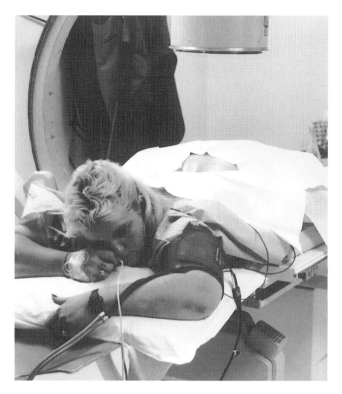

**FIGURE 9–2.**

Fluoroscopic imaging is helpful and in many cases mandatory for certain spinal procedures.

of lower back problems. The panel selected 9 of these articles for review (14,17,18,27,28,29,31, 35,37). Five other articles did not meet selection criteria but contained information used by the panel (30,33,40,41,42). They concluded that lumbar epidural injections are of no therapeutic benefit in the treatment of acute low back pain without radiculopathy. They further concluded that epidural injections are invasive and pose rare but serious potential risks. It was the opinion of the panel that epidural steroid injections may be useful as an attempt to avoid surgery.

In 1973, Dilke and colleagues studied the effect of extradural corticosteroid injection in the management of "nerve root compression syndromes associated with degenerative disc disease of the lumbar intervertebral discs" (37). Patients with pain in the distribution of the sciatic or femoral nerves accompanied by painful limitation of sciatic or femoral nerve stretch, sciatic scoliosis, and an appropriate neurologic deficit were all admitted to the hospital for participation in this study. Patients with an unclear diagnosis, bilateral disease, previous surgery, a medical history that might affect rehabilitation, or any doubt regarding the technical success of the injection were excluded from the study. One hundred patients met the selection criteria and were randomly assigned to treatment and con-

trol groups, who received 80 mg of methylprednisolone in 10 cc of normal saline via the translaminar route described by Barry and Kendall versus a superficial injection of 1 cc of normal saline into the interspinous ligament, respectively (13). All injections were performed by the same person in a double blinded manner. All participants received a graded program of physical therapy.

Variables that were assessed included duration of incapacity, relief of pain, clinical signs such as change in straight leg raise or neurologic signs, and need for other treatment such as a second injection, bracing, or surgical referral. Participants were assessed during admission and again at 3 months. The treated group showed a statistically significant decrease in analgesic requirement during admission as well as in time required before resumption of normal occupation.

Snoek and colleagues evaluated the effectiveness of extradural methylprednisolone for herniated lumbar discs (31). Patients with radiating pain in the distribution of the femoral or sciatic nerve, a neurologic deficit correlating to compression of the fourth or fifth lumbar roots or the first sacral nerve root, and myelographic findings on the appropriate side and level were included in the study. Excluded were patients with severe motor paresis, cauda equina syndrome, intolerable pain, previous lumbar surgery, known contraindications to corticosteroid therapy, and doubtful findings on myelography. Fifty-one patients were randomly divided into treatment and control groups. Both groups received a 2 cc injection into the epidural space using loss of resistance. The treatment group received 80 mg of methylprednisolone and the control group received normal saline. Seven days of bed rest were required and the participants were allowed to ambulate freely on the eighth day. Participants were assessed at 24 to 72 hours postinjection for mobility, Lasegue's test, neurologic deficit, pain, analgesic consumption, and performance in physical therapy. Further follow-up was performed between 8 and 20 months post-injection to see if they had undergone an operation. Late follow-up was by chart review, telephone interview, or letter. There was no statistically significant difference seen between the two groups at early or late follow-up. Late follow-up revealed that 14 patients from each group required surgery.

Klenerman and colleagues studied 63 patients with unilateral sciatica with or without objective neurologic findings, symptoms present for less than 6 months, and no previous hospitalization for sciatica (27). Participants were divided into four groups who randomly received a translaminar epidural injection of a 20 cc solution containing normal saline, normal saline and methylprednisolone, 0.25% bupivacaine and normal saline, or dry needling with a Touhy needle in the interspinous ligament. Patients were assessed at 2 weeks and again at 2 months by the same clinician for such variables as pain via a visual

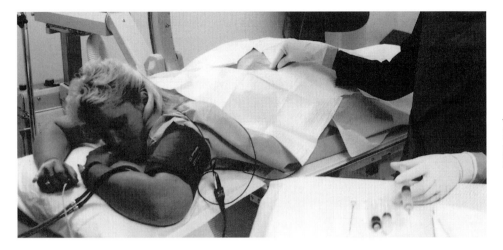

**FIGURE 9–3.**

Placing the spinal needle on the patient's skin to spot the site of injection.

analogue scale, straight leg raise, and degree of lumbar flexion. Patients were deemed failed, improved, or cured. Patients improved for each measurement but the difference between treatments was not statistically significant. They concluded that a combination of one or more of the four treatments may produce greater benefit.

In 1985, Cuckler and colleagues studied the use of epidural steroids in the treatment of lumbar pain (18). All patients with radicular pain in the lower limb were considered while patients with cauda equina syndrome or a progressive neurologic deficit were eliminated. Participants were divided into two groups. The first group had acute, unilateral sciatica with a well-defined neurologic deficit. The second group had bilateral pain, relief with change in posture, neurogenic claudication, and nonspecific neurologic deficits. All participants had failed to improve after 2 weeks of bed rest and oral anti-inflammatory agents. Patients with previous surgery participated only if their symptoms were different from the preoperative symptoms. All patients were required to have findings on CT scan, myelogram, or epidural venogram consistent with their symptoms. Seventy-three patients with a diagnosis of acute herniated nucleus pulposus or spinal stenosis were included in the study. They all received an epidural injection between the third and fourth lumbar vertebrae in the lateral decubitus position lying on the affected extremity. The treatment group received a solution of 80 mg of methylprednisolone and 5 cc of 1% procaine and the control group received a solution containing 2 cc of saline and 5 cc of 1% procaine. Participants were asked to quantitate the percentage improvement in their symptoms at 24 hours postinjection and again at 3–month intervals. Short-term success was greater than 75 percent improvement at 24 hours and short-term failure was less than 75 percent improvement at 24 hours. Long-term success was 75 percent or greater improvement in preinjection symptoms at 13–30 months. No statistically significant improvement was noted between the two groups at short- or long-term follow-up. Therefore, investigators concluded that epidural steroids have no therapeutic effect in acute or chronic neural compression syndromes.

Mathews and colleagues evaluated the treatment of back pain and sciatica using controlled trials of manipulation, sclerosant therapy, epidural injection, and traction (28). Patients were selected for the four different treatment groups based on their symptoms. Sclerosant therapy was given to patients with low backache; manipulation was provided for low backache and mechanical restriction; traction was applied for low backache and restriction of movement; and an epidural steroid injection was given to patients with low backache and sciatica with a uniradicular neurologic deficit. Local anesthetic was used as a control in the scerosant and epidural injection groups. Heat was used as a control in the manipulation and traction groups. The epidural treatment group received a caudal epidural injection of 20 cc 0.125% bupivicaine and 80 mg of methylprednisolone every other week up to three times as needed. The control group received a 2 cc injection of lidocaine over the sacral hiatus or into a tender spot. The patients were assessed at 1 and 3 months. A larger portion of the treated patients were improved at every assessment point up to 1 year with the greatest effect being at 3 months.

Dallas and colleagues compared the efficacy of epidural morphine and steroid to epidural saline and steroid (35). Twenty postlaminectomy patients with chronic low back pain diagnosed by physical and neurologic examination were included in the study. Electromyographic and radiographic examination, antinuclear antibody studies, and routine blood work were performed to complete the physical evaluation and the Minnesota Multi-Phasic Personality Inventory was performed to rule out severe depression or major psychological disorder. Patients were randomly divided into a treatment group, which received 8cc morphine sulfate followed by 80 mg

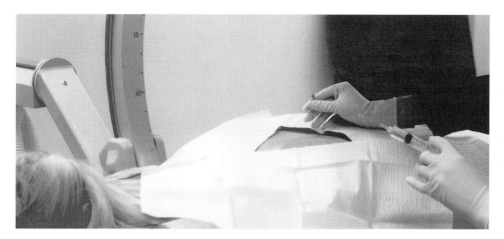

**FIGURE 9–4.**

After a skin wheal has been raised over the appropriate site, a 22 gauge 3 1/2 inch spinal needle is inserted down to the lamina under fluoroscopic guidance.

methylprednisolone, and a control group, which received 8 cc normal saline followed by 80 mg methylprednisolone. This injection was done using loss of resistance, contrast injection under image intensification, and a midline approach at the L3–4 or L4–5 interspace. A visual analogue scale (VAS) was completed by the patient prior to injection and again at 30 minutes, 2 hours, and 16 hours postinjection. Patients again completed the VAS weekly, at 1 month, and biweekly for the second month until the second injection. Two months after the first injection, the patient was given the series of injections he had not received the first time. The VAS was completed in the same way but also monthly after the second month for the next 6 months. In this study, a statistically significant number of participants obtained relief after the injection of morphine followed by steroid than with the injection of saline followed by steroid. Pain relief occurred in only 65 percent of participants and lasted 1 day to 6 weeks.

In 1988, Ridley and colleagues evaluated the effect of epidural steroids in 35 patients with pain in a sciatic nerve distribution with an appropriate neurologic deficit (29). They excluded patients whose only complaint was low back pain, leg pain, or restriction of straight leg raise; patients who had received an epidural steroid injection for the current episode of pain; and those who had previous spine surgery. The treatment group received 10 cc normal saline with 2 cc methylprednisolone into the epidural space using the translaminar method described by Barry and Kendall, while the control group received a 2 cc injection of normal saline into the interspinous ligament. The injection was repeated at 1 week if they received no benefit from the first. If no improvement was noted and placebo had been given initially, the patients were allowed to cross-over and receive the active treatment. Participants were assessed at entry and 1, 2, and 4 weeks postinjection. Long-term follow-up took place at 3 and 6 months postinjection. Changes in rest and walking pain VAS and straight leg raise were assessed. Significant improvement in both rest and walk-

ing pain was noted in the active group at 1 and 2 weeks, which was maintained up to 12 weeks. Cross-over patients noted improvement at 2 weeks postinjection. Sixty-five percent of patients maintained improvement at 24 weeks. The investigators concluded that epidural steroid injections have a useful short-term and medium-term analgesic effect and can be safely performed via the lumbar route.

In 1990, Bush and colleagues evaluated caudal epidural injections of triamcinolone and procaine for the management of intractable sciatica (17). Twenty-three patients with unilateral sciatica extending below the knee, paresthesias, and root tension signs in the form of a positive straight leg raise were included in the study. Exclusion criteria included cauda equina syndrome, presence of symptoms for less than 1 month, psychosomatic dysfunction, other serious psychopathology, and inadequate birth control in women of childbearing age. The treatment group received a caudal epidural injection of a 25 cc solution containing 80 mg of triamcinolone in normal saline and 0.5% procaine hydrochloride. The placebo group received a caudal epidural injection of 25 cc of normal saline. Each injection was repeated after 2 weeks. The patients were evaluated at each visit. They completed a symptom questionnaire and a VAS and had the angle of their straight leg raise measured by a Loebl goniometer. At 4 weeks, significant improvement was noted in the active group in straight leg raise, pain reduction, and quality of life. Many of the patients who had received treatment early in the disease process had greater relief in symptoms. The placebo group noted no significant changes. At 1 year, the placebo group had statistically significant resolution of symptoms while in the active group the earlier benefit was either maintained or improved. Comparison of the two groups no longer showed a significant difference in pain or quality of life but the treatment group continued to demonstrate a statistically significant improvement in straight leg raise compared to the control group.

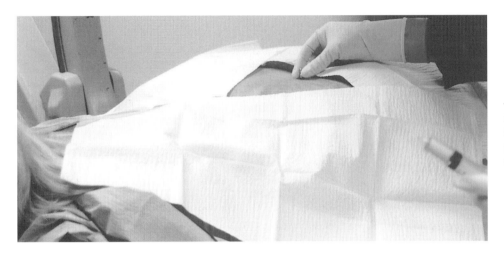

**FIGURE 9–5.**

Once the spinal needle contacts the lamina, additional local anesthesia can be given for comfort.

Breivik and colleagues compared the effect of caudal epidural injections of bupivicaine and methlyprednisolone with bupivicaine followed by saline (14). Thirty-five patients with low back pain present for several months to several years were studied. All patients had failed conservative treatment; eleven had already undergone surgery for a prolapsed intervertebral disc. All patients received either 20 cc of 0.25% bupivicaine with 80 mg depomedrol or 20 cc of 0.25% bupivicaine followed by 100 cc of normal saline via the caudal route up to three times at weekly intervals. Participants were assessed for improvement based on decrease in pain and/or paresis to a level that allowed the patient to return to work or to be rehabilitated to perform other work. Other variables assessed were Lasegue's test, deep tendon reflexes, hypesthesia/anesthesia, and sphincter disorders. Of the 16 patients in the treatment group, nine (56 percent) had considerable pain relief, with six showing objective neurologic improvement. Of the 19 patients in the control group, five (26 percent) had considerable pain relief with objective neurologic signs of improvement. Patients who did not improve after three injections were given the alternate type of injection. Seventy-three percent of the patients receiving bupivicaine and depomedrol as the second injection experienced significant improvement in pain. They concluded that up to three epidural steroid injections should be offered to persons with incapacitating low back pain when surgery is not an option. Since the authors describe neurologic abnormalities, it is assumed that "low back pain" made reference to or at least included lumbar radiculopathy.

## CRITIQUE OF LITERATURE REVIEWED BY THE AHCPR PANEL

Several study design flaws are pervasive in the medical literature regarding epidural steroid injections. Many of these flaws exsist in the literature reviewed by the panel. In order to evaluate the efficacy of a treatment like epidural steroid injections, the patient population under study must be clearly defined. Several of the studies reviewed by the panel contained a heterogeneous patient population (14,35) or patients whose pathology was not defined by an imaging study (14,17,27,28,29,35,37).

The route and volume of injection may also be important considerations in optimizing the results of L-ESI. Theoretically, success of this procedure relies on the placement of a high concentration of steroid at the target site (4). This should be optimized by placing the needle as close as possible to the target organ and injecting an adequate volume. As a result, a 20 cc caudal epidural steroid injection may not treat a right L1 radiculopathy resulting from a right posterolateral disc herniation at T12–L1 as well as a 5 cc right paramedian L-ESI at L1–2 or a 3 cc right L1 selective epidural steroid injection. The optimal volume of the injection depends in part on the

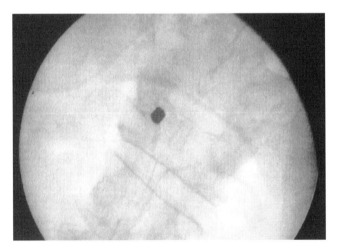

**FIGURE 9–6.**

The "en point" technique.

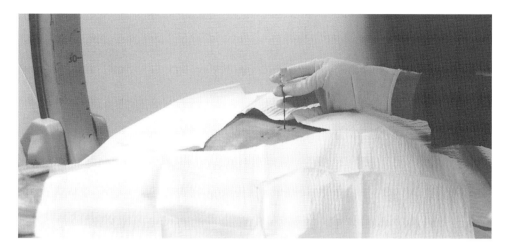

**FIGURE 9–7.**

A 3 1/2 inch 18 gauge Touhy needle replaces the spinal needle and is advanced down to the lamina, where it is subsequently "walked off" the lamina superiorly into the interlaminar space.

route of injection (4,26). In 1967, Harley demonstrated that 6 cc of contrast injected via a translaminar approach at L4–5 spread from L5 to S1 (25). This led him to suggest that more than 10 cc injected via the translaminar approach was probably unnecessary. Several of the studies reviewed by the panel did not adhere to this rationale and injected only very small volumes (31) or injected the spine at a site distant to the target organ (14,17,28).

Over the last several years, L-ESI performed without fluoroscopic guidance has also been criticized. It has been demonstrated that the "blind" placement of epidural needles results in suboptimal positioning in up to 40 percent of caudal epidurals and 30 percent of translaminar epidurals (20,21,22,33,36,43,44). Suboptimal positioning implies that the injectant does not reach its target site in sufficient volume and concentration to achieve its desired result. This may mean that the needle is placed in a nonepidural location (e.g., subarachnoid space, fascial, vascular) or an epidural location but is prevented from reaching its target site by anatomic abnormalities (central or lateral stenosis, perineural fibrosis) or variants (median raphe, periradicular cyst).

To determine the efficacy of a treament, appropriate follow-up data must be obtained. It is well known that the anti-inflammatory impact of epidurally administered methylprednisolone presents 3–7 days postinjection and lasts for 28–35 days (24). As a result, follow-up of L-ESI using methylprednisolone should be organized around this time frame. A logical follow-up protocol might be 24 hours, 1 week, 4 weeks, 8 weeks, 12 weeks, 6 months, and 12 months postinjection. Several of the studies reviewed did not adhere to a logical follow-up protocol (18,31).

## OTHER LITERATURE

There are a large number of references that have not been mentioned in this review (11,15,19,34,39,45,46,47, 48,49,50,51, 52,53,54,55,56, 57,58,59). While many have a number of design flaws, the presence of flaws does not mean that they are entirely unworthy of consideration. Most of these studies have no control group, are not blinded, and are retrospective in nature. Most are little more than a collection of anecdotes. When looked at individually, they have little value; when taken in mass, they do indicate a trend. The vast majority of these indicate a favorable short-term outcome of L-ESI in the treatment of acute lumbar radiculopathy.

The 1985 study by Helliwell and associates evaluated 39 patients with lumbar radiculopathy of at least 2 months' duration (39). Patients were excluded from the study for diagnostic uncertainty, pregnancy, previous lumbar surgery, or progressive neurologic deficit. This was a single blind, prospective study. They injected patients in the treatment group with 80 mg of methylprednisolone and 10 cc of normal saline via a translaminar route. They injected patients in the control group with 5 cc of normal saline into the interspinous ligament after appropriate local anesthesia. Only one injection was given. No other form of treatment was provided. The patients were evaluated for both subjective and objective improvements at 1 and 3 months following the injection. The treatment group showed statistically significant improvement in all variables measured at both 1 and 3 months. The authors concluded that L-ESI offered a cost-effective treatment for lumbar radiculopathy.

## RATIONALE FOR USE

Over the past several decades, compelling data have developed indicating that most disc herniations radiographically resorb on their own (4,60,61,62,63), that there is a high incidence of asymptomatic disc herniations (64,65,66), and that most patients clinically improve without surgery (62,63,67). There is also evidence of an

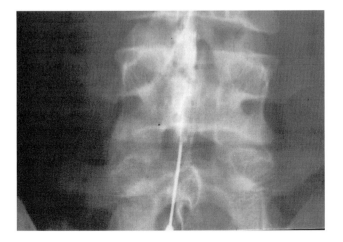

**FIGURE 9–8.**

A syringe containing air and fluid is attached to the Touhy needle and the epidural space can be entered using the "loss of resistance" technique. Contrast material can then be injected to confirm placement in the epidural space and visualize the epidural spread of fluid. The resulting "epidurogram" has a characteristic cloudlike pattern. This is followed by the injection of the steroid solution.

inflammatory basis for disc injury induced radiculopathy (53,57,68,69,70,71, 72,73,74). The anti-inflammatory property of corticosteroid is also well known. As a result, the use of L-ESI as a component of the overall treatment approach to a patient with radiculopathy seems rational. Specifically, properly placed epidural steroid should reduce the inflammatory response, thus reducing inflammatory radicular pain and potentially protecting neural structures from the degradative effects of inflammatory exudate (4,74). While this effect may be only temporizing, the self-limited nature of radiculopathy secondary to disc herniation would appear to make L-ESI an important component of a multifaceted treatment approach. As demonstrated previously, the vast preponderance of the literature is consistent regarding the short-term efficacy of L-ESI for lumbar radiculopathy. Stated another way, the object of an epidural steroid injection is not to "cure" one's back ailment but to provide temporary relief from the pain, dysfunction, and possible nerve injury while the radiculopathy resolves. Currently, there is no evidence to suggest that L-ESI increases the rate of disc herniation healing or resorption.

The literature does not support the notion that L-ESI is indicated in the treatment etiologies of low back pain without radiculopathy or radicular pain. A few of these etiologies include facet joint pain, noninflammatory disc pain, abdominal organ dysfunction, compression fracture, tumor, osteomyelitis, and metabolic dysfunction.

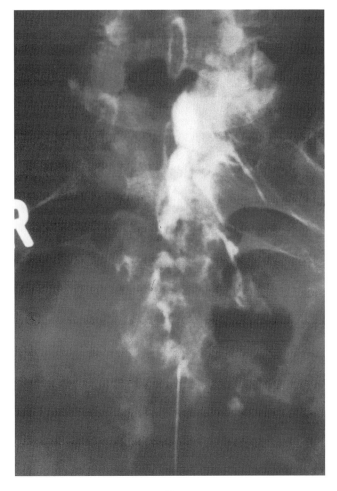

**FIGURE 9–9.**

An epidurogram via the caudal route.

## COST VERSUS HARM

The panel has suggested that epidural injections are potentially harmful. This is true but the literature suggests that the procedure is safe relative to other medical procedures. Brown reported no major complications following 500 consecutive injections (15,76). The most common complication is a spinal tap headache. This occurs when the dura mater is violated by the epidural needle and a sufficient amount of cerebrospinal fluid leaks out from the thecal sac to cause a positional headache (3,12,40,32). When affected persons assume an erect posture, they develop a throbbing headache and when they lie flat their headache substantially dissipates. The condition is almost always benign and is associated with very little morbidity. It is usually easily treated by relative rest, analgesics, and rehydration. A blood patch is occasionally necessary to help seal the rent in the dura mater. This condition occurs once in every 200 epidural injections.

Other minor complications from epidural steroid injections include transient water retention (76,77), transient congestive heart failure secondary to water retention (78), and transient hypotension (79).

Other more serious complications include epidural abscess, meningitis (80,81), and epidural hematoma. The incidence of epidural hematoma is reported to be approximately less than 1 in 4,000 (82,83), and the incidence of the other complications mentioned is so rare that it is unknown.

The panel has also suggested that epidural injections are expensive. At the time of this writing, the total cost of a lumbar epidural without fluoroscopic guidance, sedation, cardiac or vital sign monitoring, or formal recovery procedures ranges from $180 to $550 (84). A fluoroscopically directed epidural injection in an operative suite with sedation, cardiac and vital sign monitoring, and formal recovery ranges from $900 to $1,200.

This compares favorably with microdiscectomy, which has published costs ranging from $3,600 for ambulatory care to $23,000 for inpatient care and has a host of potential risks (85,86). A partial list of complications includes discitis, nerve root injury, repeat disc herniation, epidural abscess and other spinal canal infections, perineural fibrosis, and arachnoiditis. Additionally, the short- and long-term failure rates of this type of surgery are as high as 20 percent and 40 percent, respectively (87). The reported incidence of discitis following discectomy is 2 percent (88,89,90) and that of repeat disc herniation ranges from 3 percent to 19 percent (91,92,93,94). There are no reported statistics on the other complications mentioned. This procedure carries with it the inherent risks of anesthesia, which depend on the type of anesthesia used.

While epidural injections are costly and potentially harmful, their expense and complication profile compares favorably with other medical interventions.

## FURTHER STUDY

The current body of literature regarding L-ESI is deficient, as are many bodies of literature dealing with other areas of medicine. Further careful investigation should be carried out to better define indications and efficacy of epidural cortisone injections in the treatment of spine-related problems. Additional uncontrolled studies will be of limited benefit to the current body of literature.

Future study design should evaluate the efficacy of L-ESI in a population with imaging study evidence of a single-level disc herniation at a predefined level, a corresponding clinical examination, and with symptoms of a defined duration. The route of administration, volume and type of injectant, and radiographic direction should be controlled. The study should be double blinded and prospec-

tive in nature with defined cross-over permitted. The size of the study and control groups should be of adequate size to reach statistical significance. The measures of success should include both objective and subjective criteria.

Several portions of the same study can be developed. The patient population should have an MRI proven single-level disc herniaiton at L4–5 or L5–S1, no adjacent degenerative discs, no other anatomical reason for radiculopathy (e.g., central or lateral stenosis), a clincial examination consistent with L5 and/or S1 radicular pain and dysfunction, and no medical conditions that may promote or prolong the condition (e.g., diabetes mellitus). The patients should also be involved in a predefined physical therapy program that emphasizes flexibility, low-impact aerobic conditioning (e.g., stationary bike), non-disc-loading general conditioning, and stabilization activities. The first branch of study should evaluate duration of symptoms with the first layer being acute (0–3 months), the second layer being subacute (3–6 months), and the third layer being chronic (greater than 6 months). The second branch should compare the results of fluoroscopically guided translaminar injections to the blind technique of Barry and Kendall. The third branch should evaluate fluoroscopically directed translaminar, transforaminal, and caudal epidural cortisone injections. The fourth layer should compare methylprednisolone to triamcinolone and betamethasone. The fifth layer should evaluate volume of injectant with 2 cc and 10 cc volume compared for translaminar injecions, 10 cc and 20 cc volumes used for caudal injecitons, and 2 cc and 5 cc volumes for transforaminal injections at the level and side of involvement. The last branch should evaluate the efficacy of L-ESI as it relates to the size of disc injury using a predescribed classificaton system (75).

*S*ummary

Epidural injections have been employed to treat low back pain since 1901. Since that time there have been a number of drugs, routes, volumes, and indications for injection used. The body of medical literature dealing with epidural injections as a treatment for low back and related pain syndromes as a whole is in poor condition, with the vast majority of its reports being uncontrolled, retrospective, and without fluoroscopic visualization. More work needs to be done.

The panel screened 74 articles and elected to review nine. Out of the nine studies reviewed, one evaluated the effects of epidural morphine and steroid in patients with "failed back syndrome," irrespective of their clinical presentation. This study was irrelevant to the mainstream use of L-ESI for radiculopathy. The other eight studies dealt with L-ESI for radiculopathy, although one study (14) did allow postsurgical patients into the study. They were all reasonably well controlled (14,17,18,27,28, 29,31,37). Five of these studies indicated positive short-term relief of pain and recommended their use as an adjunct to the treatment of lumbar radiculopathy (14,17,28,29,37). One study indicated objective improvement at 1 year follow-up compared to controls (17). Two studies found no improvement with L-ESI over controls (18,31). These results can easily be explained by an inopportune follow-up protocol. The last study demonstrated that a greater percentage of patients in the treatment group improved than in any of the control groups but that this improvement did not reach statistical significance (27). This finding is probably due to a small sample size.

Overall, the L-ESI literature is fraught with poorly designed studies. The majority of controlled and uncontrolled studies indicate that L-ESI provides short-term benefit for patients with lumbar radiculopathy and are an important component to an overall treatment approach, but more work needs to be done.

## References

1. Mayer T, Gatchel R. *Functional restoration for spinal disorders: The sports medicine approach.* Philadelphia: Lea & Febiger, 1988.
2. Holbrook T, et al. The frequency of occurrence impact and cost of selected musculoskeltal conditions in the United States. *Amer Acad Ortho Surg* 1984.
3. Benzon H. Epidural steroid injections for low back pain and lumbosacral radiculopathy. *Pain* 1986; 24:277–295.
4. Weinstein S, Herring S. Epidural steroid injections. *NASS Contemp Concepts* 1994; Oct:1–11.
5. Cathelin F. Mode d'action de la cocaine injecte dans l'espace epidural par le procede du canal sacre. *C R Soc Biol* 1901; 53:478.
6. Pasquier M, Leri D. Injection intra-et extradurales de cocaine a dose minime dans le traitement de la sciatique. *Bull Gen Ther* 1901; 142:196.
7. Viner N. Intractable sciatica—the sacral epidural injection—an ineffective method of giving relief. *Canad Med Ass J* 1925; 15:630.
8. Robechhi A, et al. Prime esperienze clinichein campo eumatologico. *Minerva Med* 1952; 98:1259–1263.
9. Lievre J, et al. L'injection transsacree: Etude clinique et radioilogique. *Bull Soc Med* 1957; 73:1110–1018.
10. Brown J. Pressure caudal anesthesia and back manipulation. *Northw Med* 1960; 59:905–909.
11. Goebert H, et al. Painful radiculopathy treated with epidural injections of procaine and hydrocortisone acetate. Results in 113 patients. *Anesth Analg* 1961; 40:130–134.
12. Swerdlow M, Sayle-Creer W. A study of extradural medication in the relief of the lumbosciatic syndrome. *Anaesthesia* 1970; 25:341–345.
13. Barry P, Kendall P. Corticosteroid infiltration of the epidural space. *Ann Phys Med* 1962; 6:267–273.
14. Breivik H, et al. Treatment of chronic low back pain and sciatica: A comparison of caudal epidural injections of bupivicaine and methylprednisolone with bupivicaine followed by saline. In: Bonica JJ, Alber-Fessard D (eds). Advances in pain research and therapy. New York: Raven Press, 1976: 927–32.
15. Brown F. Management of discogenic pain using epidural and intrathecal steroids. *Clin Orthop* 1977; 129:72–78.
16. Brown F. Protocol for management of acute low back pain with/without radiculopathy, including the use of epidural and intrathecal steroids. In: Brown FW (ed.). *American Academy of Orthopedic Surgeons Symposium on the Lumbar Spine.* St. Louis: Mosby, 1981:126–136.
17. Bush K, Hillier S. Controlled studies of caudal epidural injections of triamcinolone plus procaine for the management of intractable sciatica. *Spine* 1991; 16(15):572–575.
18. Cuckler J, et al. The use of epidural steroids in the treatment of lumbar radicular pain. A prospective, randomized, double-blind study. *J Bone Joint Surg [Am]* 1985; 67(1):63–68.
19. Daly P. Caudal epidural anesthesia in lumbosciatic pain. *Anaesthesia* 1970; 25:346–348.
20. Dreyfuss P. Epidural steroid injections. A procedure ideally performed under fluoroscopic control and with contrast media. *International Spinal Injection Society Newsletter* 1993; 1(5).
21. Ellenburg M, et al. Epidural steroid injection: A procedure ideally performed using fluoroscopic control. *Radiology* 1988; 168:554–557.
22. El-Khoury G, et al. Epidural steroid injection: A procedure ideally performed using fluoroscopic control. *Radiology* 1988; 168:554–57.
23. Green L. Dexamethasone in the treatment of symptoms due to herniated lumbar disc. *J Neurol Neurosurg Psychiatry* 1975; 38:1211–1225.
24. Green P, et al. The role of epidural cortisone injection in the treatment of discogenic low back pain. *Clin Orthop* 1980; 153:121–125.
25. Harley C. Extradural cortisone infiltration. A follow up study of 50 cases. *Ann Phys Med* 1967; 9:22–28.
26. Heyes-Moore G. A rational approach to the use of epidural medication in the treatment of sciatic pain. *Acta Orthop Scand* 1978; 49:366–70.
27. Klenerman L, et al. Lumbar epidural injections in the treatment of sciatica. *Rhuematol* 1984; 23(1):35–38.
28. Mathews P, et al. Back pain and sciatica: Controlled trials of manipulation, traction, sclerosant, and epidural injections. *Br J Rheumatol* 1987; 26:416–423.
29. Ridley M, et al. Outpatient lumbar epidural corticosteroid injection in the management of sciatica. *Br J Rheumatol* 1988; 27(4):295–299.
30. Rocco A, et al. Epidural steroids, epidural morphine, and epidural steroids combined with morphine in the treatment of post-laminectomy syndrome. *Pain* 1989; 36(3):297–303.
31. Snoek W, Weber H, Jorgensen B. Double blind evaluation of methylprednisolone for herniated lumbar discs. *Acta Orthop Scand* 1977; 48:635–641.
32. Warr A, et al. Chronic lumbosciatic syndrome treated by epidural injection and manipulation. *Practitioner* 1972; 299:53–59.

33. White A. Injection techniques for the diagnosis and treatment of low back pain. *Orthop Clin North Am* 1983; 14(3);553–567.

34. Yates D. A comparison of the types of epidural injections commonly used in the treatment of low back pain and sciatica. *Rheumatol Rehab* 1978; 17:181–186.

35. Dallas T, et al. Epidural morphine and methylprednisolone for low back pain. *Anesthesiology* 1987; 67(3):408–411.

36. Renfrew D, et al. Correct placement of epidural steroid injections: Fluoroscopic guidance and contrast administration. *AJNR* 1991; 12:1003–1007.

37. Dilke T, Burry H, Grahame R. Extradural cortisone injection in the management of lumbosacral nerve root compression. *Br Med J* 1973; 2(867):635–637.

38. Beliveau P. A comparison of epidural anesthesia with and without corticosteroid in the treatment of sciatica. *Rheumatol Phys Med* 1971; 11:40–43.

39. Helliwell M, et al. Outpatient treatment of low back pain and sciatica by a single extradural corticosteroid injection. *Brit J Clin Pract* 1985: 228–231.

40. Kepes E, Duncalf D. Treatment of low back ache with spinal injections of local anesthetics, spinal and systemic steroids. A review. *Pain* 1985; 22(1):33–47.

41. Mandell P, et al. *Low back pain. A historical and contemporary overview of occupational, medical, and psychological issues of chronic back pain.* Thorofare, NJ: SLACK, Inc., 1989:219.

42. Mooney V. Injection studies. Role in pain definition. In: Frymore J (ed.). *The adult spine: Principles and practice.* New York: Raven Press, 1991:527–540.

43. Mehta M, Salmon N. Extradural block. Confirmation of the injection site by x-ray monitoring. *Anaesthesia* 1985; 40:1009–1012.

44. White A, Derby R, Wynne G. Epidural injections for the diagnosis and treatment of low back pain. *Spine* 1980; 5(1):78–86.

45. Bernat J. Intraspinal steroid therapy. *Neurology* 1981; 31:168–171.

46. Bokonjic R. Epidurale infiltration von Dexa-Neurobion zur Behandlung von Diskushernien. *Med Welt* 1975; 26:302–305.

47. Bonika J, et al. Peridural block, an analysis of 3,637 cases. A review. *Anesthesiology* 1957; 18:723–784.

48. Bullard J, Houghton F. Epidural steroid treatment of acute herniated nucleus pulposus. *Anesth Anag* 1977; 56:862–863.

49. Cappio M. Il trattamento idrocortisonico per via epidurale sacrale delle lombosciatalgia. *Reumatismo* 1957; 9:60–70.

50. Coomes E. A comparison between epidural anaesthesia and bed rest in sciatica. *Br Med J* 1961; 1:20–24.

51. Cyriax J. Epidural anaesthesia and bed rest in sciatica. *Br Med J* 1961; 1:428.

52. Burn J, Langdon L. Duration of action of methylprednisolone. A study in patients with lumbosciatic syndrome. *Arch Phys Med Rehabil* 1974; 53:29–34.

53. Burn J, Langdon L. Lumbar epidural injectons for the treatment of chronic sciatica. *Rheum Phys Med* 1970; 10:368–374.

54. Davidson J, Robin G. Epidural injections in the lumbosciatic syndrome. *Br J Anaesth* 1961; 33:595–598.

55. Gardener W, et al. Intraspinal corticosteroids in the treatment of sciatica. *Trans Amer Neurol Ass* 1961; 86:214–215.

56. Gordon J. Caudal extradural injections in the treatment of low back pain. *Anaesthesia* 1980; 35:515–516.

57. Ito R. The treatment of low back pain and sciatica with epidural corticosteroid injections and its pathophysiological basis. *Nippon Saikingeka Zasshi* 1971; 45:769–777.

58. Jenkins F, et al. Treatment of low back pain and sciatica with extradural analgesia and steroid injections. *Irish Med Assoc* 1979; 72:402–406.

59. Pariesien V. Conservative treatment of low back pain with epidural steroids. *J Maine Med Ass* 1980; 71:83–92.

60. Bozzao N, et al. Lumbar disc herniations: MR imaging assessment of natural history in patients treated without surgery. *Radiology* 1992; 185:135–141.

61. Delauche-Cavallier M, et al. Lumbar disc herniation. Computed tomography scan changes after conservative treatment of nerve root compression. *Spine* 1992; 17:927–933.

62. Saal J, Saal J. Nonoperative treatment of herniated lumbar intervertebral disc with radiculopathy. *Spine* 1989; 14(4):431–437.

63. Sall J, Sall J, Herzog R. The natural history of lumbar intervertebral disc extrusions treated nonoperatively. *Spine* 1990; 15(7):633–636.

64. Boden S, et al. Abnormal magnetic-resonance scans in asymptomatic patients. *J Bone Joint Surg* 1990; 72A:403–408.

65. Hitselberger W, Witten P. Abnormal myelogram in asymptomatic patients. *J Neurosurg* 1986; 28:204–206.

66. Weisel S, et al. A study of computer assisted tomography. The incidence of positive CAT scans in an asymptomatic group of patients. *Spine* 1984; 9:549–551.

67. Weber H. Lumbar disc herniation: A prospective study of prognostic factors including a controlled trial. Part 1. *Oslo City Hosp* 1978; 28:33–61.

68. Doita M, et al. Immunohistologic study of the ruptured intervertebral disc of the lumbar spine. *Spine* 1987; 12:264–268.

69. Haro H, et al. Unregulated expression of the chemokines in herniated nucleus pulposus resorption. *Spine* 1996; 21:1647–1652.

70. Hirabayashi S, et al. A dorsally displaced free fragment of lumbar disc herniation and its histologic findings. *Spine* 1990; 15:1231–1233.

71. Kang J, et al. Herniated lumbar intervertebral discs spontaneously produce matri metalloproteinases, nitric oxide, interleukin-6, and prostoglandin E2. *Spine* 1996; 21:271–277.

72. Marshall L, Trethwie E. Chemical irritation of nerve roots in disc prolapse. *Lancet* 1973; ii:230.

73. McCarron R, et al. The inflammatory effect of nucleus pulposus. A possible element in the pathogenesis of low back pain. *Spine* 1987; 12(8):760–764.

74. Saal J, et al. High levels of inflammatory phospholipase A2 activity in lumbar disc herniations. *Spine* 1990; 15(7):674–678.

75. Modic M, et al. Magnetic resonance imaging of intervertebral disc disease. *Radiology* 1984; 152:103–111.

76. Delaney T, et al. Epidural steroid effects on nerves and meninges. *Anaesth Analg Curr Res* 1980; 59:610–614.

77. Knight C, Burnell J. Stemic side effects of extradural steroids. *Anaesthesia* 1980; 35:593–594.

78. Goebert H, et al. Sciatica: Treatment with injections of procaine and hydrocortisone acetate. Results in 113 patients. *Anesth Analg* 1960; 130–134.

79. Knutsen O, Ygge H. Prolonged extradural anesthesia with bupivicaine at lumbago and sciatica. *Acta Orthop Scand* 1971; 42:338–352.

80. Dougherty J, Frazer R. Complications of intraspinal injections of steroids. *J Neurosurg* 1978; 48:1023–1025.

81. Shealy C. Dangers of spinal injections without proper diagnosis. *JAMA* 1966; 197:1104–1106.

82. Odom J, Sih I. Epidural analgesia and anticoagulant therapy: Experience with one thousand cases of continuous epidurals. *Anaesthesia* 1983; 38:550–551.

83. Rao T, El-Etr A. Anticoagulation following placement of epidural and subarachnoid catheters. *Anesthesiology* 1981; 55:618–620.

84. HealthCare Consultants of America, Inc. *HealthCare Consultants' 1996 Physicians Fee & Coding Guide,* 6th ed. Augusta: HealthCare Consultants of America, Inc., 1995.

85. Bookwalter J, et al. Ambulatory surgery is safe in radicular disease. *Spine* 1974; 19:526–530.

86. Muralikuttan K, et al. A prospective randomized trial of chemonucleolysis and conventional disc surgery in single level disc herniation. *Spine* 1992; 17:381–387.

87. Burton C. Lumbosacral arachnoiditis. *Spine* 1978; 3:24–30.

88. Bircher M, et al. Discitis following lumbar surgery. *Spine* 1988; 13:98–102.

89. Fernand R, Lee C. Post laminectomy disc space infection: A review of the literature and a report of three cases. *Clin Orthop* 1986; 209:215–218

90. Pilgaard S. Discitis (closed space infection) following the removal of the intervertebral disc. *J Bone Joint Surg* 1969; 51A:713.

91. Pappas C, Harrington T, Sontag V. Outcome analysis of 654 surgically treated lumbar disc herniations. *Neurosurgery* 1992; 30:862–866.

92. Balderston R, et al. The treatment of lumbar disc herniation: Simple fragment excision versus disc space curettage. *J Spinal Disord* 1991; 4:22–25.

93. Ebersold M, et al. Results of lumbar discectomy in the pediatric patient. *J Neurosurg* 1987; 67:643–647.

94. Lewis P, et al. Longterm prospective study of lumbosacral discectomy. *J Neurosurg* 1987; 67:49–53.

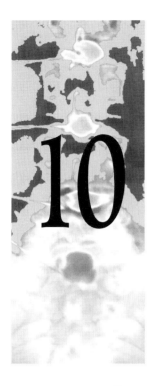

# 10 Discography

*Curtis W. Slipman, M.D.*

he Agency for Health Care Policy and Research (AHCPR) (1) developed guidelines for discography by relying on four articles published between 1968 and 1991. These were drawn from a pool of 42 publications. One reference evaluated outcomes prospectively (2), one reference was a book chapter essentially reiterating prior published reports (3), and the two remaining references reported results of discograms on normals (asymptomatic subjects) (4,5). There were no articles identified that evaluated discography in individuals with acute low back pain.

Based on their interpretation of the findings contained in these reports, the AHCPR analysis resulted in four conclusions, which warrant review:

1. Discography is "not recommended for assessing patients with acute low back pain."
2. "There is limited evidence that discography can help select patients who would benefit from spinal fusion."
3. "Interpretation is equivocal."
4. "Due to increased potential risks, CT–discography is not recommended over other imaging studies (MRI, CT) for assessing patients with suspected nerve root compression due to lumbar disc hernia."

## ANATOMY

The lumbar spine is composed of five vertebrae with an intervertebral disc interposed between adjacent vertebral bodies. A cartilaginous endplate exists between the disc and the adjacent vertebral bodies. The disc itself is comprised of a central nucleus pulposus surrounded peripherally by the annulus fibrosis. In normal young adults, the nucleus is a semi-fluid mass of mucoid material with the consistency, more or less, of toothpaste (6). The nucleus pulposus is approximately 70–90 percent water in a young healthy disc, but this percentage varies and generally decreases with age (7–12). The main constituents within the nucleus include glycosaminoglycans, proteoglycans, and collagen. Type II collagen predominates in the nucleus. Proteoglycans are the largest molecules in the body and possess an enormous capacity to imbibe water to the point of increasing their weight by 250 percent. This ability to attract and hold water results in predictable morphology. An intact nucleus is considered gel-like. Biomechanically it can display properties of either a solid or liquid substance depending on the transmitted loads and its posture (13).

The annulus fibrosis consists of collagen fibers and, in contrast to the nucleus, these are primarily Type I. These fibers are arranged in 10 to 20 concentric layers, known as lamellae, surrounding the nucleus pulposus (14,15). The orientation of the collagen fibers within each lamella is parallel and angled about 65–70° from vertical (16,17). The direction of this inclination from vertical alternates with each lamella. This alternation of the direction of fibers in consecutive lamellae is integral to the ability of the disc to resist twisting (18).

The vertebral endplate is a thin layer of cartilage located between the vertebral body and the intervertebral disc. While normally composed of both hyaline and fibrocartilage, the endplates are virtually entirely fibrocartilage in older discs. Since the intervertebral disc is the largest avascular structure in the body, it is dependent on diffusion across the endplate for nutrition and waste removal. While the disc is avascular, it is not anesthetic. Sensory information is transmitted from the outer one-third of the annulus, which is the only innervated portion of the disc (19–23). It is within this region that painful annular tears must be demonstrated during discography for the study to be considered positive.

## TECHNIQUE

Lumbar discography can be accomplished in three ways, representing a combination of two techniques and two approaches:

1. Posterolateral approach with the patient resting in the prone oblique position. A right-sided entrance site is typically employed, thereby requiring that the patient rest on his or her left side. The right hip is flexed and slightly abducted, while the right knee is flexed. Pillows are placed under the distal medial thigh to support the right leg. This leg position relaxes the right L5 nerve root, thereby minimizing the chance of needle contact during an attempt to enter the L5–S1 disc. A bolster is placed under the left flank, which will slightly tilt the pelvis and open the entrance to the L5–S1 disc.

2. Posterolateral approach with the patient prone. In contrast to the aforementioned posterolateral approach, this technique requires biplanar imaging with each needle advance as there is no safe target zone imaged.

3. Transdural approach with the patient prone. A paramedian needle entrance point is used. Extra care is taken when aligning the guide needle since the second needle will pierce the dural membrane twice prior to entering the disc space. If alignment is not accurate, repeat attempts to advance the needle will be required with each trial causing not one, but two dural punctures. Therefore, the risk of headache, nerve root injury, meningitis, and meningocele formation is theoretically increased. Consequently, a transdural approach should be reserved for instances in which the L5–S1 disc cannot be entered by the two other techniques.

Prior to positioning the patient for this test, an evaluation is required to determine which technique and approach should be used. Factors influencing this decision include patient size, patient compliance, disc space height, pelvic configuration, presence of transitional segments, and prior discectomy and/or fusion. Once this determination is made the procedure is re-explained to the patient. A sterile field is then created. A two-needle technique is used in each instance. The introducer or guide needle does not enter the disc space to obviate placement of skin flora into the nucleus. A curved two-needle technique is often needed for the posterolateral approach with the patient resting obliquely. In this case the second needle is given a gentle curve, allowing it to slip around the right S1 superior articular process and under the exiting L5 nerve root.

## HISTORICAL PERSPECTIVE ON DISCOGRAPHY GUIDELINES

In 1988, the North American Spine Society (NASS) published a position statement about discography (24). This one-page document was a consensus opinion, developed by its executive committee. Discograms were considered a procedure only for those with chronic low back pain (symptoms greater than 4 months' duration). It should be utilized only after other typical imaging studies have been performed and only as a presurgical tool; in other words, after all reasonable diagnostic and therapeutic interventions have been pursued. The document recognized that other than discography, no visualization tool offers the ability to precisely delineate disc morphology (Figure 10–1). Despite this, the committee warned that aberrant disc anatomy was not considered a sufficient determinant for a positive study. A concordant pain response during injection was emphasized as an additional criteria for a positive study.

Seven years later, NASS published an updated position paper through its diagnostic and therapeutic committee (25). In contrast to the first paper, a review of 89 articles was documented. Conclusions published in this report were consistent with the initial position paper, with some refinements:

1. Discography should only be performed by a "spine specialist experienced with the procedure."
2. Patients should be alert or "not more than mildly sedated."
3. Incidence of complications is less than 0.15 percent and 0.08 percent per patient and disc, respectively.
4. Disco-CT should be completed temporally contiguous with discography such that contrast can still be visualized.

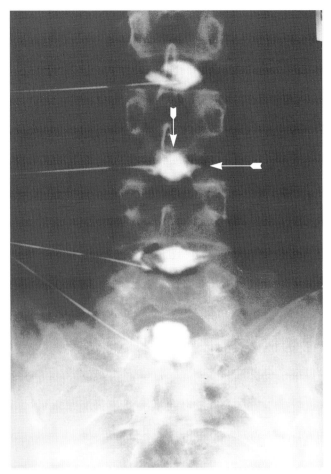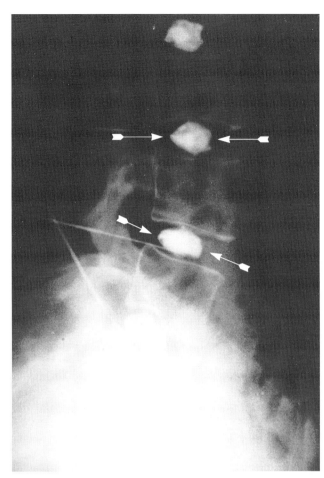

A                                  **FIGURE 10–1 A, B**                                  B

Normal four-level discogram. *A:* Posterior-anterior view. *B:* Lateral view. *Arrows* outline lateral borders of the nucleus.

As previously recommended, the selection criteria included those patients with undiagnosed intractable back pain. Additional indications were:

1. Evaluation for recurrent or lateral herniated disc.
2. Painful pseudarthrosis.
3. Painful disc within a posterior fusion.
4. Evaluate discs within and adjacent to proposed fusion level(s).
5. Ascertain whether a focal protrusion is contained prior to chemonucleolysis or minimally invasive surgery.

## REVIEW OF AHCPR CONCLUSIONS

The following discussion sequentially addresses the AHCPR conclusions with a focus on the use of discography in patients with intractable chronic back pain.

1. Discography is not recommended for patients with acute back pain.
   *Response—Agree.*

To date, there have been no published reports of discography in patients with acute low back pain. Given the general consensus that at least 90 percent of acute low back injuries resolve with minimal medical attention, it is not surprising that prospective clinical studies employing discography in the acute setting have been conducted. Nevertheless, the lack of any scientific inquiry remotely suggesting the value of discography for acute injuries does not necessarily lead to the conclusion that discography is an unreasonable tool to evaluate acute spine pain. Although the clinical application is currently nonexistent in the aforementioned setting, there appear to be important research applications.

Three standards have been applied in validating discography:

1. Comparison with normals or asymptomatic volunteers (4, 5);
2. Cadaveric studies (26–28); and
3. Correlation with surgical outcome (fusion) (29–36).

None represent an ideal reference standard due to their respective inherent limitations.

Performing a discogram on an asymptomatic subject does not represent a true control. While the morphology of any disc can be determined in an asymptomatic or symptomatic individual, concordant pain provocation cannot. Reproduction of a patient's usual pain is only possible if symptoms are present prior to performing discography. A similar analysis is applicable to cadaveric studies.

Using studies of outcomes following fusion to determine the validity of discography in diagnosing symptoms of discogenic disease assumes that this therapeutic intervention is the appropriate solution. Although there is general consensus that this is the correct surgical intervention in selected cases, much controversy continues concerning the correct type of fusion to be offered. More importantly, a fundamental flaw exists in the argument that a therapeutic intervention validates a diagnostic tool. At best, the use of such outcome studies can be viewed as predictive of the result expected from this intervention. Herein lies the conflict. The general notion is that discography identifies painful discs. Results from fusion are then scrutinized as a means of proving that a discogram truly revealed the painful disc(s). Perhaps the utility of discography should be categorized into two distinct categories: first, as an indicator of a painful disc; second, as an outcome predictor of lumbar fusion, each of which should be investigated separately.

To date, there are no available diagnostic tests that determine the location of symptomatic discs except possibly discography. In 1989, Nachemson predicted that discography would become obsolete due to the advent of MRI (37). Focal protrusions (herniated discs) are better visualized with MRI. Furthermore, MRI has the ability to reveal disc degeneration. While MRI can demonstrate disc degeneration, it cannot identify a "painful" disc. Several studies have highlighted the fallacy of relying on MRI to prove a diagnosis of degenerative disc disease as the cause of back pain (2,38–41). It has also been demonstrated that normal appearing discs on MRI may be the source of low back pain as defined by discography (38, 42). The concept of employing other visualization studies prior to ordering discography is widely accepted. Patients about to undergo discography are defined as those individuals who have intractable back pain for which no specific diagnosis has been defined with other conventional radiologic imaging (25).

2. There is limited evidence that discography can help select patients who would benefit from spinal fusion. *Response—disagree.*

Several studies have been conducted to address the question of predictive value.

In 1988, Colhoun and colleagues presented results of a prospective study evaluating the predictive value of provocative discography in a homogeneous population of patients with back and nonradicular leg pain (30). An overall sensitivity and specificity of 90.3 percent and 43 percent was obtained, respectively. One hundred thirty-seven patients (89 percent) with positive discograms achieved successful fusion. In contrast, only 52 percent of patients with negative discography obtained satisfactory symptom relief postoperatively. AHCPR accepted this single article to develop its guidelines concerning the predictive value of discography. A limitation of this study, according to AHCPR, is that 18 percent of patients did not have fusions, but laminectomies and/or discectomy. While this does represent a methodological flaw, an 18 percent figure is not accurate; only 6 percent (13 of 195) of patients underwent a surgical procedure other than fusion.

In 1988, Blumenthal and co-workers reported their results of a prospective study investigating the outcomes of anterior lumbar interbody fusion on 34 consecutive chronic back pain patients (29). All had single-level disease without a history of prior back surgery. Allograft was used for all but seven cases. Successful results were defined as return to work or normal activities using no more than nonsteroidal anti-inflammatory agents. Overall, 74 percent achieved a good result, but only 73 percent fused.

In 1990, Kozak and colleagues retrospectively evaluated simultaneous combined anterior and posterior fusion (33). A subgroup of patients never previously operated on and having positive provocative discography were separately analyzed. Twenty-one of 26 patients (81 percent) obtained a satisfactory result. Of those with single-level disease, 89 percent (8 of 9) reported a satisfactory result.

In 1991, Linson retrospectively analyzed outcomes of 51 consecutive chronic back pain patients with positive provocative discograms undergoing anterior or combined anterior and posterior fusions (31). Seventy-eight percent of patients with single-level disease without prior surgery undergoing anterior interbody fusion reported symptom improvement, while 85 percent of those with prior surgery improved. Only patients with failed back surgery and multilevel disease received combined procedures. Sixty-nine percent reported improvement. This study relied solely on Oswestry Disability Index scores to measure outcomes.

In 1992, Newman and Grinstead retrospectively reviewed 36 consecutive previously unoperated patients with concordant provocative discography who underwent anterior interbody fusion (43). Thirty-one (86 percent) had a successful result. Despite the use of an independent interviewer, conclusions from this study are limited, as outcome criteria were vague.

In 1993, Bernard published retrospective data of patients undergoing lumbar fusion (44). Of the 45 included patients, 34 underwent discography. A discogram was considered conclusive if the "radiographic abnormality correlated positively with the patient's clinical evaluation and surgical findings." Discography was positive in 32 patients (94 percent). An overall success rate of 82 percent was reported with a follow-up of at least 2 years. This study did not separate the outcome of those with positive discograms, so no specific conclusion can be drawn concerning the predictive value of discography.

In 1994, Wetzel and co-workers reported a retrospective review of 48 chronic back pain patients with positive discograms who underwent various types of lumbar fusion (32). Twenty-three percent had previous lumbar surgery. There were 8 single, 26 double, 13 triple, and 1 quadruple level fusions. Forty-six percent had a satisfactory result and 48 percent had successful arthrodesis. Of the 23 patients who achieved solid fusion, there were 22 patients with satisfactory results, representing the entire pool of satisfactory outcomes.

In 1995, Rhyne and colleagues presented results of 36 patients with positive provocative discograms who did not undergo surgery (45). The Roland and Morris disability scale, visual analogue scale, and Millon pain scale were used to measure outcome. Improvement was observed in 67 percent. Two significant methodological flaws must be detailed. First, this study relied on patient memory of their disability, functional status, and pain. Initial questionnaires were not completed prior to discography but at the time of this retrospective study, on average 3.5 years later. Second, there was a selection bias. Eight of 36 (22 percent) did not have surgery due to insurance denial. The remaining 78 percent idiosyncratically determined that surgery was not their appropriate course.

In 1995, Lee and co-workers retrospectively reviewed the results of discectomy and posterior lumbar interbody fusion in a consecutive group of 62 previously unoperated chronic back pain patients with positive provocative discograms (34). Satisfactory clinical results were obtained in 89 percent, while 93 percent returned to work.

In 1996, Parker and colleagues presented prospective data of patients who underwent provocative discography and subsequent posterolateral fusion (46). Twenty-two of 23 had positive discograms. Strict outcome criteria were used and follow-up ranged from 24 to 84 months. Only 39 percent achieved an excellent or good result. An interesting association between success and work was identified.

All subjects who obtained an excellent or good result were unemployed less than 3 months or were working prior to surgery, while 84 percent of the subjects with a poor result had been unemployed at least 6 months prior to surgery.

Although none of the cited references offer results from a prospective, blinded, randomly assigned study, they do suggest that discography is a good predictor of outcome following lumbar fusion for patients with intractable chronic low back pain. The predictive value of discography may be further enhanced by a better understanding of at least two issues. First, as identified by Parker and colleagues, work history is an important associated factor (46). Whether employment is causal or only an associated variable must be determined with further study. Second, combining psychological assessment may improve the predictive value of discography (47).

3. Interpretation is equivocal.
   *Response—disagree.*

The determination by AHCPR that interpretation of discography is equivocal is based on Holt's 1968 study of asymptomatic inmates and Walsh's 1990 study (4,5). This was surprising, given the repeated and extensive criticism of the current applicability of Holt's work. The shortcomings of this study include failure to use concordant pain response and disc morphology as criteria for a positive discogram; inconsistencies between statements and reported data; the use of a highly irritant contrast; lack of CT scan; and concerns about accuracy of needle placement (48). In contrast, Walsh's work showed high interrater reliability and agreement (5). Specifically, an adjusted percent agreement on discographic representation of disc morphology was 96 percent. Interrater reliability for pain intensity and pain behavior was 99 percent and 93 percent, respectively. There was 100 percent agreement as to whether the patient described significant pain. Finally, there was 88 percent agreement between observers about pain similarity. Walsh's work unequivocally establishes the reliability of discography, which is antithetical to the conclusions obtained by AHCPR.

4. Disco–CT should not be employed to work up nerve root compression, thereby avoiding the complications potentially associated with discography.
   *Response—disagree.*

It is not evident which data, research, or publication was used to arrive at this judgment. Of the four references cited, only the 1991 chapter by Gill and Jackson addresses this issue (3). In contrast to the AHCPR, the authors concluded that CT–discography more accurately defines foraminal, far-lateral, and recurrent herniations as compared to myelography, myelo–CT, and unenhanced CT scan. Gill and Jackson cited three references that substantiated their position: Grenier and co-workers, 1991; Jackson and co-workers, 1987; and Jackson and co-workers, 1989. In 1994, Bernard compared the value of Gd–MRI and disco–CT for recurrent disc protrusions (49). Using surgery as the gold standard, two blinded radiologists retrospectively reviewed the imaging studies of 33 patients. In each instance, the accuracy, sensitivity, and specificity was higher for disco–CT, albeit by a small percentage difference.

The AHCPR guidelines describe two potential serious complications of discography: discitis and disc herniation following disc injection.

In 1962, Collis reported one case of discitis following the performance of discography in 1,014 patients (0.1 percent) at 2,187 levels (0.05 percent) (50). In 1973, Patrick reviewed records of 123 patients and 341 disc injections (51). He described two serious complications. One involved a subsequent herniation, and the other appeared to be a case of discitis. The only frequent complication involved spinal headaches. Patrick used a transdural technique accounting for the common occurrence of headache. In 1987, Fraser and colleagues reported an incidence of discitis of 1.9 percent (4 of 210) per patient and 1 percent (4 of 417) per disc level when using a two-needle technique (52). In 1988, Guyer and colleagues reviewed records of 2,014 patients and 6,042 disc injections (53). An incidence of discitis of 0.1 percent per patient and 0.05 percent per disc was reported. In 1991, Simmons reported one case of discitis among 164 and 465 consecutive patients and disc levels, respectively. This translates to an incidence of 0.6 percent per patient and 0.02 percent per disc level (40). In 1988, Johnson retrospectively compared discograms of patients who underwent this procedure on two separate occasions (54). There was no evidence that the first discogram created any injury to the disc.

Since MRI is neither invasive nor exposes the patient to radiation, it is the study of choice to work up nerve root compression. Disco–CT should be reserved for the setting of radicular complaints, positive tension signs, and equivocal or negative MRI and CT scan.

## RESEARCH RECOMMENDATIONS

Three research proposals are discussed here. One adresses the natural history of lumbar discogenic disease. The other two focus on specific AHCPR recommendations.

1. Conduct a longitudinal prospective study of consecutive acute lower spine pain patients undergoing discography. This would provide data on the incidence of discogenic disease in acute low back pain and its natural history. One potential limitation of such investigation centers on the validity of discography in accurately assessing those who truly experience discogenic pain. Several authors have suggested monitoring pain responses during injection rather than solely describing disc morphology. This makes the study a subjective rather than an objective diagnostic tool (37). Demonstrating the validity of discography represents a serious and difficult issue to resolve. Unlike MRI in detecting focal protrusions, surgery cannot be employed as the gold standard. Additionally, no pathognomonic finding indicative of a "bad disc" can be found during spinal fusion.

2. To clarify the predictive value of discography, a multicenter, double blinded discography performed by experienced discographers on patients with intractable back pain greater than leg pain of at least 6 months' duration should be conducted. Disc morphology, manometric measurements, and pain response during injection would be recorded. Those individuals with single-level abnormalities would receive one of four interventions. Group 1 would receive no medical care. Group 2 would participate in a medically supervised graded exercise regimen. Group 3 would undergo a posterior fusion. Group 4 would undergo combined posterior and anterior interbody fusion. This study would also answer the question of which of these treatments is best for individuals with a positive discogram. In this instance, discography is employed as a predictor of therapeutic care. The results could also be used to suggest, but not establish, the natural history of degenerative disc disease.

3. Conduct a multicenter, prospective study recording the incidence of any side effects and/or complications following discography. If this project includes only members of a particular specialty, the data should be available to other types of spine experts performing discography for comparison.

## CASE STUDIES

*Case 1*

A previously athletic 45-year-old female had a chief complaint of daily low back and bilateral anterior thigh pain. During the three years before presentation, numerous lengthy attempts of appropriate conservative measures had been undertaken without success. Sitting continued to be the primary provocative factor leading to her inability to work. An MRI demonstrated disc dessication at L5–S1, and a small central focal protrusion (Figure 10–2) did not provide a definitive diagnosis. Discography revealed a fissured concordantly painful disc at L5–S1 and normal nonpainful discs at L3–4 and L4–5 (Figure 10–3). CT–disco revealed a rent extending from the dorsal aspect of the nucleus

**FIGURE 10–2A, B**

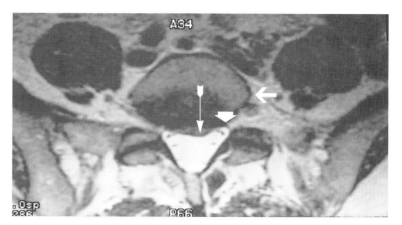

*A*: Lumbar MRI demonstrates disc desiccation at L5–S1 with minimal loss of disc height and some bulging beyond the dorsal border of the adjacent vertebrae on the mid-sagittal T2W window *(arrow)*. *B*: Axial section at L5–S1 reveals this bulge is a central focal protrusion *(arrow)*. Left S1 ventral and dorsal rootlets *(arrowhead)*, left L5 nerve root *(white arrow)*.

A

B

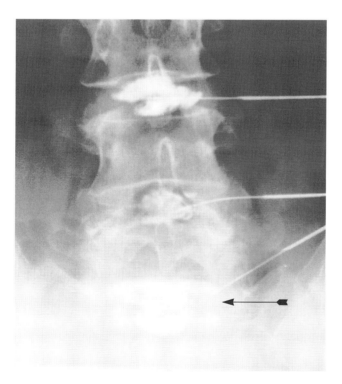

**FIGURE 10–3**

Three-level discogram. Posterior-anterior views reveal normal lobular discs at L3–4 and L4–5. At L5–S1 a fissured pattern is demonstrated *(arrow)*.

through the outermost posterior annular fibers ending at the 4 o'clock and 8 o'clock positions (Figure 10–4). A posterior fusion was performed with full pain relief and return to her active pre-morbid lifestyle.

### Case 2

A 49-year-old professional was 8 months status post right L4–5 hemilaminectomy and discectomy when he developed severe back pain and mild right anterior thigh pain. The leg symptoms did not extend beyond the proximal one-half of the thigh. Examination revealed no dermatomal or myotomal deficits, symmetric and intact reflexes, and negative root tension signs including reverse straight leg raise. MRI demonstrated a small right focal protrusion at L3–4 (Figure 10–5). Conservative measures failed to provide symptom reduction. Discography demonstrated a discordantly painful fissured disc at L3–4 (Figure 10–6) and a concordantly painful fissured disc at L4–5. The concordant pain was reported as a 96/100 using a visual analogue scale. CT–disco revealed a right focal protrusion at L3–4 (Figure 10–7) and extravasation of contrast at L4–5 (Figure 10–8). A posterolateral fusion at L4–5 resulted in complete back and leg pain relief.

## Summary

Provocative discography represents an important clinical tool for a variety of patients with low back pain despite the continued controversy regarding its usefulness (55,56). It is recommended:

1. For chronic and intractable low back pain (25);
2. For radicular pain, positive tension signs, and equivocal imaging studies, particularly for the previously operated spine (25, 49);
3. To evaluate discs adjacent to impending fusion level for spondylolisthesis, pseudarthrosis, segmental instability (25,57–58); and
4. Prior to chemonucleolysis or minimally invasive spine surgery (MISS) (25).

It must be emphasized that this procedure is only applicable to chronic and not acute low back pain, with the exception of patients undergoing chemonucleolysis or MISS.

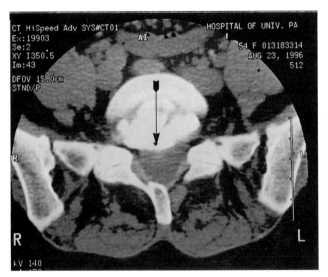

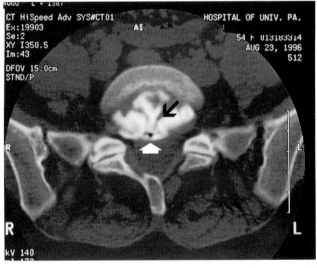

A                                    **FIGURE 10–4A, B**                                    B

CT–disco at L5–S1. *A:* Soft tissue. *B:* Bone windows reveal a fissured disc and a small central focal protrusion *(arrow)*. A midline posterior rent extends from the nucleus to the outer margins of the annulus *(white arrow)*. An air bubble introduced during injection of contrast is identified at 6 o'clock (arrowhead).

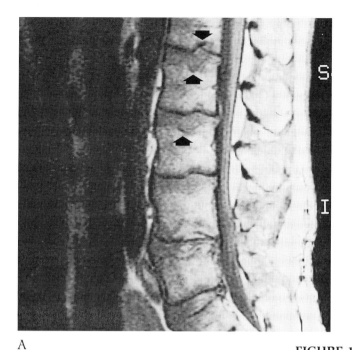

A

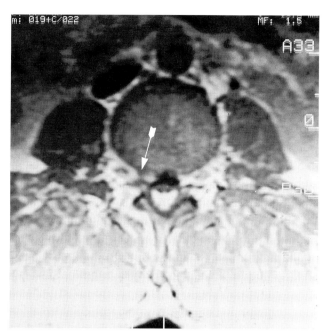

B

**FIGURE 10–5A, B**

*A:* T1W sagittal view of a lumbar MRI reveals multilevel disc disease; multiple endplate fractures (Schmorl's nodes) *(black arrowhead),* desiccation and loss of disc height at L4–5. *B:* Contrast enhanced T1W axial section of L3–4 demonstrates a right focal protrusion *(arrow).*

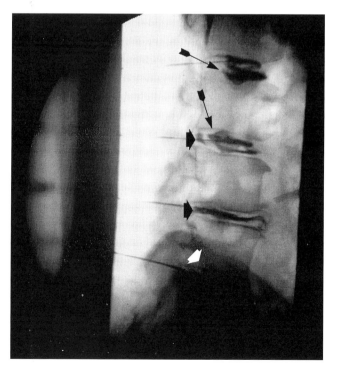

A

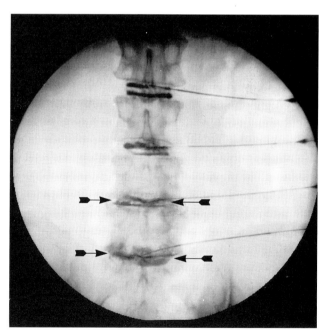

B

**FIGURE 10–6A, B**

Four-level discogram. *A:* A midline posterior or posterolateral rent *(black arrow)* is demonstrated at L3–4, L4–5, and L5–S1 as contrast extends beyond normal nuclear margins *(white arrows)* on the lateral view. *B:* Posterior-anterior projection. Contrast extends beyond the nucleus to fill the lateral annular margins at L4–5 and L5–S1 *(black arrowhead).*

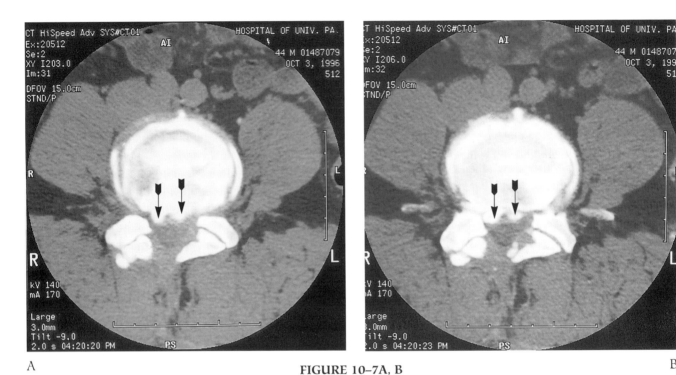

A                              **FIGURE 10–7A, B**                              B

*A* and *B:* Sequential soft tissue windows of CT–disco at L4–5. Contrast extends into the epidural space, which is bi-lobed, smoothly contoured, and well marginated *(arrow).* This abnormality may represent pouching of granulation tissue, caused by pressure of injection, at the site of surgery or a retained/recurrent focal protrusion.

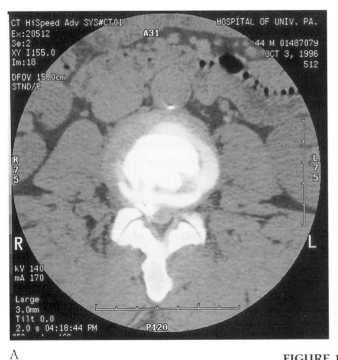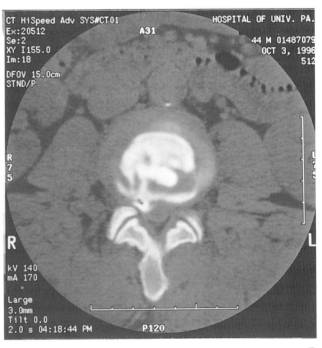

A                              **FIGURE 10–8A, B**                              B

*A.* CT-disco at L3-4 demonstrating a right focal protrusion on the soft tissue window. *B.* A tear extending from the nucleus to the outer rim of the annulus is seen at the 6:30 position with a few small air bubbles on the bone window.

# References

1. Bigos S, Bowyer O, Broon G, et al. Acute low back problems in adults. Clinical Practice Guideline No. 14. AHCPR Pub 95–0642.. U.S. Dept. of Health & Human Services, 1994.

2. Buirski G. Magnetic resonance signal patterns of lumbar discs in patients with low back pain: A prospective study with discographic correlation. *Spine* 1992; 10:1199–1204.

3. Gill K, Jackson RP. CT–discography. In: Frymoyer JW (ed.). *The adult spine: Principles and practice.* New York: Raven Press, 1991:443–456.

4. Holt EP Jr. The question of lumbar discography. *J Bone Joint Surg [Am]* 1968; 4:720–726.

5. Walsh TR, Weinstein JN, Spratt KF, Lehmann TR, Aprill C, Sayre H. Lumbar discography in normal subjects: A controlled, prospective study. *J Bone Joint Surg [Am]* 1990; 7:1081–1088.

6. Bogduk N, Twomey LT. *Clinical anatomy of the lumbar spine.* Melbourne: Churchill Livingstone, 2:12.

7. Beard HK, Stevens RL. Biochemical changes in the intervertebral disc. In: Jayson MIV (ed.). *The lumbar spine and backache.* London: Pitman, 1980:407–436.

8. Gower WE, Pedrimi V. Age-related variation in protein polysaccharides from human nucleus pulposus, annulus fibrosus and costal cartilage. *J Bone Joint Surg [Am]* 1969; 51A:1154–1162.

9. Naylor A. Intervertebral disc prolapse and degeneration. The biochemical and biophysical approach. *Spine* 1976; 1:108–114.

10. Naylor A, Shental R. Biochemical aspects of intervertebral discs in aging and disease. In: Jayson MIV (ed.). *The lumbar spine and backache.* New York: Grune & Stratton, 1976:317–326.

11. Puschel J. Der wassergehalt normaler und degenierieter zwischenwirbel-scheiben. *Beitr Path Anat* 1930; 84: 123–130.

12. Schmorl G, Junghanns H. *The human spine in health and disease.* New York: Grune & Stratton, 1971;2:18.

13. Iatridis JC, Weidenbaum N, Setton LA, Mow VC. Is the nucleus pulposus a solid or a fluid? Mechanical behaviors of the nucleus pulposus of the human intervertebral disc. *Spine* 1996; 21:1174–1184.

14. Armstrong JR. *Lumbar disc lesions.* Edinburgh: Churchill Livingstone, 1965; 3:13.

15. Taylor JR. The development and adult structure of lumbar intervertebral discs. *J Man Med* 1990; 5:43–47.

16. Hickey DS, Hukins SWL. X-ray diffraction studies of the arrangement of collagen fibers in human fetal intervertebral disc. *J Anat* 1980; 131:81–90.

17. Hickey DS, Hukins SWL. Relation between the structure of the annulus fibrosis and the function and failure of the intervertebral spine. *Spine* 1980; 5:100–116.

18. Bogduk N, Twomey LT. *Clinical anatomy of the lumbar spine.* Melbourne: Churchill Livingstone;2:125.

19. Bogduk N. The innervation of the lumbar spine. *Spine* 1983; 8:286.

20. Bogduk N, Twomey LT. *Clinical anatomy of the lumbar spine.* New York: Churchill Livingstone;2:161.

21. Hirsch C, Ingelmark BE, Miller M. The anatomical basis for low back pain. *Acta Orthop Scand* 1963; 33:1–17.

22. Jackson HC, Winkelmann RK, Bickel WH. Nerve endings in the human lumbar spinal column and related structures. *J Bone Joint Surg [Am]* 1966; 48A:1272–1281.

23. Malinsky J. The ontogenetic development of nerve terminations in the intervertebral discs of man. *Acta Anat* 1959; 38:96–113.

24. North American Spine Society. Position Statement on Discography. 1988.

25. Guyer RD, Ohnmeiss DD. Contemporary concepts in spine care. Lumbar discography. Position statement from the North American Spine Society and Therapeutic Committee. *Spine* 1995; 18:2048–2059.

26. Adams MA, Dolan P, Hutton WC. The stages of disc degeneration as revealed by discograms. *J Bone Joint Surg [Br]* 1986; 68:36–41.

27. Yasuma T, Ohno R, Yamauchi Y. False-negative lumbar discograms: Correlation of discographic and histologic findings in postmortem and surgical specimens. *J Bone Joint Surg [Am]* 1988; 70:1279–90.

28. Yu SW, Haughton VM, Sether LA, Wagner M. Comparison of MR and discography in detecting radial tears of the annulus: A post-mortem study. *AJNR* 1989; 10:1077–81.

29. Blumenthal SL, Baker J, Dossett A, Selby DK. The role of anterior lumbar fusion for internal disc disruption. *Spine* 1988; 5:566–569.

30. Colhoun E, McCall IW, Williams L, Pullicino VNC. Provocation discography as a guide to planning operations on the spine. *J Bone Joint Surg [Br]* 1988; 2:267–71.

31. Linson MA, Williams H. Anterior and combined anteroposterior fusion for lumbar disc pain: A preliminary study. *Spine* 1991; 2:143–145.

32. Wetzel FT, LaRocca SH, Lowery GL, Aprill CN. The treatment of lumbar spinal pain syndromes diagnosed by discography: Lumbar arthrodesis. *Spine* 1994; 7: 792–800.

33. Kozak JA, O'Brien JP. Simultaneous combined anterior and posterior fusion: An independent analysis of a treatment for the disabled low-back pain patient. *Spine* 1990; 4:322–328.

34. Lee CK, Vessa P, Lee JK. Chronic disabling low back pain syndrome caused by internal disc derangements: The results of disc excision and posterior lumbar interbody fusion. *Spine* 1995; 3:356–361.

35. Simmons EH, Segil CM. An evaluation of discography in the localization of symptomatic levels in discogenic disease of the spine. *Clinical Orthopaedics and Related Research* 1975; 108:57–69.

36. Weatherly CR, Prickett CF, O'Brien, JP. Discogenic pain persisting despite solid posterior fusion. *J Bone Joint Surg [Br]* 1986; 1:142–143.

37. Nachemson A. Editorial comment: Lumbar discography—where are we today? *Spine* 1989; 6:555–557.

38. Horton WC, Daftari TK. Which disc as visualized by magnetic resonance imaging is actually a source of pain? A correlation between magnetic resonance imaging and discography. *Spine* 1992; 6:S164–S171.

39. Jensen MC, Brant-Zawadzki MN, Obuchowski N, Modic MT, Malkasian D, Ross JS. Magnetic resonance imaging of the lumbar spine in people without back pain. *New Engl J Med* 1994; 2:69–73.

40. Simmons EH, Emery SF, McMillin JN, Landa D, Kimmich S. Awake discography: A comparison study with magnetic resonance imaging. *Spine* 1991; 6:S216–S221.

41. Boden SD, Davis DO, Dina TS, Patronas NJ, Wiesel SW. Abnormal magnetic-resonance scans of the lumbar spine

in asymptomatic subjects: A prospective investigation. *J Bone Joint Surg [Am]* 1990; 72:403–408.

42.  Zucherman J, Derby R, Hsu K, Picetti G, Kaiser J, Schofferman J, Goldthwaite N, White A. Normal magnetic resonance imaging with abnormal discography. *Spine* 1988; 12:1355–1359.

43.  Newman MH, Grinstead EL. Anterior lumbar interbody fusion for internal disc disruption. *Spine* 1992; 17:831–3.

44.  Bernard TN Jr. Lumbar discography and post-discography computerized tomography: Refining the diagnosis of low-back pain. *Spine* 1990; 15:690–707.

45.  Rhyne III AL, Smith SE, Wood KE, Darden II BV. Outcome of unoperated discogram-positive low back pain. *Spine* 1995; 20:1997–2001.

46.  Parker LM, Murrell SE, Boden SD, Horton WC. *Spine* 1996; 21:1909–1917.

47.  Block AR, Vanharanta H, Ohnmeiss DD, Guyer RD. Discographic pain report: Influence of psychological factors. *Spine* 1996; 21:334–338.

48.  Simmons JW, Aprill CN, Dwyer AP, Brodsky AE. A reassessment of Holt's data on: "The question of lumbar discography." *Clinical Orthopaedics and Related Research* 1988; 237:120–124.

49.  Bernard TN Jr. Using computed tomography/discography and enhanced magnetic resonance imaging to distinguish between scar tissue and recurrent lumbar disc herniation. *Spine* 1994; 24:2826–2832.

50.  Collis JS, Gardner WJ. Lumbar discography: An analysis of one thousand cases. *J Neurosurg* 1962; 19:452–461.

51.  Patrick BS. Lumbar discography: A five year study. *Surg Neurol* 1973; 1:267–273.

52.  Fraser RD, Osti OL, Vernon-Roberts B. Discitis after discography. *J Bone Joint Surg [Br]* 1987; 69B:26–35.

53.  Guyer RD, Collier R, Stith W, et al. Discitis after discography. *Spine* 1988; 12:1352–1354.

54.  Johnson RG. Does discography injure normal discs? An analysis of repeated discograms. *Spine* 1989; 4:424–426.

55.  Bogduk N, Modic MT. Controversy: Lumbar discography. *Spine* 1996; 21:402–404

56.  Nachemson A, Zdeblick TA, O'Brien JP. Controversy: Lumbar disc disease with discogenic pain. What surgical treatment is most effective? *Spine* 1996; 21:1835–1838

57.  Errico TJ. The role of discography in the 1980s (letter). *Radiology* 1988; 162:285

58.  Murtagh FR, Arrington JA. Computer tomographically guided discography as a determinant of normal disc level before fusion. *Spine* 1992; 17:826–830.

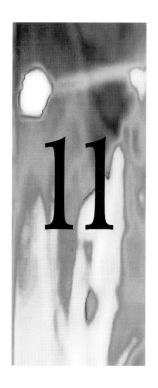

# 11 Diagnostic Nerve Root Blocks

*Curtis W. Slipman, M.D.*

iagnostic selective nerve root blocks are commonly used injections for patients with acute or chronic low back pain. The test should be ordered when a diagnosis is unavailable with other investigative techniques. It is frequently needed in a patient with buttock, lateral thigh, and lateral calf pain who has a normal MRI, normal EMG, and has failed a reasonable period of physical therapy. When used in this manner, diagnostic selective nerve root blocks represent a critical element in a diagnostic algorithm. In contrast, an individual who has back, lateral thigh, and pretibial pain, positive root tension signs, focal weakness of the gluteus medius and extensor hallucis longus, and an L4–5 ipsilateral posterolateral focal protrusion would not be a candidate for this test. In this case, a diagnosis of an L5 radiculopathy is apparent. Ordering a diagnostic selective nerve root block (SNRB) would be unnecessary.

## ANATOMY

Each lumbar nerve root leaves the thecal sac and exits the osseous confines of the spine immediately underneath its respective pedicle. For example, the L4 nerve root travels under the L4 pedicle, exiting between the L4 and L5 vertebral bodies. As the ventral and dorsal rootlets begin to join together as the nerve root, they remain enclosed by dura and cerebrospinal fluid. This relationship between CSF and nerve root ends once the dorsal root ganglion (DRG) is formed. Lateral to the DRG neither the dural or subarachnoid membranes can be found. Since in nearly every instance the DRG is located medial to or at the mid-point of the neural foramen, dural puncture can be avoided by penetrating the needle tip at or proximal to the 6 o'clock position (Figure 11–1).

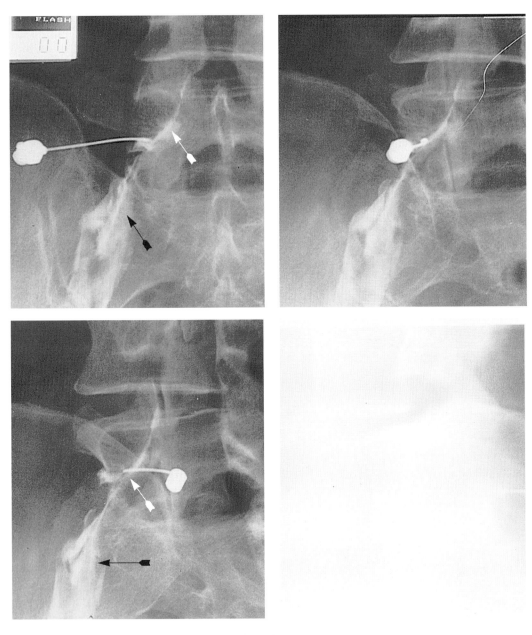

**FIGURE 11–1**

Four views of an L5 SNRB. Posterior-anterior projection demonstrates needle tip at 6 o'clock position *(top left)*. Oblique views *(top right and bottom left)* demonstrate contrast outlining the L5 root *(white arrow)* and the lumbosacral plexus *(black arrow)*. Lateral view *(bottom right)* shows needle tip at superior tip of the neural foramen where the nerve root exits.

## TECHNIQUE

This procedure should be performed with fluoroscopic guidance to ensure that only the nerve root and not the epidural space, adjacent nerve roots, or other structures are anesthetized (Figure 11–2) (1). Contrast is infused to demonstrate appropriate needle placement and injectate flow (Figure 11–3). Immediately thereafter, a small aliquot (0.5 to 1.0 cc) of local anesthetic is injected. During the interval of local anesthetic effect, the patient is assessed to determine the extent of pain relief. When at least 80 percent symptom reduction is obtained, this is considered a

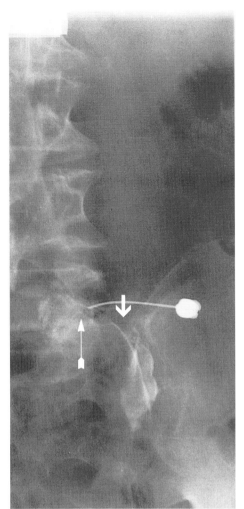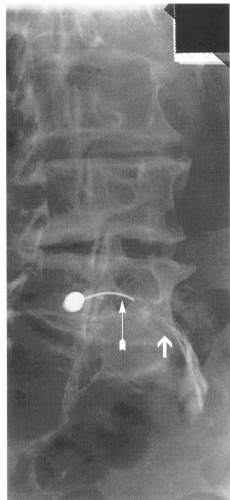

**FIGURE 11–2**

Single needle technique for an L5 SNRB. Posterior–anterior view *(left)* and oblique view *(right)* demonstrate 1.5 cc. of contrast outlining the L5 root in its foraminal *(arrow)* and extraforaminal *(large arrow)* location.

positive block, while lesser relief is deemed negative. The next step in the diagnostic algorithm should be pursued following a negative response. A positive block leads to the formulation of a specific diagnosis, thereby leading to a change in the rehabilitative treatment plan.

## AHCPR GUIDELINES

The Agency for Health Care Policy Research (AHCPR) guidelines for acute low back pain are based on 360 cited references (2). Of these publications, only one refers to selective nerve root blocks (SNRB) (3). This 1983 chapter by White is an overview of various lumbar injection

procedures, of which a page and a half are devoted to lumbar nerve blocks. White's chapter is quoted for reasons other than their discussion about SNRB since there is no mention of SNRB in the AHCPR guidelines. The paucity of clinical publication about selective nerve root blocks and the omission of the few studies evaluating this procedure may have led to the repudiation of diagnostic SNRB by the AHCPR. Table 11–1 summarizes the data reported by these omitted studies.

In 1971, Macnab and co-workers revealed the value of diagnostic SNRB in the preoperative evaluation of any patient with negative imaging studies and clinical findings of root irritation (4). They found the observation of contrast flow helpful, but not conclusive. Relief of usual

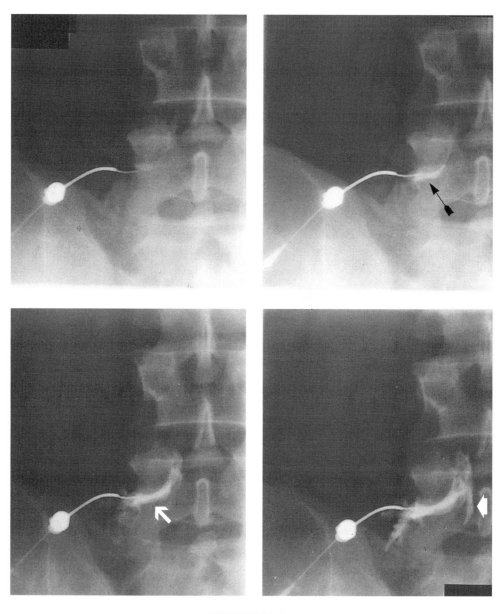

**FIGURE 11–3**

Double needle technique for an L5 SNRB. Pattern of contrast flow is demonstrated with four sequential posterior–anterior images. Top left image identifies proper needle placement. As contrast is injected, 0.5 cc *(arrow)* and 1.0 cc *(large arrow)*, the L5 root is clearly outlined in the neural foramen. Note how the root closely follows the medioinferior and inferior boundaries of the L5 pedicle. With additional contrast instillation, 1.3 cc, the epidural space is outlined *(arrowhead)*.

symptoms following injection of local anesthetic (1.0 cc of 2 percent Xylocaine) was the main determinant for diagnosis confirmation. The impression created by these anecdotal reports was that diagnostic SNRB was of greater value in predicting outcome for patients without prior surgery versus those previously operated on.

In 1973, Schutz and colleagues reported that of 15 patients with a positive diagnostic SNRB, 13 (87 percent) had a corroborative lesion uncovered during surgery (5). This retrospective paper did not provide information about outcomes.

In 1974, Krempen and Smith reported surgical

**TABLE 11–1**
*Articles reporting results of surgery performed on the basis of a diagnostic selective nerve root block*

| AUTHOR | YEAR | POSITIVE BLOCK & SURGERY | SURGICAL CONFIRMATION (%) | SURGICAL OUTCOME (%) |
|--------|------|--------------------------|---------------------------|----------------------|
| Schultz | 1973 | 15 | 87 | ? |
| Krempen | 1974 | 16 | 100 | 100 |
| Haueisen | 1985 | 41*/46 | 93*/94 | ? |
| Kikuchi | 1988 | 86 | ? | 100 |
| Dooley | 1988 | 45 | 98 | 64 |
| | | | | Herniated nucleus pulposus |
| | | | | 100 |
| | | | | Spinal stenosis |
| | | | | 82 |
| | | | | Epidural fibrosis |
| | | | | 71 |
| | | | | Arachnoiditis |
| | | | | 8 |
| Stanley | 1990 | 19 | 95 | ? |
| Akkerveeken | 1993 | ? | 100 | ? |

* Tension signs included

results of 16 patients who had a positive diagnostic SNRB (6). All had a corroborative lesion. In this group of failed back surgery patients, good or excellent leg pain relief was obtained in 100 percent. Contrast flow was considered helpful in many, but not all, instances.

In 1980, Tajima and colleagues published operative findings in 106 patients who underwent diagnostic/therapeutic SNRB (7). They concluded that radiculography provided important diagnostic information, as did response to local anesthetic infiltration. A number of limitations in this paper must be highlighted. First, a volume of 3.0 cc of a mixture of steroid and 1.0% Xylocaine was infused. It is generally accepted that no more than 1.0 cc should be used to prevent inadvertent anesthesia of the sinovertebral nerve, furcal nerve, or adjacent nerve roots. Second, outcome was not systematically reported. Third, there was no comparison of the utility of radiculography versus response to local anesthetic injection.

In 1985, Haueisen and co-workers retrospectively analyzed SNRB, electromyography, and myelography results in 55 patients who had a positive diagnostic SNRB (concordant symptom reproduction, full symptom relief, and loss of any tension sign) (8). In 38 of 41 (93 percent) who had surgery, a corroborative lesion was identified. If loss of a positive tension maneuver was dropped from the definition of a positive block, surgical confirmation

was achieved in 43 of 46 (94 percent). Myelography and electromyography correctly revealed the lesion in 24 percent and 38 percent, respectively. There was one false-negative (1.8 percent) and three false-positives (6 percent) for diagnostic selective nerve root block.

In 1988, Kikuchi and Hasue correlated results of myelography and SNRB with surgical findings and outcomes (9). A total of 119 patients were treated. Eighty-six underwent surgery, and all had complete symptom relief. While myelography correctly identified the level of the lesion, contrast patterns during SNRB localized the area of abnormality more precisely. Case reports were included to underscore their conclusions.

In 1988, Dooley and colleagues retrospectively analyzed response to diagnostic SNRB and outcomes following surgery (10). Forty-four of 46 patients in whom concordant symptom provocation during nerve root stimulation and complete symptom relief following local anesthetic infiltration was achieved had confirmation of pathology at surgery (one patient was not operated on). Of the nine patients with a herniated disc, 100 percent obtained complete leg pain relief and 78 percent had complete back pain relief. Seventeen had stenosis, with 14 (82 percent) describing complete symptom relief. The remaining 19 patients had arachnoiditis or epidural fibrosis. Eight percent of the former and 71 percent of the latter obtained symptom relief. Patients in whom typical symptoms were provoked during SNRB without symptom relief after local anesthetic injection ultimately had root level pathology, but at multiple levels. There were only four patients in this group, thereby precluding any definitive statements. When SNRB evoked unfamiliar pain, surgery either failed to demonstrate corroborative pathology or the outcome was poor.

In 1990, Stanley and co-workers conducted a prospective study in which 50 consecutive patients underwent SNRB (11). Nineteen of 20 patients who had concordant symptom provocation during nerve root stimulation and complete symptom relief following local anesthetic infiltration had subsequent surgery. Eighteen (95 percent) had surgical confirmation. These results were superior to radiculography or CT scan. Outcomes were not reported.

In 1992, Nachemson scrutinized the literature on low back care (12). He believed most interventions had not yet been proven. Nevertheless, he indicated that diagnostic selective nerve root block provided important prognostic information about surgical outcome.

In 1993, van Akkerveeken reiterated data from his 1989 thesis regarding sensitivity, specificity, and predictive values for diagnostic SNRB (13,14). A positive block required concordant symptom reproduction during root stimulation and full relief following local anesthetic infusion. Of those patients with complete leg pain relief, surgery confirmed a lesion in 100 percent. A sensitivity and specificity of 100 percent and 90 percent was reported, respectively. A positive predictive value of 95 percent was obtained for diagnostic SNRB in relation to surgical outcome. More information about the methodology is required before any firm conclusions can be drawn from these seemingly impressive values.

In 1995, Derby and co-workers retrospectively assessed the value of SNRB for predicting surgical outcome (15). Seventy-one of 78 consecutive patients with leg pain greater than back pain, who underwent an epidural or SNRB within 1 month prior to surgery and achieved at least 80 percent postinjection symptom reduction, were studied. Patients were then divided according to steroid response. A positive response was arbitrarily determined to require at least 50 percent symptom reduction for at least 1 week. For those patients with symptoms greater than 1 year, a positive steroid response predicted a positive surgical outcome, while a negative one indicated that the opposite would occur. A sensitivity of 85 percent, specificity of 95 percent, negative predictive value of 95 percent, and positive predictive value of 85 percent were obtained. One important limitation of this study must be highlighted; results were dependent on patient memory. Patients were asked to recollect information about steroid response and surgery an average of 8 months after the intervention (16).

## RESEARCH RECOMMENDATIONS

Several projects should be undertaken to demonstrate the value of diagnostic SNRB in acute or chronic back pain. Four research ideas applicable to acute injuries and current clinical applicability of SNRB follow.

QUESTION: *What is the sensitivity and specificity of fluoroscopically guided diagnostic SNRB to demonstrate radicular pain?*

To answer this question, a prospective double blind study evaluating patients with symptoms of an acute radiculopathy, positive tension signs, and an imaging study demonstrating a corroborative focal protrusion should be conducted. Local anesthetic or normal saline would be injected about the involved root or one of two uninvolved roots. The order of medication injected and nerve root addressed would be done randomly. Visual analogue scores would be recorded pre- and post-block. Sensitivity, specificity, and false-positive values for response to SNRB could then be obtained. Hard copies of the radiculogram would be compared by two independent observers for purposes of assessing reproducibility of contrast patterns, interrater reliability, and intrarater reliability.

QUESTION: *What is the minimal volume required to achieve anesthesia?*

To answer this question, a prospective double blind study evaluating patients with symptoms of an acute radiculopathy, positive tension signs, and an imaging study demonstrating a corroborative focal protrusion should be carried out. Various volumes of 2% Xylocaine would be infused to determine the minimal injectate required.

QUESTION: *Is concordant symptom production consistently achieved during nerve root provocation and is it necessary?*

To answer this question, a prospective single blind study evaluating patients with symptoms of monoradicular claudication and an imaging study demonstrating a corroborative lateral stenotic lesion should be completed. Two successive SNRBs of the involved or an uninvolved root would be randomly performed. Subjects would complete pre- and post-block visual analogue scales. Mooney pain drawings would be administered pre-block, immediately post-block to record distribution of root provocation, and at 30 minutes to assess symptom relief.

QUESTION: *Is diagnostic SNRB safe?*

To answer this question, a multicenter prospective study recording the incidence of any side effects and/or complications following SNRB should be conducted. If this project includes only members of a particular specialty, the data will be available for comparison to other types of spine experts performing SNRB. Preliminary investigation of this question has begun. In one study, a retrospective analysis using an independent reviewer of more than 250 consecutive lumbar selective nerve root blocks revealed no major complications (17). A prospective study using independent interviewers demonstrated no short- or long-term complications in over 350 consecutive SNRBs (18). These two studies demonstrate that fluoroscopically guided lumbar SNRB is a safe procedure when performed or supervised by an experienced spine physician.

It must be emphasized that fluoroscopic guidance is essential when performing an SNRB. Potential complications can be minimized by viewing exactly where the needle tip is located and diagnostic accuracy is enhanced. There are instances in which vascular injection occurs despite a negative aspiration in four quadrants. Presumably the large differential in diameter of the vascular structure injected and the needle leads to a high negative pressure with ensuing vascular wall collapse during aspiration. Such an occurrence would lead to a false-negative block as the local anesthetic would be delivered into the circulatory system rather than into the perineural sheath. Furthermore, it is impossible to predict the pattern of flow of injected substances during SNRB (3,19). Observing where the contrast medium travels during fluoroscopy allows the needle to be oriented for precise target delivery.

### CLINICAL RECOMMENDATIONS

Diagnostic selective nerve root block may be beneficial in the following circumstances:

1. Buttock with or without back pain unresponsive to oral agents and physical therapy, and negative imaging studies.
2. Thigh pain with or without proximal symptoms, unresponsive to oral agents and physical therapy, negative imaging studies, and no acute findings with electrodiagnostic testing.
3. Calf or pretibial pain with or without proximal symptoms, unresponsive to oral agents and physical therapy, negative imaging studies, and no acute findings with electrodiagnostic testing.
4. Knee or ankle pain of inexplicable etiology, unresponsive to oral agents.

A positive response to a diagnostic selective nerve root block may not lead to detection of a previously undiagnosed lesion, as suggested by the previously referenced studies. In many instances radicular pain results from a biochemical rather than a biomechanical process accounting for the negative imaging studies (20, 21). Therapeutic selective nerve root block should be performed for these patients.

## Summary

A review of the aforementioned overlooked studies suggests that diagnostic selective nerve root blocks represent an integral component in the evaluation of acute low back pain. A more definitive statement cannot be made due to limitations in the methodology employed in each of the studies. All studies, save for Stanley's, were retrospective. Although Stanley conducted a prospective study, outcomes were not reported. Standardized outcome tools to assess blocks or surgery were not used.

## References

1. Slipman CW. Injection techniques. In: Grabois M, Garrison SJ, Hart KA, Lehmkuhl LD, eds. *Physical medicine and rehabilitation: The complete approach.* Boston: Blackwell Science:1997.
2. Bigos S, Bowyer O, Broon G, et al. Acute low back problems in adults. Clinical Practice Guideline No. 14. AHCPR Pub. 95–0642. U.S. Dept. of Health & Human Services:1994.
3. White AH. Injection techniques for the diagnosis and treatment of low back pain. *Orthop Clin North Am* 1983; 14:553–567.
4. Macnab I. Negative disc exploration: An analysis of the causes of nerve root involvement in sixty-eight patients. *J Bone Joint Surg [Am]* 1971; 53A:5891–5903.
5. Schutz H, Lougheed WM, Wortzman G, Awerbuck BG. Intervertebral nerve-root in the investigation of chronic lumbar disc disease. *Can J Surg* 1973; 16:217–221.
6. Krempen JF, Smith BS. Nerve root injection: A method for evaluating the etiology of sciatica. *J Bone Joint Surg [Am]* 1974; 56A:1435–1444.
7. Tajima T, Furukawa K, Kuramochi E. Selective lumbosacral radiculography and block. *Spine* 1980; 1:68–77.
8. Haueisen DC, Smith BS, Myers SR, Pryce ML. The diagnostic accuracy of spinal nerve injection studies. *Clin Orthop Rel Res* 1985; 198:179–183.
9. Kikuchi S, Hasue M. Combined contrast studies in lumbar spine disease: Myelography (peridurography) and nerve root infiltration. *Spine* 1988; 13:1327–1331.
10. Dooley JF, McBroom RJ, Taguchi T, Macnab I. Nerve root infiltration in the diagnosis of radicular pain. *Spine* 1988; 13:79–83.
11. Stanley D, McLaren MI, Euinton HA, Getty CJM. A prospective study of nerve root infiltration in the diagnosis of sciatica: A comparison with radiculography,

computed tomography, and operative findings. *Spine* 1990; 6:540–543.

12. Nachemson A. Newest knowledge of low back pain: A critical look. *Clin Orthop Rel Res* 1992; 279:8–20.

13. van Akkerveeken PF. Lateral stenosis of the lumbar spine. Thesis. University of Utrecht, 1989.

14. van Akkerveeken PF. The diagnostic value of nerve root sheath infiltration. *Acta Orthop Scand* 1993; 64:61–63.

15. Derby R, Kine G, Saal JA, Reynolds J, Goldthwaite N, White AH, Hsu K, Zucherman J. Response to steroid and duration of radicular pain as predictors of surgical outcome. *Spine* 1992; 6:S176–S183.

16. Derby R. Personal communication.

17. Slipman CW, Meyers JS, Chou LH, Sterenfeld EB, Abrams S. Complications of fluoroscopically-guided spinal injections. *Arch Phys Med Rehabil* 1995; 76:1032.

18. Huston CW, Slipman CW, Meyers JS, Yang ST, Anghel BN. Side effects and complications of fluoroscopically guided nerve root injections. *Arch Phys Med Rehabil* 1996; 77:937.

19. Purcell-Jones G, Pither CE, Justins DM. Paravertebral somatic block: A clinical, radiographic, and computed tomographic study in chronic pain patients. *Anesth Analg* 1989; 68:32–39.

20. Hasue M. Pain and the nerve root: An interdisciplinary approach. *Spine* 1993; 18:2053–2058.

21. Saal J. The role of inflammation in lumbar pain. *Spine* 1995; 20:1821–1827

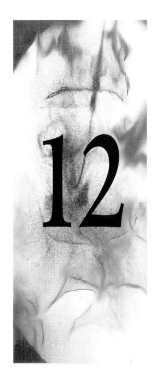

# 12 Lumbar Facet Injections

*Paul Dreyfuss, M.D., and Susan Dreyer, M.D.*

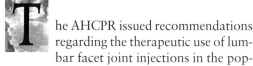he AHCPR issued recommendations regarding the therapeutic use of lumbar facet joint injections in the population of patients with acute low back pain (1). The common use of facet joint injections as a diagnostic tool in patients with subacute or chronic low back pain was not addressed by the AHCPR. A more comprehensive consensus regarding the role of facet joint injections in the diagnosis and treatment of low back pain was published as a "Current Concepts" series in the journal *Spine* (2).

This chapter aims to critique the AHCPR guidelines, especially in regard to their limitations. In review, the AHCPR guidelines state "facet joint injections are invasive and not recommended for use in the treatment of patients with acute low back problems." The guidelines summarize: (1) facet injections "do not appear to be effective for treating acute low back pain"; (2) "no studies have adequately investigated the efficacy of facet joint injections for patients with acute low back problems"; (3) "facet joint injections are associated with rare potential serious complications" (1).

The strength of the scientific evidence reviewed by the AHCPR was reported as "C," which is defined as the existence of limited research-based evidence to support the guideline statement. Seventeen articles were screened, but only five randomized controlled studies met their methodologic review criteria. Only two other papers contained information used by the panel, but these papers did not meet AHCPR methodology criteria (1).

As background for our critique of the AHCPR guidelines, we review the history, anatomy, mechanics, pathology, clinical presentation, differential diagnosis, diagnostic studies, and treatments for facet pain with an emphasis on intra-articular, corticosteroid facet joint injections. We examine in detail the five therapeutic intra-articular corticosteroid injection studies the AHCPR used to justify their recommendations (3,4,5,6,7). With this backround information, we discuss the conclusions drawn by the AHCPR. Additional recommendations regarding the application of facet joint injections in the modern practice of spine care are presented. We suggest future studies and base our own conclusions on a broader appraisal of the literature (2).

## INTRODUCTION

Low back pain (LBP) describes an ubiquitous symptom complex with a number of etiologies. Lifetime incidence of LBP ranges between 60 percent and 90 percent (8,9,10) and is the leading cause of disability in people younger than 45 years of age (11). Historically, much of LBP has been attributed to lumbar disc herniations (12). However, other possible etiologies include pain due to intrinsic and extrinsic disc disease, the sacroiliac joints, spinal stenosis, ligaments, muscles, viscerogenic and other nonspinal causes. The posterior, paired joints of the spinal column are commonly called *facet joints*, more formally and precisely *zygapophyseal joints*, and briefly, *z-joints*. Pain can emanate from these joints. The nociceptive capacity of these joints has been well established through anatomic, provocative, and clinical studies.

Eliminating sensation from a z-joint has been proposed as a way to allow an examiner to determine if that joint is responsible for the patient's pain. Injections of local anesthetic into the z-joint or around its nerve supply are clinical methods of eliminating pain from focal areas such as z-joints. The anatomic accessibility of the z-joints and their nerve supply makes diagnostic blocks particularly appealing.

Based on responses to single blocks, the prevalence of lumbar z-joint pain in patients with low back pain ranges from 7.7 percent to 75 percent (3,13–26). The wide variation in reported prevalence rates may reflect selection bias, variable population subsets referred to individual clinicians, or placebo responses. The lower prevalence rates were reported in larger samples with fewer inclusion criteria. However, even in the studies reporting a low prevalence, the authors acknowledge the existence of lumbar z-joint mediated pain (23,25,27,28).

Using the comparative, double block protocol, the prevalence of z-joint mediated chronic low back pain is 15 percent as diagnosed at two tertiary American spine centers (29). In an older (median age 59 years) population of patients referred to a rheumatologist in Australia, the prevalence of chronic z-joint pain was 40 percent. This study employed extra-articular placebo injections using normal saline in addition to sequential intra-articular z-joint blocks using bupivacaine (30). Hence, this clinical entity of z-joint mediated LBP cannot be denied or ignored. Double block or placebo-controlled injection techniques have not been applied to a population with acute low back pain; thus, the prevalence of z-joint pain in acute (<3 months) low back pain is unknown.

## HISTORY

In 1911, Goldthwaite first recognized lumbar z-joints as a potential source of back pain (31). In 1933, Ghormley coined the term *facet syndrome* (32). In 1976, Mooney and Robertson used fluoroscopy to document the precise location of their intra-articular lumbar z-joint injections in asymptomatic volunteers; these injections of hypertonic saline caused back and lower extremity pain (22) (Figure 12–1). Mooney and colleagues were also the first to document relief of low back and lower extremity pain in patients after injection of local anesthetic into the lower lumbar z-joints (22).

## Anatomy

The lumbar z-joints are paired, true synovial joints that comprise the posterolateral articulation between vertebral levels. Each joint is comprised of a larger, posteriorly and medially facing concave superior articular process from the inferior vertebral level of the joint and a reciprocally oriented anteriorly and laterally facing inferior articular process from the superior vertebral level (Figure 12–2). The 10 lumbar z-joints form the posterior portion of the intervertebral foramina. Each joint's morphology approximates between a C and J shape (33). Usually, the more superior lumbar z-joints are oriented in the sagittal plane while the lower lumbar z-joints are oriented at 45 degrees

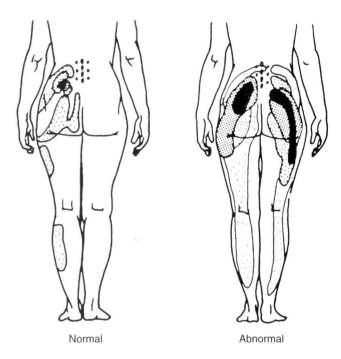

Normal                    Abnormal

**FIGURE 12–1**

Pain referral patterns produced by intra-articular injections of hypertonic saline in asymptomatic (normal) and symptomatic (abnormal) patients. (Reprinted with permission from Mooney V, Robertson J: The facet syndrome. *Clin Orthop* 1976; 115:149–56)

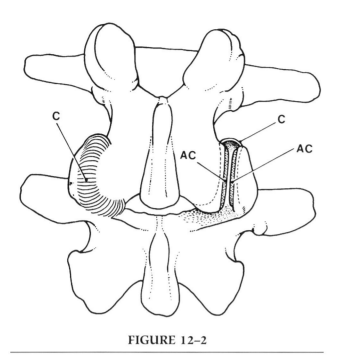

**FIGURE 12–2**

Posterior view of the lumbar zygapophyseal joints. AC denotes the articular cartilage and C the joint capsule. (Reprinted with permission from Bogduk N, Twomey LT. *Clinical anatomy of the lumbar spine,* 2nd ed. London: Churchill Livingstone, 1991)

with respect to the sagittal plane, such that the posterior aspect of the joint is located laterally. The most inferior joints may approach a frontal plane orientation (33)

Lumbar z-joints are true synovial joints that contain hyaline cartilage, a synovial membrane, a fibrous capsule, nociceptive fibers from the medial branches of the dorsal rami (33,34,35,36,37), and a joint space with a potential capacity of 1–2 cc (38) (Figure 12–2). Each lumbar z-joint is innervated by two medial branches of the dorsal rami from that level and the level above (39,40). For example, the L4/5 lumbar z-joints are innervated by both the L4 and L3 medial branches.

The fibrous lumbar z-joint capsule is 1 mm thick and attaches 2 mm from the articular margins (41,42). The capsule serves to limit bending forces and resists a backward sliding motion during extension (41). The capsule is richly innervated with nociceptive and autonomic nerve fibers (43,44,45). Mechanoreceptors have been demonstrated in rabbit lumbar z-joint capsules (46,47), and substance P has been isolated in degenerative lumbar z-joint subchondral bone (48). The synovium may contain nociceptors (44,45), although these synovial nerves may serve only to regulate blood flow (49,50)

At the superior and inferior ends of the z-joint capsule are two subcapsular recesses within which are fibroad-

ipose meniscoids that project into the joint. Teleologically, it has been suggested that they protect exposed cartilaginous articular surfaces during movement (33,36). Capsular redundancy at the superior and inferior portions of the lumbar z-joint creates two subcapsular recesses (33).

## Mechanics125

Lumbar z-joints limit motion between vertebrae and, at times, assist in axial weight bearing (37,51–55). The more sagittally oriented lumbar z-joints limit axial rotation, while the more coronal ones limit shearing forces. Full forward flexion occurs through sliding of the inferior articular process in relation to the superior articular process by 5–7 mm (33). In lordotic postures, the lumbar z-joints bear an average of 16 percent of the axial load and in the presence of lumbar spondylosis, up to 70 percent of the compressive load (51,52,56). Maximal pressure in the lumbar z-joints occurs during extension (51). Hyperextension can cause an inferior articular process to slide past a superior articular process to contact the subjacent laminae (56).

The lumbar z-joints assist the disc in resisting compressive forces in lordotic postures. The z-joints' capsular ligaments protect the posterior anulus of the disc from excess torsion and flexion stress (33,52)

## Pathology

The ability of the lumbar z-joints to cause pain has been well established clinically (22,29,57–61). Additionally, anatomic (33,40) and histologic (43–45,48) studies have documented the rich innervation of the lumbar z-joints. Despite these studies, which reproduce (or alleviate) back and leg pain with lumbar z-joint stimulation (or analgesia) and the supportive anatomic and histologic findings, the precise cause of most lumbar z-joint pain remains unknown.

Hyperextension increases the load borne by the lumbar z-joints and stretches the capsule. This mechanical deformation may stimulate the nociceptors in the joint's capsule (34,56). Microtrauma, such as small articular fractures, have been proposed to cause post-traumatic lumbar z-joint pain. Microfractures not readily apparent on routine x-rays occasionally can be detected with stereoradiography (62). Lumbar z-joint fractures, capsular tears, splits in the articular cartilage, and hemorrhage have all been documented on postmortem studies of trauma victims who had normal x-rays (63). However, correlation of these findings with LBP was not established.

Osteoarthritis is another proposed cause of lumbar z-joint pain, but radiographic changes of osteoarthritis are equally common in symptomatic and asymptomatic patients (64,65).

Other theories on lumbar z-joint pain include meniscoid entrapment and extrapment (36,66), synovial impingement (67), chondromalacia facetae (68), joint subluxation (69), "restriction" to normal articular motion from soft tissue or articular causes (33,69,70), and capsular and synovial inflammation (33). Occasionally, the lumbar z-joints are affected by systemic arthritides such as rheumatoid arthritis and ankylosing spondylitis (71,72). No studies have explored the prevalence of lumbar z-joint pain in this population using lumbar z-joint analgesic injections. Other rarities such as villo-nodular synovitis, synovial cysts, and infection are potential sources of lumbar z-joint pain (73,74,75)

## DIFFERENTIAL DIAGNOSIS

Disc disease, nerve root compression, sacroiliac joint syndrome, primary or secondary myofascial syndromes, and nonspinal etiologies may all mimic lumbar z-joint pain. Nonspinal disorders including gastrointestinal disorders, genitourinary, or gynecologic sources can usually be distinguished on clinical grounds and with supportive laboratory investigations. A number of algorithms have been reported and are useful in diagnosing nonspinal etiologies of LBP (76,77).

## CLINICAL PICTURE

Initially, the clinician must base his presumptive diagnosis of lumbar z-joint pain on a constellation of historical and physical findings after fracture, infection, neoplasm, viscerogenic referred pain, isolated muscular/ligamentous pain, sacroiliac joint pain, nerve root pain, and intrinsic and extrinsic discogenic pain sources have been reasonably excluded. No noninvasive pathognomonic finding or constellation of findings can definitively distinguish lumbar z-joint mediated pain from other sources of LBP (26,27,28,37,58,78). The diagnosis of lumbar z-joint pain remains one of exclusion and confirmation by analgesic injections.

### Signs and Symptoms

The clinical presentation of lumbar z-joint mediated back pain appears to overlap considerably with the presentation of LBP due to other etiologies. Although patients with lumbar z-joint pain are neurologically intact, they can demonstrate pain-inhibited weakness, subjective nondermatomal extremity sensory loss, and other sensory complaints as far distal as the foot (17,58).

The largest study of provocative, historical, and other tests for lumbar z-joint pain involved 390 LBP patients (28). Patients were selected from a population of over 2,500 for their localized lower back pain, normal neurologic exam and ability to participate in lumbar z-joint injections. The authors report that their study population undoubtedly included patients with back pain due to other etiologies, including discogenic disease. Postoperative patients and patients with spondylolysis, spondylolisthesis, and scoliosis were all included as long as they presented with local lumbar pain and a normal neurologic exam. The response of this mixed population to either unilateral or bilateral L4–5 or L5–S1 lumbar z-joint injections was evaluated with regard to 127 potentially predictive variables. Older age, prior history of LBP, absence of leg pain, absence of exacerbation by Valsalva, normal gait, absence of "muscle spasm," and maximal pain on extension after forward flexion all correlated significantly with post-injection relief. However, none of these variables were unique to the group of patients responding to lumbar z-joint injections (28). The most significant flaws in this study were failure to definitively diagnosis lumbar z-joint pain and inclusion of patients with pain of other etiologies. The 30 patients who achieved complete pain relief post-injection were perhaps the patients with true lumbar z-joint pain. The investigators report that there were no unique identifiable features even in this group, but do not report details of this subanalysis.

Because of the potential for placebo response to injections, a recent, prospective, cross-sectional, analytical study required physiologic analgesic responses to two separate and distinct anesthetic injections (double block protocol) to be included in the group diagnosed with true lumbar z-joint pain (58). The clinical features of this group were compared with those who did not achieve pain relief after both anesthetic blocks. Despite the rigorous selection criteria, no clinical symptom or sign reliably predicted those with true lumbar z-joint pain versus those who did not respond to each of the anesthetic blocks in a physiologic fashion (58). Pain production/relief with sitting, standing, or walking did not predict those who would respond to lumbar z-joint injections versus those who did not (58). Nor was there a statistically significant difference between responders and nonresponders with pain provocation on flexion, extension, rotation, rotation plus extension, or straight leg raising (58). The major flaw in this study was that it included only 26 patients with definite lumbar z-joint pain and this group was further subdivided by presenting signs and symptoms. The net result is a study biased toward not detecting significant differences.

## DIAGNOSIS

To date, there are no pathognomonic, noninvasive radiographic, historical, or physical examination findings that allow one to definitively identify lumbar z-joints as the source of low back and referred lower extremity pain (28,35,37). Magnetic resonance imaging, CT, dynamic bending films, and radionuclide bone scanning do not reliably predict symptomatic lumbar z-joints (18,24,26,57,79,80,81). Single photon emission computed tomography (SPECT) is currently under investigation as a means to identify symptomatic, metabolically active z-joint pathology but is not recommended for routine use (82,83). Spinal CT has not yet been studied in symptomatic lumbar z-joints.

Even though there are no noninvasive pathognomonic findings in z-joint mediated pain, one must still approach diagnostic blocks in a rational and systematic fashion. Each clinician still relies on a constellation of physical examination findings to guide which levels to initially investigate. One method begins with investigation of potentially painful z-joints at the sites of maximal tenderness upon deep palpation, at levels where mechanical, segmental provocation causes concordant pain and/or at levels demonstrating palpable "articular restriction" (70) in light of other segmental findings such as facilitated muscle tone. If localizing signs are absent, L4–5 and L5–S1 z-joints should be considered first for injection as these levels are more commonly involved (37,58).

## Imaging Studies

There are no pathognomonic diagnostic imaging studies in symptomatic lumbar z-joints and as in other causes of LBP, the imaging studies must be closely correlated with the clinical presentation. Pain is a subjective experience. The presence of an anatomic abnormality is not diagnostic of pain from that abnormality. A cost-effective screening test with high specificity and sensitivity for lumbar z-joint pain is lacking. Cost constraints and the overall benign nature of lumbar z-joint pain may limit the search for such a test. However, because diagnostic tests are typically undertaken to exclude more ominous causes of LBP, the spinal practitioner must be aware of the potential findings. Radiographs, computed tomography (CT), CT/myelography, bone scans, SPECT, and MRI provide additional diagnostic information when used in a judicious and logical manner. Imaging studies only provide anatomical information and cannot independently determine whether a particular structure is painful (57,84,85,86).

Degenerative joints are not always painful (18,26,85), but some studies report that severely degenerated joints are more likely symptomatic (13,14,20). Others document that even advanced degenerative joint changes on computed tomography (CT) or magnetic resonance imaging (MRI) are not always painful (18,26,85,87). Even using placebo-controlled z-joint blocks, CT was found to poorly discriminate patients with and without z-joint mediated pain (57). More than half of persons aged 40 or older have evidence of lumbar z-joint arthropathy on CT scans (85). Whether such degenerative findings account for a given patient's pain complex requires clinical correlation, with selective analgesic injections of the suspected structures. Furthermore, the absence of degenerative or pathologic lumbar z-joint changes on plain radiographs, CT, MRI, bone scan, or SPECT scan does not exclude the potential for lumbar z-joint mediated pain (14, 21,24, 26,37,57, 81,82,83). Radiographically normal lumbar z-joints can be painful, as evidenced by excellent pain relief from intra-articular joint blocks in patients with normal CT and/or plain films (13,19,21,24,26,37,68)

Analogous to the high incidence of lumbar z-joint abnormalities on advanced spinal imaging, the prevalence of disc abnormalities on CT or MRI scans rises with age (84). Therefore, radiographic evidence of disc pathology is not a contraindication to lumbar z-joint injection procedures if the clinical evaluation provides sufficient cause to investigate the lumbar z-joints and not the discs (24,26).

Diagnostic, fluoroscopically confirmed, intra-articular anesthetic injections may relieve low back and lower extremity pain even in the presence of structural abnormalities of the intervertebral disc on CT or MRI (24,26)

## Diagnostic Injections

Analgesia from injection of local anesthetic into the lumbar z-joints or at their nerve supply has been accepted as the standard for diagnosis of z-joint pain (Figures 12–3 and 12–4). Because no reliable, noninvasive diagnostic tools exist for the accurate diagnosis of lumbar z-joint mediated pain, and because the clinical features of lumbar z-joint pain and other anatomical entities overlap, fluoroscopically guided lumbar z-joint injections of local anesthetics are commonly employed methods for isolating or excluding the lumbar z-joints as the source of back and leg pain (6,35). Either intra-articular or medial branch blocks can be used in the diagnostic workup (6,35,88,89) (Figures 12–3 and 12–4). Physiologic analgesia is the underlying principle; pain relief following blockade of the nociceptive fibers implicates the blocked structure as the source of pain (90,91,92,93). Therefore, analgesia following local anesthetic blocks of the lumbar z-joint or its nerve supply (two medial branch nerves) indicates that the pain emanates from the blocked joint(s). However, because analgesic blocks rely on the patient's subjective response, they are prone to false-positive responses. The patient's desire to obtain relief and the physician's enthusiasm for a procedure inadvertently encourage such false-positive responses. False-positive responses may be greatly

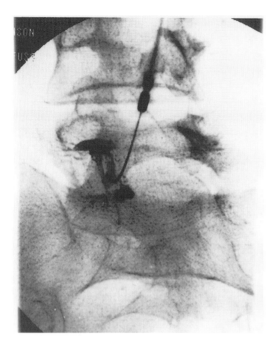

**FIGURE 12–3**

L5–S1 zygapophyseal joint arthrogram with contrast filling the superior and inferior capsular recesses.

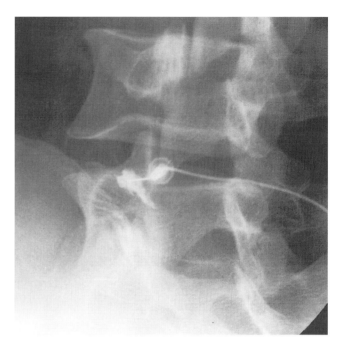

**FIGURE 12–4**

Oblique radiograph demonstrating contrast injection prior to a L4 medial branch block at the mid-position of the nerve as it lies between the L5 transverse process and superior articular process.

diminished when a control injection is employed. In order to avoid subjecting patients to inert injections as a control, comparative anesthetic blocks have been advocated (90,91,92,93). The principle of comparative local anesthetic blocks is based on controlled, double blind, randomized studies demonstrating the significantly longer duration of action of bupivacaine compared with that of Xylocaine (94,95,96). Duration of pain relief should reflect the pharmacokinetics and half-life of the local anesthetic employed. For example, pain relief after an injection of bupivacaine should outlast the analgesia obtained after an injection of lidocaine. The double block diagnostic paradigm requires two separate lumbar z-joint injections (intra-articular lumbar z-joint injections or medial branch blocks), each employing a different local anesthetic. Only patients who accurately report different durations of substantial analgesia with the different anesthetics are then considered to be true responders. This double block paradigm is thought to exclude false-positive and placebo responses to a single injection (97). Analgesia after a single session of lumbar z-joint injections has a 32 percent placebo response rate and a 38 percent false-positive rate (59,97). However, even this rigorous double block paradigm approach may have limitations in completely excluding placebo responders, but remains supe-

rior to single diagnostic blocks (98). Only a placebo injection can best detect a placebo response (98)

If the intent of the lumbar z-joint procedure is purely diagnostic, anesthetic alone should be used. If diagnostic inquiry is the only goal, medial branch blocks can be performed in lieu of intra-articular blocks with equal diagnostic sensitivity (6,34,35,37,58,88). The target accuracy of medial branch blocks has been validated (88). When joint entry cannot be obtained, medial branch blocks can still provide diagnostic information. The specifics of lumbar z-joint block techniques can be found elsewhere (37,89,99)

## TREATMENT

Controlled, prospective studies comparing treatment and natural history of lumbar z-joint pain are lacking and are desperately needed to guide the practitioner in selecting the most appropriate and cost-effective program. Conservative care of acute LBP includes lumbar z-joint mediated low back and leg pain; confirmation of the exact pain generator is usually not required because most episodes of LBP are self-limited (100,101). Initial care is prescribed based on a presumptive diagnosis established by considering the mechanism of injury, pain patterns, physical findings, and imaging results. Conservative care of acute LBP, including lumbar z-joint pain, may include oral non-narcotic analgesics and anti-inflammatory medications, modalities, traction, instruction in body mechanics, education, selective strengthening, flexibility training, specialized manual physical therapy, aerobic conditioning, and time.

General principles of rehabilitation apply when treating lumbar z-joint mediated LBP. Flexibility and strength deficits should be identified and corrected. Education and training with respect to proper body mechanics, posture, and proprioception are essential. Early mobilization and physiologic stresses promote soft tissue healing through optimal alignment of collagen fibers (102) while preventing the deleterious effects of immobilization including atrophy, weakening of ligaments, and impaired joint nutrition (103). Rehabilitation goals for lumbar z-joint injuries include complete return of function, full pain-free range of motion, "normal" flexibility and strength, and education for prevention of future injury.

Specific individual care should be provided based on a detailed clinical evaluation rather than a generic prescription based on a standard algorithm. Unfortunately, there is not one single prospective controlled study on the efficacy of any treatment for proven (via analgesic response to double blocks) lumbar z-joint pain. Furthermore, there are no studies assessing the efficacy of medication, physical therapy (modalities, flexibility/exercise), manual therapy (manipulation and other direct/indirect joint/soft tissue mobilization techniques), psychological intervention, or miscellaneous treatments employed alone or in combination with potentially therapeutic lumbar z-joint blocks in those patients with lumbar z-joint pain diagnosed by even single diagnostic blocks. The studies evaluating treatment of LBP of lumbar z-joint origin documented by analgesia after single diagnostic blocks involve assessing the efficacy of isolated corticosteroid lumbar z-joint injections (3), posterior lumbar fusion (27,104,105), and radiofrequency denervation (106,107).

The authors advocate confirming a clinical suspicion of lumbar z-joint pain with diagnostic lumbar z-joint injection procedures only after a minimum of 4 weeks of appropriate, directed conservative care has failed to bring relief (2,108). This allows for natural history to be an effective "treatment" that is reported to resolve 80–90 percent of acute low back pain in 4 to 6 weeks (109,110). If pain is substantially inhibiting progress in physical therapy, earlier use of lumbar z-joint injection procedures may help focus therapies on a specific level and provide adequate analgesia to facilitate participation (111). Treatment of subacute and chronic LBP is potentially more efficacious when an anatomic diagnosis is established and a multidisciplinary team approach is undertaken. Isolating the pain generator is critical to the development of scientific treatment protocols for LBP of various etiologies. Ultimately, this will yield specific rather than empiric therapeutic interventions.

## Lumbar Z-Joint Injections

### Therapeutic Injection

The therapeutic effect of intra-articular lumbar z-joint corticosteroids remains presumptive. The need for a potent anti-inflammatory agent in lumbar z-joint pain is controversial. In fact, immunohistochemical evaluation of lumbar z-joint tissues removed from patients with lumbar spondylosis has failed to demonstrate inflammatory cells (50). The effects of steroids on intracapsular inflammation is only presumptive based on known anti-inflammatory actions of steroids at other sites. There have not been any formal studies that address the mechanism of corticosteroid action within the z-joint, nor have there been any formal studies that have documented intracapsular inflammation in those suffering from z-joint pain. Despite the uncertainty of their action, several investigators endorse their use (5,14,15,16,19,20,21,22). In addition to their anti-inflammatory effects, corticosteroids may exert regulatory effects on the cellular responses within the microenvironment of bone itself (112) or may exert an inert effect such as lavage of the joint's surface that could be provided with other agents such as saline.

No long-term side effects from intra-articular z-joint injections using corticosteroids have been reported (3,4,15,17,18,19,21, 22,25,27,28,113). The appropriate dose remains empiric. Several studies suggested that long-term relief is more common, but not restricted to those with demonstrable degenerative changes in the lumbar z-joints (13,14,18). In open trials, patients with and without significant z-joint degeneration or disc pathology have had long-term success from z-joint injection (19,20,21,24). No common factors have been identified in these open clinical studies to predict which patients will have prolonged benefit from instillation of steroids into the z-joints.

Open, uncontrolled clinical studies evaluating the long-term relief of back and leg pain from isolated intra-articular lumbar z-joint steroids report variable relief in 18 percent to 63 percent of subjects (4,13,14, 16,19,20,21,24). However, due to the open study design the results are inherently biased toward favorable outcomes. The variability of results may represent heterogeneity of patient populations and lack of uniform post-injection rehabilitation programs. The rates reported were for populations of patients with chronic LBP who received injections and not just those individuals who responded favorably to an initial diagnostic injection of local anesthetic.

The response to lumbar z-joint corticosteroid injections in pathologically distinct subgroups such as patients with spondyloarthropathies or spondylolysis affecting the lumbar z-joints has not been studied in a controlled fashion or even in large open trials. One uncontrolled study reported relatively long-term benefit from lumbar z-joint corticosteroids in 5 of 11 patients (45 percent) with presumed symptomatic spondylolysis (113).

### Controlled Lumbar Z-Joint Injection Studies

Only five studies of intra-articular corticosteroid lumbar z-joint injections have been performed to compare the results to those of a similar group not receiving intra-articular steroids (3,4,5,6,7). These include the studies the AHCPR carefully reviewed to reach their guideline conclusions.

1. The study by Lilius included patients with greater than 3 months' duration of unilateral, nonradicular LBP who failed to respond to medication and physical therapy (4). Twenty-seven patients with pain despite previous discectomy were also included. Patients were prospectively randomized into three treatment groups: intra-articular lumbar z-joint injection with cortisone and local anesthetic, intra-articular injection with saline alone, or pericapsular injection of cortisone and local anesthetic. At 1 hour post-injection, 70 of the 109 patients (64 percent) achieved pain relief. Thirty-six percent achieved pain relief lasting 3 months. No statistically significant difference in response rate between the groups was found. Thus, no benefit could be attributed to the corticosteroid.

Although reported as randomized and controlled, the research design contained several flaws and met only four of the 32 criteria proposed for reporting of randomized controlled trials (114). The four criteria met were: stating the unit of assignment, adequately presenting summary data, reporting the actual probability values, and appropriately interpreting the probability values. Problems with this study were not limited to the method of reporting, but also included several design flaws. First, the selection criteria were overly broad. Lumbar z-joint mediated pain was the presumptive diagnosis but no attempt was made to confirm the diagnosis with anesthetic lumbar z-joint injections. Thus, the study population was not pure lumbar z-joint pain. Second, the volumes (3–8 cc) injected "into" the lumbar z-joints were excessive. Maximum lumbar intra-articular volumes have been estimated at 2 cc. Larger volumes of anesthetics may cause extravasation onto other pain-sensitive structures in the epidural space, intervertebral foramen, and paraspinal tissues, resulting in a loss of both diagnostic and therapeutic specificity. Inject-

ing 8 cc of saline into a space that physiologically holds only 2 cc may cause significant mechanical effects that can potentially modulate pain responses (115). Third, failure to exclude placebo responders from any of the groups dilutes any potential difference between groups. Finally, large standards of deviation for the variables measured and suboptimal outcome measures further limit the statistical power of this study.

2. Carette reported that a randomized, prospective, controlled study on treatment of lumbar z-joint pain concluded that intra-articular methylprednisolone lumbar z-joint injections "have very little efficacy in patients with LBP" (3). This study met the majority (22 of 32) of the criteria for reporting of randomized controlled trials (114). The criteria not met included a failure to report how successful the blinding method was and whether blinding was maintained during data entry. Patients were selected based on an analgesic response of greater than 50 percent relief with a single intra-articular lidocaine block (58 percent of 101 patients). These patients were then randomized to receive either intra-articular saline or intra-articular methylprednisolone. Initial follow-up was at 1 month post-injection when 20 patients (42 percent) in the methylprednisolone group had substantial pain reduction compared to 16 patients (33 percent) in the saline group. The difference was not statistically significant. At 6 months 46 percent of the methylprednisolone group and 15 percent of the saline group continued to experience marked pain relief. The difference was statistically significant (p = 0.002) but was attributed to increased co-intervention in the methylprednisolone group.

Although well-designed, Carette's study is not without limitations. Failure to exclude placebo responders may account for the relatively high incidence of patients with presumed lumbar z-joint pain compared to other false-positive/placebo-controlled prevalence studies showing a 15–40 percent prevalence. A mixed subject population that includes both patients with the disease and patients without the entity in question contaminates the group being studied; the number of placebo responders included proportionately dilutes the findings of the true responses and will make detecting a difference between the study and control group more difficult. Additionally, a selection criterion of only 50 percent reduction in pain after single blocks may allow for those with combined painful entities rather than pure lumbar z-joint pain. Another design flaw was the assumption that intra-articular saline is a true placebo; others propose that intra-articular saline may have a therapeutic effect as it may break painful adhesions or modulate local nervous system loops. Furthermore, saline is known to provide pain relief in excess of that expected from placebo in other pain syndromes including myofascial pain and reflex sympathetic dystrophy. Additionally, there was no assessment of differences between groups during the phase of maximum corticosteroid bioavailability (first 2 weeks) post-block.

Finally, the effects of intra-articular lumbar z-joint corticosteroids were evaluated in isolation and not as part of a comprehensive conservative treatment plan provided equally to both groups. In fact, when co-intervention occurred (22 percent in the corticosteroid vs. 12.5 percent in the saline group), there was some indication of significant benefit from the combination. The co-interventions largely took place 1 month or greater after the active injections. Marked or very marked pain relief in 46 percent of the methylprednisolone group after 6 months is substantial considering that these were patients with pain for greater than 6 months. The investigators attempted to discount the effects of the co-interventions, but even found that when a "worst case analysis" was performed by assuming that none of the patients with co-interventions had improved after 6 months regardless of the study group, there was still statistical significance (p = 0.05), with the corticosteroid group more improved. When in those patients who had co-interventions the results of the last evaluation (before co-interventions) was substituted for all subsequent evaluations, statistical significance was lost (p > 0.05). These data perturbations only indirectly reinforce the concept that co-interventions (even 1 month after injection) may be truly synergistic with injected corticosteroids. Potentially, the analgesic effects of lumbar z-joint injections serve as a window of opportunity for progression through a previously intolerable active conservative treatment. Optimally, co-interventions would be concentrated in the first 2–3 weeks after injection.

3. Lynch reported a controlled treatment trial on lumbar z-joint pain that was prospective but not randomized or blinded (5). In this study 50 patients with chronic (greater than 6 months) LBP with focal paraspinal tenderness and increased pain on hyperextension, no "true motor weakness or anesthesia," systemic arthropathy, spondylosis, or spondylolisthesis were included in the study. Lumbar z-joint injections were attempted at the level considered to be symptomatic and the level above. Intra-articular placement of the corticosteroid without anesthetic was attempted in all 50 patients; however, in 15 patients the needle was noted to be extra-articular on injection of both joints and in eight others, only one of the two injections was confirmed to be intra-articular upon injection of the contrast agent. The extra-articular injections were then used as a control group to which the intra-articular group was compared. Total pain relief occurred in 9 of 27 patients who received intra-articular corticosteroids in both joints compared to none of 15 patients who received only extra-articular corticosteroids. Only two patients in the intra-articular group did not obtain at least partial benefit, whereas seven of the 15

control patients had no pain relief. The authors concluded that intra-articular injections were far more effective than extra-articular corticosteroids.

The limitations of Lynch's study include lack of randomization, poor outcome assessment tools, failure to select patients with isolated z-joint pain as determined by diagnostic injections, failure to blind the examining physician, the use of a physiologically active agent (periarticular steroids) for the control, and no controlled monitoring or structuring of co-interventions.

4. Marks compared the effects of intra-articular anesthetic/corticosteroid versus medial branch blocks (6). The study concluded that "facet joint injections and facet nerve blocks may be of equal value as diagnostic tests, but neither is a satisfactory treatment for chronic low back pain." Eighty-six chronic LBP patients were randomized to z-joint injections with anesthetic/corticosteroid or medial branch blocks. Follow-up was performed at 30 to 60 minutes and at 1 and 3 months post-block. A four-point subjective pain scale was used for follow-up assessment. There was no statistical difference between the groups immediately post-block or at 3 months, but at 1 month the intra-articular injection group was more improved than the medial branch block group and was significant (p < 0.05). Marks's study is limited by not selecting patients with established z-joint pain by analgesic blocks; failure to have a blinded, independent observer; poor limited outcome assessment tools; no assessment during the phase of maximal corticosteroid bioavailability; no control or placebo group; no control or monitoring of co-interventions; and not providing structured co-interventions following blocks.

5. Nash compared z-joint injections versus medial branch blocks (7). The study concluded that "neither treatment was of any significant benefit." Sixty-seven patients were randomized to either lumbar z-joint injections or medial branch blocks with only a 1 month follow-up. Assessment included work status, pain level, and drug intake. There was no appreciable difference in evaluations between the groups at follow-up. This study is limited by not establishing a diagnosis of z-joint pain prior to randomization and not assessing for the diagnosis after the blocks. Thus, potentially all patients in the study had a diagnosis other than z-joint pain, making the study invalid. Furthermore, there was no blinded observer, poor assessment tools, no asessment during the phase of maximum corticosteroid bioavailability, no control or placebo group, and no control, monitoring, or structuring of co-interventions.

## Rebuttal

In review, the AHCPR guidelines summary statement was that "facet joint injections are invasive and not recommended for use in the treatment of patients with acute low back problems." Within the AHCPR's summary of findings section on facet injection, the panel made the following additional points: (1) facet injections "do not appear to be effective for treating acute low back pain"; (2) "no studies have adequately investigated the efficacy of facet joint injections for patients with acute low back problems"; and (3) "facet joint injections are associated with rare potential serious complications" (1)

We agree that no studies have adequately investigated the efficacy of facet joint injections for patients with acute low back problems and that facet joint injections are associated with rare potential serious complications. There are absolutely no randomized, controlled comparision studies that have assessed in isolation, or as part of a rehabilitation program, corticosteroid facet joint injection in those with low back pain of less than 3 months' duration. However, because facet joint injections have not been formally evaluated in acute low back pain, it cannot be confidently stated that they "do not appear to be effective in the treatment of acute low back pain." This statement has yet to be refuted or validated by scientific inquiry. One must remember that the absence of proof is not the proof of absence.

The AHCPR panel did review the one study that reported a complication from a lumbar facet injection (116) and appropriately acknowledged the rarity of potential, serious complications from this injection procedure.

Agreeably, z-joint injections should not be performed for acute LBP that is of 4 weeks' or less duration. After 4 weeks (no spontaneous resolution of LBP), z-joint and medial branch nerve injections are valuable diagnostic functional and physiologic tests. The AHCPR completely ignored the documented, validated diagnostic ability of facet joint injection procedures. An anatomic diagnosis is the basic foundation for the formulation of an effective treatment plan, scientifically validated or not. Ignoring this basic tenet of medicine, to make a diagnosis is nothing more than planned ignorance. Electing not to accept the ability to make a diagnosis of the pain generator with facet joint injection procedures because the definitive outcome studies are yet to be performed is ludicrous. At the least, documenting the facet joints as the pain source can prevent unnecessary (inappropriate) treatments aimed at the wrong presumed pain generator, such as an asymptomatic disc herniation.

The use of z-joint corticosteroid injections in treatment isolation has not been validated via randomized controlled studies in acute or chronic LBP. As commonly accepted, they may have therapeutic value in the context of a comprehensive treatment protocol in low back pain rather than as an isolated treatment modality. However, this is yet to be scientifically validated. Facet joint injections are commonly used to facilitate aggressive, conservative care that previously failed or could not be performed due to pain such as advanced manual physical therapy (111). The AHCPR guidelines acknowledge that one "therapeutic objective of facet joint injections is temporary relief from motion-limiting pain so the patient may proceed into an appropriate exercise program." Interestingly, as discussed previously, Carette's study (3) indirectly suggests that co-interventions following intra-articular corticosteroid facet injections can improve outcome more than expected from the injection alone.

## Future Studies

Additional studies should explore the relevance of false-positive and placebo responses to z-joint injections as they relate to the resolution of symptoms and improvement of function with various treatments. Individuals who obtain excellent relief from intra-articular steroids, saline, or anesthetic should be studied to determine characteristics that distinguish them from other patients with LBP. Studies should compare intra-articular saline/anesthetic against extra-articular or muscular injections in a controlled, blinded fashion to establish whether intra-articular saline imparts a therapeutic benefit (via mechanical effects) apart from a placebo response.

Previous studies evaluating the effectiveness of intra-articular steroids and anesthetics have used these injections in isolation or have not carefully controlled concomitant therapies. Future studies should address whether or not intra-articular anesthetic and anesthetic/corticosteroid injections followed by a more aggressive conservative program during the period of relative analgesia increases long-term efficacy. A post-injection conservative program may employ, for example, physical therapy and/or joint mobilization/manipulation (111)

The therapeutic role of z-joint injections should be evaluated in the subpopulations of acute, subacute, and chronic low back pain patients, i.e., pain of less than 4 weeks' duration, 1 to 6 months' duration, and more than 6 months' duration. All studies should be randomized and controlled and should assess whether facet injections impart any advantage with and/or without particular controlled co-interventions during the state of anesthesia and/or corticosteroid analgesia. The natural history must be established for proven z-joint pain to allow comparisions of various interventions with the natural history in these various subsets. The true anatomic specificity of anesthetic agents injected needs to be determined, including comparisons of the target accuracy of medial branch blocks with that of intra-articular injections. Evaluating whether stronger anesthetic agents in smaller volumes into the lumbar z-joints or around the medial branch nerves achieve a more specific, solid blockade remains to be determined.

## Costs and Harms of Lumbar Facet Injections

In competent hands and with the use of fluoroscopy, the risks of lumbar facet injections are minimal. Fluoroscopy virtually eliminates the risk of nerve root contact or inadvertent needle placement into the epidural, subdural, or subarachnoid spaces. Essentially, the only risks are those inherent to any needle placed through the skin into the deeper soft tissue spaces: bleeding, local soreness, hematoma, reaction to the injected medications, and infection. Although possible, infection has never been reported following lumbar facet joint injections using appropriate sterile technique. There is only one case report in the literature regarding any complications from lumbar facet injections (116).

The costs of lumbar facet injections vary with the number of joints injected and the physician and facility charges. To our knowledge, typical total charges (physician and facility fees) for 2–4 lumbar facet joint injections range from $500 to $1,700.

## Facet Joint Injection Recommendations

The contemporary concepts series of reviews published in *Spine* was orchestrated by the North American Spine Society (NASS) and "expresses a consensus representing general views of current practice and should not be used to dictate care of patients to the exclusion of innovation or tailoring to special circumstances." The following seven recommendations, as stated in the contemporary concepts review on lumbar zygapophyseal joint injections (2), are based on a much broader review of the literature than that used by the AHCPR. The AHCPR reviewed only 17 papers and accepted only five randomized controlled studies that met their methodologic standards to justify their recommendation. They did not review a plethora of papers that had clinical relevance yet failed to meet their methodologic standards. The seven recommendations that follow are based on review of 89 basic science and clinical papers (2).

1. The primary role of z-joint injections is diagnostic. Intra-articular z-joint injections and medial branch blocks are able to provide a specific anatomic diagnosis of z-joint mediated pain. Intra-articular z-joint injections and medial branch blocks are thought to have equal diagnostic specificity.

2. Lumbar z-joint injection procedures should be reserved for those patients with low back pain who fail to respond to a directed, conservative treatment trial and have had pain for at least 4 weeks. Earlier use of injections in routine cases is not justified as the natural history of acute low back pain is one of spontaneous resolution.

3. The therapeutic benefit of z-joint injections remains controversial. If employed, their potential benefit for the individual case needs to be carefully weighed. If used at all, they should be used to facilitate more aggressive conservative care and not as an isolated treatment. Certainly, if prolonged response to intra-articular steroids does not occur after the first injection, no further administration of corticosteroids is indicated. There is no role for a "series" of z-joint injections given without regard to patient response to the initial cortisone injection.

4. Injections should be performed only under fluoroscopic guidance. Contrast medium should be used for both intra-articular z-joint injections and medial branch blocks to ensure appropriate subsequent injectant spread. Minimal sedation, if any, should be used. Intravenous access is not routinely required, but should be immediately available if not established at the onset of the injection.

5. Normal or abnormal imaging should not be used solely to determine the need or lack thereof for z-joint injection procedures. In most cases either radiographs or advanced imaging will have been obtained as part of the diagnostic workup and allow the physician to exclude potential contraindications to injection procedures.

6. There are no known pathognomonic findings in low back pain of z-joint origin. Patients selected for diagnostic z-joint injections must provide informed consent and joints must be blocked in a systematic fashion. Although not proven to be of diagnostic benefit, many physicians start at the level with localizing signs. Others begin with the more commonly involved L4–5 and L5–S1 joints.

7. Patients who respond to initial z-joint block(s) are candidates for a second injection with a different local anesthetic. Excellent physiologic relief after both blocks provides the most accurate criterion for diagnosis of z-joint mediated pain outside of placebo-controlled injections. Patients who achieve reproducible, time appropriate analgesia after both sets of z-joint blocks are potential candidates for additional procedures such as medial branch neurotomy.

# Summary

Much remains to be learned regarding the lumbar z-joints and their role in low back pain. Despite excellent studies demonstrating the nociceptive ability of these joints, there is a paucity of good scientific studies defining the optimal treatment for lumbar z-joint pain. The fact that the AHCPR review process found only five studies that met their methodologic criteria highlights the lack of scientific data proving or disproving the efficacy of lumbar z-joint injections. The guidelines are further weakened by their narrow focus on only acute low back pain, which severely limits the application of the guidelines to the typical clinical practice with a mixture of acute, subacute, and chronic low back pain patients.

The AHCPR guidelines support the consensus among practicing spine specialists that lumbar facet injections are not routinely indicated in the treatment of acute low back pain. The larger question remains: what is the optimal treatment of lumbar facet pain and what role do facet injections play in patients with more recalcitrant back pain? The AHCPR guidelines do not offer any direction. Furthermore, the guidelines fail to examine the diagnostic role of lumbar z-joint injections. We have attempted to provide insight into the guideline's deficiencies while citing the limitations of the available data.

## References

1. Bigos S, Bowyer O, Braen G, et al. Acute Low Back Problems in Adults. Clinical Practice Guideines, No. 14. AHCPR Publication No 95–0642. Rockville, MD: Agency for Health Care Policy and Research, Public Health Service, U.S. Department of Health and Human Services. December 1994.
2. Dreyfuss PH, Dreyer SJ, Herring SA. Lumbar zygapophyseal (facet) joint injections. *Spine* 1995; 20: 2040–2047.
3. Carette S, Marcoux S, Truchon R, et al. A controlled trial of corticosteroid injections into the facet joints for chronic low back pain. *New Engl J Med* 1991; 325:1002–1007.
4. Lilius G, Laasonen EM, Myllynen P, et al. Lumbar facet joint syndrome: A randomised clinical trial. *J Bone Joint Surg* 1989; 71B:681–690.
5. Lynch MC, Taylor JF. Facet joint injection for LBP. *J Bone Joint Surg [Br]* 1986; 68B:138–141.
6. Marks R, Houston T. Facet joint injection and facet nerve block—a randomized comparison in 86 patients. *Pain* 1992 49:325–328.
7. Nash TP. Facet joints—intra-articular steroids or nerve block? *Pain Clinic* 1990; 3(2):563–564
8. Bierung-Sorenson F. Physical measurements as risk indicators for low back trouble over a one year period. *Spine* 1984; 9:106–119.
9. Frymoyer JW, Pope MH, Clements JH, et al. Risk factors in LBP. An epidemiological survey. *J Bone Joint Surg [Am]* 1983; 65:213–218.
10. Svensson H, Vedin A, Wihelmsson C, Andersson GBJ. LBP in relation to other diseases and cardiovascular risk factors. *Spine* 1983; 8:277–285.
11. Pope MH, Andersson GBJ, Frymoyer JW, Chaffin DB (eds.). *Occupational LBP. Assessment, treatment and prevention.* St. Louis: Mosby, 1991.
12. Mixter WJ, Barr JS. Rupture of the intervertebral disc with involvement of the spinal canal. *N Engl J Med* 1934; 211:210.
13. Carrera GF. Lumbar facet joint injection in low back pain and sciatica: Preliminary results. *Radiology* 1980; 137:665–667.
14. Carrera GF, Williams AL. Current concepts in evaluation of the lumbar facet joints. *CRC Crit Rev Diagn Imag* 1984; 21:85–104.
15. Destouet JM, Gilula LA, Murphy WA, Monsees B. Lumbar facet joint injection: Indication, technique, clinical correlation and preliminary results. *Radiology* 1982; 145:321–325.
16. Destouet JM, Murphy WA. Lumbar facet block: Indications and technique. *Orthop Review* 1985; 14:57–65.
17. Fairbank JCT, Park WM, McCall IW, O'Brien JP. Apophyseal injection of local anesthetic as a diagnostic aid in primary low-back pain syndromes. *Spine* 1981; 6:598–605.
18. Helbig T, Lee CK. The lumbar facet syndrome. *Spine* 1988; 13:61–64.
19. Lau LSW, Littlejohn GO, Miller MH. Clinical evaluation of intra-articular injections for lumbar facet joint pain. *Med J Aust* 1985; 143:563–565.
20. Lewinnek GE, Warfield CA. Facet joint degeneration as a cause of low back pain. *Clin Orthop* 1986; 213: 216–222.
21. Lippit AB. The facet joint and its role in spine pain: Management with facet joint injections. *Spine* 1984; 9:746–750.
22. Mooney V, Robertson J. Facet joint syndrome. *Clin Orthop* 1976; 115:149–156.
23. Moran R, O'Connell D, Walsh MG. The diagnostic value of facet joint injections. *Spine* 1986; 12:1407–1410.
24. Murtagh FR. Computed tomography and fluoroscopy guided anaesthesia and steroid injection in facet syndrome. *Spine* 1988; 13:686–689.
25. Raymond J, Dumas JM. Intra-articular facet block: Diagnostic tests or therapeutic procedure? *Radiology* 1989; 151:333–336.
26. Revel ME, Listrat VM, Chevalier XJ, et al. Facet joint block for low back pain: Identifying predictors of a good response. *Arch Phys Med Rehabil* 1992; 73:824–828.
27. Jackson RP. The facet syndrome: Myth or reality? *Clin Orthop* 1992; 279:110–121.
28. Jackson RP, Jacobs RR, Montesano PX. Facet injection in low back pain: A prospective statistical study. *Spine* 1988; 13:966–971.
29. Schwarzer AC, Aprill CN, Derby R, Fortin J, Kine G, Bogduk N. The relative contributions of the disc and zygapophyseal joint in chronic low back pain. *Spine* 1994; 19:801–806.
30. Schwarzer AC, Wang SC, Bogduk N, McNaught PJ, Laurent R. Prevalence and clinical features of lumbar zygapophyseal joint pain: A study in an Australian population with chronic low back pain. *Ann Rheum Dis* 1995; 54(2):100–106
31. Goldthwait JE. The lumbosacral articulation: An explanation of many cases of lumbago, sciatica and paraplegia. *Boston Med Surg J* 1911; 164:365–372.
32. Ghormley RK. Low back pain with special reference to the articular facets, with presentation of an operative procedure. *JAMA* 1933; 101:1773–777.
33. Bogduk N, Twomey LT. *Clinical anatomy of the lumbar spine.* 2nd ed. London: Churchill Livingstone, 1991
34. Bogduk N, Long DM. Percutaneous lumbar medial branch neurotomy. A modification of facet denervation. *Spine* 1980; 5:193–200.

35. Bogduk N. Back pain: Zygapophyseal blocks and epidural steroids. In: Cousins MJ, Bridenbaugh PO (eds.). *Neural blockade in clinical anaesthesia and management of pain.* 2nd ed. Philadelphia: JB Lippincott, 1989: 263–267.

36. Bogduk N, Engel R. The menisci of the lumbar zygapophyseal joints. A review of their anatomy and clinical significance. *Spine* 1984; 9:454–460.

37. Derby R, Bogduk N, Schwarzer A. Precision percutaneous blocking procedures for localizing spinal pain. Part 1: The posterior lumbar compartment. *Pain Digest* 1993; 3:89–100.

38. Glover JR. Arthrography of the joints of the lumbar vertebral arches. *Orthop Clin North Am* 1977; 8:37–42.

39. Bogduk N. Innervation of the lumbar spine. *Spine* 1983; 8:286–293.

40. Bogduk N, Wilson AS, Tynan W. The human lumbar dorsal rami. *J Anat* 1982; 134:383–397.

41. Cyron BM, Hutton WC. The tensile strength of the capsular ligaments of the apophyseal joints. *J Anat* 1981; 132:145–150.

42. Yahia LH, Garzon S. Structure of the capsular ligaments of the facet joints. *Ann Anat* 1993; 175:185–188.

43. Ashton IK, Ashton BA, Gibson SJ, et al. Morphological basis for back pain: The demonstration of nerve fibers and neuropeptides in the lumbar facet joint capsule but not in the ligamentum flavum. *J Orthop Res* 1992; 10:72–78.

44. Giles LG, Hasrvey AR. Immunohistochemical demonstration of nociceptors in the capsule and synovial folds of human zygophpyseal joints. *Br J Rheumatol* 1987; 26:362–364.

45. Giles LGF, Taylor JR. Innervation of the lumbar zygapophyseal joint folds. *Acta Orthop Scand* 1987; 58:43–46.

46. Avramov AI, Cavanugh JM, Ozaktay CA, et al. The effects of controlled mechanical loading on group II, III and IV afferent units from the lumbar facet joint and surrounding tissue. An in vitro study. *J Bone Joint Surg* 1992; 74:1464–1471.

47. Yamashita T, Cavanaugh JM, El-Bouhy AA, et al. Mechanosensitive afferent units in the lumbar facet joint. *J Bone Joint Surg* 1990; 72:865–870.

48. Beaman DN, Graziano GP, Glover RA, Wojtys EM, Chang V. Substance P innervation of lumbar spine facet joints. *Spine* 1993; 18:1044–1049.

49. Gronblad M, Korkala O, Konttinen YT, et al. Silver impregnation and immunohistochemical study of nerves in lumbar facet joint plical tissue. *Spine* 1991; 16:34–38.

50. Konttinen YT, Gronblad M, Korkala O, et al. Immunohistochemical demonstration of subclasses of inflammatory cells and active, collagen-producing fibroblasts in the synovial plicae of lumbar facet joints. *Spine* 1990; 15:387–390.

51. Dunlop RB, Adams MA, Hutton WC. Disc space narrowing and the lumbar facet joints. *J Bone Joint Surg [Br]* 1984; 66B: 706–710.

52. Adams MA, Hutton WC. The mechanical function of the lumbar apophyseal joints. *Spine* 1983; 8:327–330.

53. Hickey DS, Huskins DWL. Relation between the structure of the annulus fibrosus and the function and failure of the intervertebral disc. *Spine* 1980; 5:100–116.

54. Taylor JR, Twomey LT. Age changes in lumbar zygapophyseal joints—observations on structure and function. *Spine* 1986; 11:739–745.

55. Twomey LT, Taylor JR. Sagittal movements of the human vertebral column: A quantitative study of the role of the posterior elements. *Arch Phys Med Rehabil* 1983; 64: 322–325.

56. Yang KH, King AI. Mechanism of facet load tranmission as a hypothesis for low back pain. *Spine* 1984; 9: 557–565.

57. Schwarzer AC, Wang S, O'Driscoll D, Harrington T, Bogduk N, Laurent R. The ability of computed tomography to identify a painful zygapophyseal joint in patients with chronic low back pain. *Spine* 1995; 20:907–912.

58. Schwarzer AC, Aprill CN, Derby R, Fortin J, Kine G, Bogduk N. Clinical features of patients with pain stemming from the lumbar zygapophyseal joints. Is the lumbar facet syndrome a clinical entity? *Spine* 1994; 19:1132–1137.

59. Schwarzer AC, Wang S, Laurent R, McNaught P, Brooks PM. The role of the zygapophyseal joint in chronic low back pain. *Aust NZ J Med* 1992; 22:185.

60. Hirsch D, Ingelmark B, Miller M. The anatomical basis for low back pain. *Acta Orthop Scand* 1963; 33:1–17.

61. McCall IW, Park WM, O'Brien JP. Induced pain referral from posterior lumbar elements in normal subjects. *Spine* 1979; 4:441–446.

62. Sims-Williams H, Jayson MIV, Baddely H. Small spinal fractures in back patients. *Ann Rheum Dis* 1978; 37: 262–265.

63. Twomey LT, Taylor JR, Taylor M. Unsuspected damage to lumbar zygapophyseal (facet) joints after motor vehicle accidents. *Med J Aust* 1989; 151:210–217

64. Lawrence JS, Sharp J, Ball J, Bier F. Osteoarthritis. Prevalence in the population and relationship between symptoms and X-ray changes. *Ann Rheum Dis* 1966; 25: 1–24.

65. Magora A, Schwartz TA. Relation between the low back pain syndrome and X-ray findings. *Scand J Rehab Med* 1976; 8:115–125.

66. Bogduk N, Jull G. The theoretical pathology of the acute locked back: A basis for manipulative therapy. *Man Med* 1985; 1:78–82.

67. Kraft GL, Leventhal DH. Facet synovial impingement. *Surg Gynec Obst* 1951; 93:439–443.

68. Eisentein SM, Parry CR. The lumbar facet arthrosis syndrome. *J Bone Joint Surg* 1987; 69B:3–7.

69. Schafer RC, Faye LJ. *Motion palpation and chiropractic technic.* 2nd ed. Huntington Beach, CA: The Motion Palpation Institute, 1990

70. Faye LJ, Wiles MR. Manual examination of the spine. In: Haldeman S (ed.). *Principles and practice of chiropractic.* 2nd ed. San Mateo, CA: Appleton & Lange, 1992: 301–318.

71. Ball J. Enthesopathy of rheumatoid and ankylosing spondylitis. *Ann Rheum Dis* 1971; 30:213–223.

72. Jayson MIV. Degenerative disease of the spine and back pain. *Clin Rheum Dis* 1976; 2:557–584.

73. Campbell AJ, Wells IP. Pigmented villonodular synovitis of a lumbar vertebral facet joint. *J Bone Joint Surg* 1982; 64A:145–146.

74. Hemminghytt S, Daniels DL, Williams AL, et al. Intraspinal synovial cysts: Natural history and diagnosis by CT. *Radiology* 1982; 145:375–376.

75. Rush J, Griffiths J. Suppurative arthritis of a lumbar facet joint. *J Bone Joint Surg* 1989; 71B:161–162.

76. Deyo R. Early diagnositc evaluation of LBP. *J Gen Intern Med* 1986; 1:328–338.

77. Wiesel S, Feffer H, Rothman R. A prospective evaluation of a standardized diagnostic and treatment protocol. *Spine* 1984; 9:199–203.

78. Schwarzer AC, Derby R, Aprill CN, Fortin J, Kine G, Bogduk N. Pain from the lumbar zygapophyseal joints: A test of two models. *J Spinal Disorders* 1994; 7:331–336.

79. Haas M, Nyiendo J, Petersen C, et al. Lumbar motion trends and correlation with low back pain. Part I: A roentgenological evaluation of coupled motion in lateral bending. *J Manip Physiol Ther* 1992; 15:145–158.

80. Haas M, Nyiendo J. Lumbar motion trends and correlation with low back pain. Part II: A roentgenological evaluation of quantitative segmental motion in lateral bending. *J Manip Physiol Ther* 1992; 15:224–234.

81. Raymond J, Dumas JM, Lisbona R. Nuclear imaging as a screening test for patients referred for intra-articular facet block. *J Can Assn Radiol* 1984; 35:291–292.

82. Ryan PJ, Di Vadi L, Gibson T, Fogelman I. Facet joint injection with low back pain and increased facetal joint activity on bone scintigraphy with SPECT: A pilot study. *Nuclear Medicine Communications* 1992; 13:401.

83. Schwarzer AC, Scott AM, Wang S, Hoschl R, Wiseman JC, Cooper RA, Laurent R. The role of bone scintigraphy in chronic low back pain: Comparison of SPECT and planar images and zygapophyseal joint injection. *Aust NZ J Med* (Abstract) 1992; 22:185.

84. Jensen M, Brant-Zwawadzki M, Obuchowski N. Magnetic resonance imaging of the lumbar spine in people without back pain. *New Engl J Med* 1994; 2:69–73.

85. Wiesel SW, Tsourmas N, Feffer HL, et al. A study of computer assisted tomography I: The incidence of positive CAT scans in an asymptomatic group of patients. *Spine* 1981; 9:549–551.

86. Herzog R. Selection and utilization of imaging studies for disorders of the lumbar spine. *Phys Med Rehab Clin North Am* 1991; 2:7–59.

87. Bough B, Thakore J, Davies M, Dowling F. Degeneration of the lumbar facet joints: Arthrography and pathology. *J Bone Joint Surg* 1990; 72B:275–276.

88. Dreyfuss P, Schwarzer AC, Lau P, Bogduk P. Specificity of lumbar medial branch and L5 dorsal ramus blocks: A computed tomography study. *Spine* 1997; 22:895–902.

89. Dreyfuss P, Lagattuta F, Kaplansky B, Heller B. Zygapophyseal joint injection techniques in the spinal axis. In: Lennard T (ed.). *Physiatric procedures in clinical practice*. Philadelphia: Hanley & Belfus, 1995: 206–226.

90. Barnsley L, Lord S, Bogduk N. Comparative local anaesthetic blocks in the diagnosis of cervical zygapophyseal joint pain. *Pain* 1993; 55:99–106.

91. Boas RA. Nerve block in the diagnosis of LBP. *Neurosurg Clin North Am* 1991; 2:807–816.

92. Bonica JJ. Local anesthesia and regional blocks. In: Wall PD, Melzack (eds.). *Textbook of pain*. 2nd ed. Edinburgh: Churchill Livingstone, 1989:724–743.

93. Bonica JJ, Buckley FP. Regional analgesia with local anesthetics. In: Bonica JJ (ed.). *The management of pain*. Vol. 2. Philadelphia: Lea & Febiger, 1990:1883–1966.

94. Moore D, Brindenbaugh P, et al. Bupivacaine for peripheral nerve block: A comparision with mepivacaine, lidocaine and tetracaine. *Anesthesiology* 1970; 32:460–463.

95. Rubin A, Lawson D. A controlled trial of bupivacaine: A comparison with lignocaine. *Anaesthesia* 1968; 23:327–331.

96. Watt M, Ross D, Atkinson R. A double blind trial of bupivacaine and lignocaine. *Anaesthesia* 1968; 23:331–337.

97. Schwarzer AC, Aprill CN, Derby R, Fortin J, Kine G, Bogduk N. The false positive rate of uncontrolled diagnostic blocks of the lumbar zygapophyseal joints. *Pain* 1994; 58:195–200.

98. Lord SM, Barnsley L, Bogduk N. The utility of comparative local anesthetic blocks versus placebo-controlled blocks for the diagnosis of cervical zygapophyseal joint pain. *Clin J Pain* 1995; 11:208–213.

99. Dreyer SJ, Dreyfuss P, Cole A. Zygapohyseal (facet) joint injections: Intra-articular and medial branch block techniques. In: Weinstein S (ed.). *Injection techniques: Principles and practice. Physical medicine and rehabilitation clinics of North America*. Vol. 6, No. 4. Philadelphia: WB Saunders, 1995:715–742.

100. Vallfors B. Acute, subacute and chronic LBP: Clinical symptoms, absenteeism, and working environment. *Scand J Rehab Med* 1985; 11(Suppl):1–98.

101. Anderson G, Svensson H-O, Oden A. The intensity of work recovery in LBP. *Spine* 1983; 8:880–884.

102. Kellet J. Acute soft tissue injury—a review of the literature. *Med Sci Sports Exerc* 1986; 18:489–500.

103. Herring S. Rehabilitation of muscle injuries. *Med Sci Sports Exerc* 1990; 22:453–456.

104. Esses SI, Moro JK. The value of facet blocks in patient selection for lumbar fusion. *Spine* 1993; 18:185–190.

105. Tsang IK. Perspective on low back pain. *Curr Opin Rheumatol* 1993; 5:219–223.

106. Lora J, Long D. So-called facet denervation in the management of intractable back pain. *Spine* 1976; 1:121–126.

107. Ogsbury JS, Simon RH, Lehman RAW. Facet "denervation" in the treatment of low back syndrome. *Pain* 1977; 3:257–263.

108. Dreyer SJ, Dreyfuss PH. Low back pain and the zygapophyseal (facet) joints. *Arch Phys Med Rehabil* 1996; 77:290–300

109. Anderson GBJ, Svensson H-O, Oden A. The intensity of work recovery in low back pain. *Spine* 1983; 8:880–884.

110. Vallfors B. Acute, subacute and chronic low back pain: Clinical symptoms, absenteeism, and working environment. *Scand J Rehab Med* 11(Suppl):1–98.

111. Dreyfuss P, Michaelsen M, Horne M. MUJA: Manipulation under joint anesthesia/analgesia: A treatment approach for recalcitrant low back pain of synovial joint origin. *J Manip Physiol Ther* 1995; 18:537–546.

112. Russell R. Cellular regulatory mechanisms that may underlie the effects of corticosteroids on bone. *Br J Rheumatol* 1993; 32S:6–10.

113. Maldague B, Mathurin P, Malghem J. Facet joint arthrography in lumbar spondylolysis. *Radiology* 1981; 140:29–36.

114. The Standards of Reporting Trials Group. A proposal for structured reporting of randomized controlled trials. *JAMA* 1994; 272(24):1926–1931.

115. Wyke B. Articular neurology—a review. *Physiotherapy* 1981; 58:563–580.

116. Thomson SJ, Lomax DM, Collet BJ. Chemical meningism after lumbar facet joint block with local anaesthetic and steroids. *Anaesthesia* 1991; 46(7):563–564.

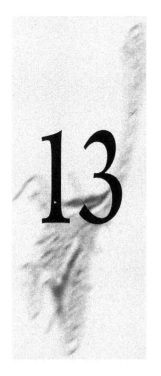

# 13 The Sacroiliac Joint

*Christopher Huston, M.D.*

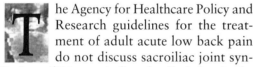

The Agency for Healthcare Policy and Research guidelines for the treatment of adult acute low back pain do not discuss sacroiliac joint syndrome (SIJS). Sacroiliitis was indirectly alluded to in the section discussing the use of bone scan (1,2). The sacroiliac joint has been demonstrated to be a source of low back pain by provocation studies and anesthetic relief with fluoroscopically guided sacroiliac joint block (SIJB) (3,4,5).

The incidence of acute sacroiliac joint syndrome is unknown. Mierau and co-workers (6) attempted to prospectively establish the incidence of sacroiliac joint (SIJ) dysfunction and low back pain in school children. Diagnosis of SIJS was based on a positive Gillet test, which was positive in 29.9 percent and 41.5 percent of the 6–12 and 12–17 age groups, respectively. Of those with a positive Gillet test, 64.7 percent had a history of low back pain. Mierau and co-workers concluded that there is a relationship between SIJ dysfunction and low back pain. Unfortunately, a positive Gillet test has not been shown to be diagnostic of SIJ dysfunction. The inter-rater reliability of this test has been questioned (7). The incidence of sacroiliac dysfunction cannot be determined from this study.

## ANATOMY

The sacroiliac joint is an auricular-shaped diarthrodial joint with a joint capsule, synovial fluid, and hyaline cartilage on the sacral side and fibrocartilage on the iliac side. The cartilage is 2–3 times thicker on the sacral side (8,9,10,11).

The fibers of the joint capsule blend anteriorly and posteriorly with the supporting ligaments. The anterior sacroiliac ligament is weak and thin. Posteriorly, the interosseous ligament is adjacent to the articular cartilage. The ligament consists of short bands connecting the iliac and sacral joint surfaces. Interwoven with the interosseous ligament, the next layer of the posterior ligamentous complex is the posterior sacroiliac ligament (Figure 13–1). The posterior ligamentous complex has cranial and caudal divisions. The cranial group of the posterior ligamentous complex becomes taut with standing as the sacrum moves ventrally (12). During weight bearing, the vertically transmitted force is resisted by the caudal group (12). Other ligaments also affect the stability of the SIJ.

The sacrotuberous ligament originates from the anterior and posterior iliac spine and sacral 3–5 segments and inserts on the ishcial tuberosity (13). The sacrospinous ligament originates from the last two sacral segments and the first coccygeal segment inserting on the

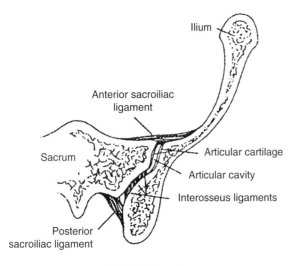

**FIGURE 13–1**

Anterior and posterior ligaments of the SIJ. (From Bernard TN, Jr, Cassidy JD. The sacroiliac joint syndrome. Pathophysiology, diagnosis, and management. In: Frymoyer JW, Ducker TB, Hadler NM, Kostuik JP, et al., eds. *The adult spine. Principles and practice.* New York: Raven Press, 1991:2107–2130; with permission.)

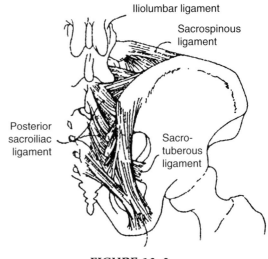

**FIGURE 13–2**

Sacrotuberous and sacrospinous ligaments. (From Bernard TN, Jr, Cassidy JD. The sacroiliac joint syndrome. Pathophysiology, diagnosis, and management. In: Frymoyer JW, Ducker TB, Hadler NM, Kostuik JP, et al., eds. *The adult spine. Principles and practice.* New York: Raven Press, 1991: 2107–2130; with permission.)

tip of the ischial spine (Figure 13–2). These ligaments limit posterior SIJ movement (13). The iliolumbar ligament is composed of several ligaments. The superior iliolumbar ligament extends from the intertranverse ligament of L4 and L5 and inserts on the ilium. The anterior and posterior iliolumbar ligaments originate from the transverse process of L5 and insert on the sacrum and ilium. The inferior iliolumbar ligament originates from the transverse process, inserts in the iliac fossa, and fuses with the anterior sacroiliac ligament (14). The long dorsal sacroiliac ligament originates from the posterior superior iliac spine and adjacent ilium and inserts on the lateral crest of S3 and S4 segments and occasionally to S5 (15).

The piriformis, biceps femoris, and gluteus maximus have fibrous connections to the sacrotuberous ligaments and may induce tension on the ligament (Figure 13–3) (16). The quadratus lumborum, erector spinae, gluteus maximus, gluteus minimus, piriformis, iliacus, and latissimus dorsi have fibrous expansions that blend anteriorly and posteriorly with the SIJ ligaments (17). The long dorsal sacroiliac ligament has fibrous connections with the gluteus maximus, erector spinae, and thoracodorsal fascia (15). These muscles may provide stability to the SIJ by affecting the sacroiliac joint ligaments.

The sacroiliac joint is innervated by the posterior rami of the lumbosacral roots (18). Anteriorly, the joint

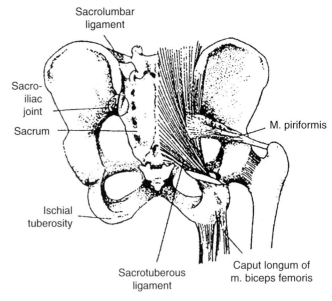

**FIGURE 13–3**

Fibrous connections of the biceps femoris and piriformis to the sacrotuberous ligament. (From Vleeming A, Stoeckart R, Snijders CJ. The sacrotuberous ligament: A conceptual approach to its dynamic role in stabilizing the sacroiliac joint. *Clin Biomech* 1989; 4:201–203; with permission.)

receives innervation variably from L3–S2 and the superior gluteal nerve (19). Posteriorly, joint innervation has been reported from S1–2 (19) and L4–S3 (20). The lumbosacral trunk is in close proximity to the SIJ and may be displaced by osteophytes from the SIJ (21,22).

An accessory SIJ has been reported to be present in 13–35.8 percent of individuals (23,24). The accessory SIJ has been found in the region of lateral sacral tuberosity at the level of the S2 foramen and medial to the posterior superior iliac spine. The incidence of an accessory SIJ increases with age and is higher in Caucasians compared to African-Americans.

With aging, a variety of degenerative changes take place in the SIJ (8,9,10,11,13,25). Degenerative changes may be present in the third decade (8,13) With advancing age, progressive degenerative changes are seen (8,10,13). By the fifth decade, degenerative changes were present in 91 percent of males and 77 percent of females (13). Bony anklyosis was present in 51 percent of males and 5.8 percent of females (13). Over the age of 60 years, degenerative changes were seen in all specimens. Bony anklyosis was seen in 82 percent of males and 30 percent of females (13). These changes should be kept in mind when interpreting radiologic studies of the SIJ.

## BIOMECHANICS

The forces of the lower extremities are transmitted to the trunk through the sacrum. With weight bearing, the upper sacrum is forced downward and anteriorly, wedging into the ilia (26). The SIJ and supporting ligaments are subjected to these forces. The interosseous ligament resists the anterior displacement and tendency for the ilia to be displaced laterally. The pubic bones offer anterior stability to the SIJ (14). Abnormalities in motion at the SIJ have been postulated to be associated with low back pain. This concept created controversy regarding whether the SIJ moves and if clinicians could detect aberrant motion. From this, various investigators measured motion at the SIJ.

Egund and co-workers (27) implanted tantalum balls into the ilium and sacrum adjacent to the SIJ. Utilizing stereophotogrammetry, the motion of the SIJ was measured in four volunteers. Two degrees of maximum motion and 2 mm of gliding were seen. Sturesson and co-workers (28), utilizing a similar technique, found motion of 1–3 degrees and translation up to 1.6 mm, with 90 percent of rotation occurring in an $x$ axis.

Other investigators have utilized stereophotogrammetry with skin markers or without markers, which may have resulted in overestimates of the degrees of motion in the SIJ (29,30). Motion has been measured with varying loads until bony or ligamentous failure occurred.

Miller and co-workers (31), in cadaveric studies, noted small displacements (0.5 mm and 1.9 degrees) with loading of the SIJ in various directions. Loading the SIJ until failure resulted in fractures to the sacrum except in torsion tests with ligamentous failure. In torsion tests, force was applied to the anterior ligamentous complex instead of the stronger, posterior ligamentous complex. Rothkotter and Berner (32) performed an in vitro study of load required for SIJ failure in fresh cadavers. They found that the ligaments and interlocking effect of the articular surface provided SIJ stability. They also noted that only a small degree of displacement occurs under physiologic joint loading.

Sturesson and colleagues (28) evaluated motion of SIJ with changes in position. With supine to stand, the ilia rotated posteriorly relative to the sacrum. Additionally, there was widening of the posterior aspect of the joint. With stand to prone hyperextension, the ipsilateral ilium rotated anteriorly. The contralateral side also rotated anteriorly but to a lesser extent. Sturesson and co-workers (28) state that the ilia and sacrum move as a unit linked by the pelvic ring. With nutation, gliding motion of the SIJ of approximately 2 mm has been demonstrated (27). Nutation is anterior rotation of the sacrum relative to the ilia, and counternutation is posterior rotation of the sacrum (15).

With nutation and counternutation, sagittal rotation and translation occurs. With nutation, the axis of rotation is through the iliac tubercle at S2 (27). With different motions, the axis of rotation may vary (33). The motion of the sacroiliac joint has not been completely characterized. Lavignolle and co-workers (34) concluded from a biomechanical study that motion of the SIJ is still a mystery.

Vleeming and co-workers (35) evaluated the affect of the sacrotuberous ligament on the SIJ. Tension applied to the sacrotuberous ligament decreased rotation with nutation. The biceps femoris has connections with the sacrotuberous ligament and may affect nutation and counternutation. These investigators believed that the connection of the gluteus maximus to the sacrotuberous ligament was relatively unimportant. They concluded that biceps femoris flexibility and strength may affect the SIJ. Vleeming and co-workers (15) studied tension to the long dorsal sacroiliac ligament in cadavers. The ligament became tense with counternutation, loading the erector spinae, and tension to the sacrotuberous ligament. Tension decreased with nutation, loading the latissimus dorsi and the gluteus maximus. Loading the biceps femoris had no effect on the ligament. Vleeming and colleagues (15) state that understanding the dynamics of the sacrotuberous ligament, long dorsal sacroiliac ligament, and surrounding muscles with nutation and counternutation is important in understanding low back pain from the SIJ.

## PATIENT HISTORY

Individuals with sacroiliac joint syndrome present with pain over the sacral sulcus with or without referral into the buttock (36,37,38,39,40). Fortin and co-workers (41) utilized fluoroscopically guided sacroiliac joint blocks (SIJB) with provocation to map pain referral from the SIJ. A vertical area of 3 x 10 cm just inferior to PSIS was experienced by all volunteers (Figure 13–4, A and B) (41). SIJS pain may refer to various aspects of the lower extremity, given the multiple levels of innervation of this joint. Areas of radiation may include the posterior thigh (38,42,43), inner thigh (42), below the knee (38,42,43), groin (4,43), abdomen (44), and scapula (37). Schuchman and Cannon (45) found 68 percent of those with SIJS had lower extremity symptoms.

SIJS may occur acutely from trauma with transmission through the hamstring (42). It may also occur with sudden heavy lifting (36,37,46), prolonged lifting and bending (43), torsional strain (43), arising from a stooped position (46), fall onto a buttock (39), or rear-end motor vehicle accident with the ipsilateral foot on the brake (39). SIJS may occur from repetitive shear or torsional forces

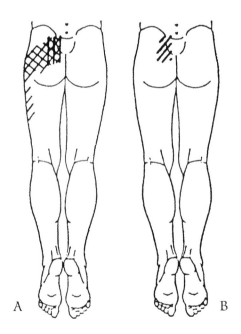

**FIGURE 13–4A, B**

Mapping of provoked pain from SIJB. *A:* Common to all volunteer subjects. *B:* Composite of referred pain for all volunteer subjects. (From Fortin JD, Dwyer AP, West S, Pier J. Sacroiliac joint: Pain referral maps upon applying a new injection/arthrography technique. Part I: Asymptomatic volunteers. *Spine* 1994; 19:1475–1482; with permission.)

to the SIJ, as occurs in sports such as figure skating, golf, and bowling (39).

Pain in SIJS may be aggravated by pressure to the sacral sulcus as with sitting (20,42) or lying on the affected side (42,43). Pain worsens with riding in a car (20), weight bearing on the affected side with standing or walking (42), Valsalva (42), and trunk flexion with legs straight (40). Trunk flexion in a seated position with the knees flexed does not aggravate SIJS because tension on the hamstring is reduced (40). Pain is mitigated with weight bearing on the opposite leg with the ipsilateral leg flexed (42). Walking and standing have also been stated to alleviate symptoms (20).

Schwarzer and co-workers (4) found pain referred to the groin was the only complaint statistically significant for a positive SIJB in 43 consecutive patients with low back pain. Patients were diagnosed with SIJS by fluoroscopically guided SIJB. Dreyfuss and co-workers (47) were unable to reproduce this result. Furthermore, Dreyfuss and co-workers (47), in a prospective study utilizing fluoroscopically guided SIJB, did not find any historical factor statistically significant to predict SIJS. This study did not blind the examiner and performance of SIJB, which may be important in reducing bias.

History is important to rule out other conditions that result in low back pain with or without lower extremity symptoms and other causes of sacroiliac joint pain. Individuals with a sudden increase in physical activity may develop stress reactions or fractures involving the SIJ (48,49). Bone scan was positive in these case reports of military recruits and athletes.

Rheumatologic conditions may affect the SIJ. Sacroiliitis occurs with seronegative spondyloarthropathies, gout (50,51), and familial Mediterranean fever (52).

Infection may involve the SIJ with such organisms as *Pseudomonas aeruginosa, Staphylococcus aureus, Cryptococcus, Mycobacterium tuberculosis,* and *Treponema pallidum* (53,54,55,56,57,58). History of intravenous drug abuse and immunosuppression should raise suspicions. Women in the postpartum period may present with pyogenic sacroiliitis (58). While roentgenograms may demonstrate cortical erosions early, on plain films are often negative (54,55,56,57). Bone scan and sedimentation rate are useful diagnostic tests. Fluoroscopically guided SIJ aspiration or biopsy with culture confirms the diagnosis.

Neoplasm may involve the SIJ and mimic SIJS (59). The pelvis accounts for 40 percent of bony metastasis and is second only to the spine (59). The most frequent tumors of the SIJ are giant cell tumors, chondrosarcomas, and metastases (60). Pigmented villonodular synovitis of the SIJ has been reported (61).

Metabolic conditions such as hyperparathyroidism, Fanconi's syndrome, and renal osteodystrophy may affect the SIJ (51,62).

## PHYSICAL EXAMINATION

Various physical examination maneuvers are utilized in the diagnosis of SIJS, including tests of SIJ mobility and pain provocation (Figures 13–5, 13–6, 13–7, 13–8, and 13–9 A, B). Mobility tests focus on establishing whether the SIJ is hypo- or hypermobile. Recent studies have raised concern about the validity of mobility testing (17) and physical examination tests (47).

Potter and Rothstein (7) prospectively determined

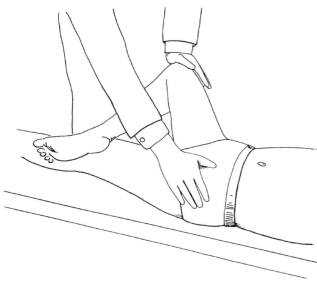

**FIGURE 13–5**

Patrick's test. Flexion, abduction, external rotation, and extension force applied to produce SIJ pain.

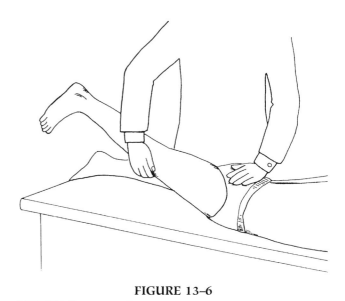

**FIGURE 13–6**

Yeoman's test. Examiner's hand placed over SIJ with hyperextension of the ipsilateral hip to produce SIJ pain.

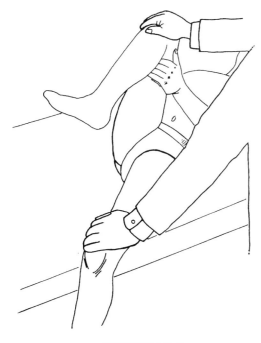

**FIGURE 13–7**

Gaenslen's test. Hyperextension force applied to the hip with the pelvis and lumbar spine held fixed by extreme flexion of the contralateral hip to produce SIJ pain.

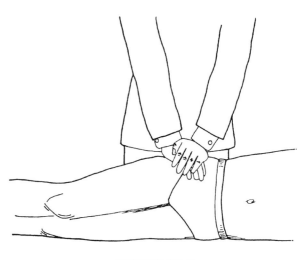

**FIGURE 13–8**

Iliac compression test. Downward force applied to iliac crest to provoke SIJ pain.

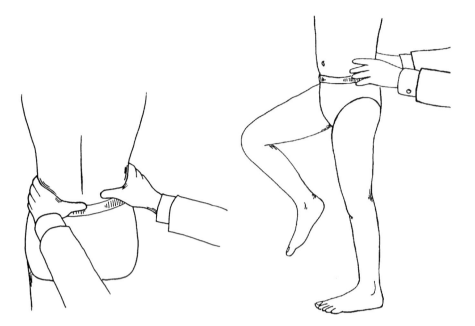

**FIGURE 13–9 A, B**

Gillet test. Thumb placed over S2 and PSIS. Subject flexes ipsilateral hip. Normally, PSIS moves inferiorly. Positive test is superior movement or lack of descent of PSIS. Test with poor interrater reliability.

interrater reliability in 13 SIJ tests: palpation in standing and sitting of iliac crests, PSIS, and ASIS; standing Gillet; standing flexion test; sitting flexion test; supine iliac gapping test; supine long sitting test; side-lying iliac compression test; and prone knee flexion test. The tests were performed on 17 subjects. Eight experienced physical therapists were paired and performed the 13 tests in the same order. Interrater reliability was less then 70 percent for all of the tests. Subject's body habitus and the physical therapist's years of experience made no difference in interrater reliability. The authors concluded that tests for sacroiliac joint position and mobility are not reliable.

Dreyfuss and co-workers (63), in a prospective, single blind study of 101 asymptomatic and 26 low back pain subjects, evaluated the specificity of the standing flexion, seated flexion, and Gillet test. The false-positive rates for the standing flexion, seated flexion, and Gillet tests were 13 percent, 8 percent, and 16 percent, respectively. In the asymptomatic group, 20 percent were positive for one of the three screening tests. The authors concluded that the specificity of these tests is not ideal.

Slipman and co-workers (64) performed a prospective study concerning the predictive value of SIJ stress tests in the diagnosis of SIJS. Fifty consecutive patients who described pain over the sacral sulcus with three positive provocative tests underwent fluoroscopically guided SIJB. Twenty-nine had at least 80 percent relief comparing pre- and post-block visual analogue scale. The positive predictive value for the provocative maneuvers was 0.58. Subjects with pain over the sacral sulcus with less than three provocative maneuvers had a 0.97 negative predictive value (65). The authors concluded that physical

examination alone is inadequate to diagnose SIJS.

Maigne and co-workers (66) prospectively evaluated the significance of provocative tests for diagnosing SIJS in 54 subjects who underwent fluoroscopically guided SIJBs using a double block protocol. A positive block with a short-acting anesthetic agent was repeated with a long-acting anesthetic agent as a confirmatory block. Nineteen had a positive initial block with 10 positive confirmatory blocks. The seven provocative maneuvers tested were not statistically significant for predicting a positive double block.

Dreyfuss and co-workers (47) evaluated the value of physical examination and history in diagnosing SIJ pain. A panel from nine disciplines considered to be experts in sacroiliac joint pain decided on 12 tests most likely to be reliable in the diagnosis of SIJ dysfunction. The 12 tests were pain drawing depicting pain over SIJ, buttock, or groin; subjects pointing within 2 inches from PSIS as maximal site of pain; sitting with partial elevation of the buttock on the affected side; Gillet test; thigh thrust; Patrick's test; Gaenslen's test; midline sacral thrust; sacral sulcus tenderness; and joint play. A physician and chiropractor independently and sequentially performed all physical examination tests. Test results were compared to a gold standard of 90 percent relief of pain from a fluoroscopically guided SIJB utilizing 2% lignocaine and Celestone Soluspan. Sixty-eight patients underwent unilateral SIJB and 17 underwent bilateral SIJB. None of the 12 tests were found to be diagnostically sound, whether performed by a chiropractor or by a physician. The authors concluded that physical examination tests for SIJ pain are not of diagnostic value.

It is unlikely that examiners can detect 1–3 mm or 1–3 degrees of SIJ motion (17). The improbability of detecting SIJ motion on physical examination and lack of interrater reliability suggest that further research is needed before mobility tests can be considered of value in the diagnosis of SIJS. Furthermore, the studies of Slipman (64), Maigne (66), and Dreyfuss and colleagues (47) raise speculation about the value of current physical examination tests in the diagnosis of SIJS. In these studies, blinding of the examiner and physician performing the SIJB would be preferable to reduce bias.

## IMAGING STUDIES

### Plain Films

Degenerative changes on SIJ radiographs may be seen in asymptomatic individuals over the age of 50 years (67,68). These findings are in agreement with anatomic studies performed on cadavers of different age groups (8,9,10,13,25). Studies concerning inter- and intrarater reliability demonstrate large variability in interpretation of radiographic findings of sacroiliitis (69,70,71). The use of plain films in acute sacroiliac joint syndrome cannot be supported from these findings. Furthermore, various investigators have found SIJ plain films not to be helpful in the diagnosis of acute SIJS (42,43). Only the study of LaBan and coworkers (72) has suggested that plain films may be of benefit. However, their study was retrospective, not blinded, and of small sample size; whether diagnosis was based on fluoroscopically guided SIJB was not indicated. Their findings of motion at the pubic symphysis with single leg standing in an asymptomatic population is unknown.

Plain films should be reserved for the evaluation of other conditions affecting the SIJ. Roentgenograms may be helpful in the evaluation of osteitis condensans illi, Reiter's syndrome, psoriatic arthritis, ankylosing spondylitis, rheumatoid arthritis, infection, gout, hyperparathyroidism, and COPD (73). Plain films are also useful in the evaluation of neoplasia and trauma.

### Scintigraphy

Use of scintigraphy in the evaluation of sacroiliac disorders is mainly to evaluate for inflammatory, infectious, metabolic, or traumatic conditions. Quantitative scintigraphy was developed to improve detection of abnormalities in the sacroiliac joints. Uptake of radiotracer over the sacroiliac joint is compared to uptake over the sacrum or femur. The result is reported as the sacroiliac joint/sacral (SIJ/S) ratio or index. The optimum time of scanning is at least 3.5 hours after injection (74), with no difference in the use of 99mTc-methylene diphosphonate and 99mTc-dicarbocypropane

diphosphonate in the evaluation of sacroiliitis (75). Studies concerning the use of scintigraphy in sacroiliac joint disorders have mainly been concerned with the early detection of sacroiliitis in rheumatologic conditions.

Quantitative bone scan may be positive when plain films are normal or equivocal (76,77). Bone scan sensitivity has been reported as ranging from 38 percent to 65 percent (76,77,78). Because of low sensitivity, the value of quantitative bone scan as a screening test for early sacroiliitis has been questioned (2). In active sacroiliitis patients under the age of 30 years, bone scan has been negative (1). A positive bone scan has not been proven to be specific for sacroiliitis (78,79). Another difficulty with quantitative scintigraphy in sacroiliitis is overlap between normals and symptomatic patients (79,80). The use of quantitative bone scan in the early detection of sacroiliitis is controversial.

Slipman and co-workers (81) prospectively evaluated scintigraphy in SIJS. The diagnosis of SIJS was confirmed with a positive fluoroscopically guided SIJ block. Because bone scan sensitivity was low, they concluded that bone scan was not an effective screening tool in SIJS (81). Based on this study, lack of supporting studies, and the controversy with use in sacroiliitis, scintigraphy is currently not justified in the diagnosis of SIJS. Bone scan is of value in the diagnosis of septic sacroiliitis (82,83,84) and stress reactions and fractures of the SIJ (48,49).

### Computed Tomography

No prospective or retrospective studies evaluating the use of computed tomography in SIJS were identified in the English literature. The use of computed tomography in the evaluation of sacroiliitis has been studied. Computed tomography is more sensitive than plain films in sacroiliitis (85,86).

The value of CT in sacroiliac disorders is in providing increased bony detail when plain films are equivocal, especially in detection of early sacroiliitis or sacral fracture with trauma. CT is of use in the diagnosis of a variety of conditions affecting the SIJ, including diffuse idiopathic skeletal hyperostosis, Behçet's syndrome, and hyperparathyroidism (87,88,89). The use of CT in the diagnosis of acute sacroiliac joint syndrome is currently not indicated. One study was performed in asymptomatic subjects demonstrating normal degenerative findings with aging (90). These findings should be kept in mind when interpreting CT in patients.

### MRI

Two studies with differing results evaluated MRI along with other imaging studies in sacroiliitis. Hanly and co-workers (78) found a sensitivity of 54 percent, whereas

Battafarano and co-workers (77) reported a sensitivity of 100 percent. Further studies are required to evaluate MRI in sacroiliitis. No studies concerning MRI in SIJS were found in a Medline search of the English literature. Studies concerning abnormal findings in an asymptomatic population along with those suffering from SIJS need to be performed.

## SACROILIAC JOINT BLOCK

### Diagnostic Sacroiliac Joint Block

Sacroiliac joint block may be diagnostic or therapeutic. In diagnostic SIJB, anesthetic agent is introduced into the SIJ under fluoroscopic guidance. Confirmation of placement is established with radiologic contrast agent (Figure 13–10). At least 75 percent resolution of the patient's pain over the ipsilateral SIJ is considered diagnostic of pain emanating from the SIJ (4).

Haldeman and Soto-Hall (91) report on the use of 20–30 cc of procaine injected into the sacroiliac joint for

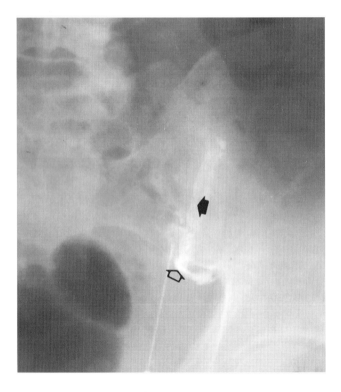

**FIGURE 13–10**

Sacroiliac joint block. Needle placed in joint. *Solid arrow* demonstrates contrast with arthographic pattern. *Open arrow* demonstrates contrast in the inferior recess of the joint capsule.

the diagnosis and treatment of SIJ strain. The injections were performed without the use of radiologic confirmation and probably represent periarticular injections. The article is of historical interest in introducing the concept of anesthetic injections to diagnose SIJS.

Norman and May (92) describe the usefulness of sacroiliac joint block in the diagnosis of sacroiliac joint pain mimicking intervertebral disk syndrome. Norman utilized 2 cc local anesthetic into the SIJ with radiologic confirmation. Norman and May report in their 10 years of practice that this was helpful in 300 cases in treating patients with question of SIJS versus herniated nucleus pulposus.

Miskew and co-workers (53) describe the use of fluoroscopy to obtain access to the SIJ. Eight subjects underwent aspiration of the SIJ under fluoroscopy for suspected infection. Seven of the cultures were positive. One negative aspiration was later found to be infected at surgery. The infection was in the superior aspect of the joint and cannulation was inferiorly. The authors report the joint can be loculated separating the superior from the inferior portion of the joint.

Hendrix and co-workers (93) describe a fluoroscopic technique for aspiration or injection of the SIJ. They also measured the radiation exposure with the technique. In females and males, gonad exposure was 40–60 mR/minute and 10–15 mR/minutes, respectively. Skin exposure was 1,200–3,000 mR/minute for both sexes. By comparison, an AP scout film results in gonad exposure of 150–200 mR and 20–30 mR in females and males, respectively. Skin exposure is 500–650 mR. Hendrix and co-workers (93) report that their technique can be performed more rapidly than the technique described by Miskew and colleagues (53) with less radiation exposure. Maugars and co-workers (94) report fluoroscopy time was less than one minute to perform bilateral SIJB utilizing the Hendrix technique.

Fortin and co-workers (3) utilized provocation on SIJB to establish a diagnosis of SIJS. Fifty-four consecutive patients with low back pain lasting greater than 2 weeks referred for discography or facet joint block completed pain drawings. Two blinded examiners reviewed the drawings to correlate with pain maps of SIJ pain developed from earlier work (41). Sixteen subjects had pain drawings suggestive of SIJ pain as agreed by both examiners. These 16 subjects underwent SIJB; all had provocation of pain. With anesthetic injection, two experienced complete relief and 10 had greater than 50 percent relief. The authors concluded that the pain drawing was of benefit in determining candidates for SIJB. The authors further concluded that provocation of symptoms of SIJB is important. Diagnosis of SIJ pain with provocation of symptoms but without relief from anesthetic agent has been questioned (95,96).

Schwarzer and co-workers (4) utilized fluoroscopically guided diagnostic SIJB with pain provocation versus relief from anesthetic agent in the evaluation of chronic low back pain in 43 consecutive subjects . Relief of at least 75 percent of pain over the SIJ and buttock with 1 ml of 2% lignocaine was a positive block. Additionally, provocation of concordant pain with injection of contrast agent prior to anesthetic injection was recorded.

There was a negative correlation between relief of pain and failure to provoke pain or reproduction of similar but not exact pain. While relief of pain occurred more frequently in those with exact reproduction of pain, the association was not statistically significant. The authors concluded that pain relief with anesthetic agent is diagnostic and pain provocation is not diagnostic of SIJ pain.

False-positive and false-negative rates for diagnostic SIJB have not been established. One reason this remains unanswered is lack of a gold standard for comparison to diagnostic SIJB. The false-positive rate could be evaluated with control blocks utilizing either saline or an anesthetic agent with a different half-life (4). In using two anesthetic agents with different half-lives, the duration of symptom relief is compared with the half-life of the anesthetic agent for an appropriate response. The individual performing the injection should be blinded to the patient's clinical status. An independent evaluator blinded to the agent utilized and the patient's clinical status records the result of the injection.

False-negative studies may occur with faulty needle placement. Individuals need to be experienced or formally trained in the performance of SIJB and interpretation of the arthographic patterns to minimize this error. False-negatives may theoretically occur if loculations exist in the joint separating the anesthetic agent from the painful portion of the joint (53). Ethical consideration of subjecting patients to extra radiation with a second injection procedure and use of a placebo injection (saline) has presented difficulty in pursuing this needed research.

## Therapeutic Sacroiliac Joint Block

Norman and May (92) report on the successful management of sacroiliac joint pain utilizing SIJB with hydrocortisone and radiologic confirmation of needle placement. Norman did not report actual results of the 300 cases he treated over 10 years.

Maugars and co-workers (94) utilized corticosteroid injection of the SIJ in patients with seronegative spondyloarthropathy. This was a retrospective study of 22 patients who underwent 42 injections in 24 procedures. Sacroiliac joint blocks were done with fluoroscopic guidance utilizing the technique of Hendrix. The patients had an average age of 33 years (range 18–55), and SIJ mean symptom duration of 17 months (range 1–96 months). All subjects had buttock pain, 10 with thigh pain, 4 with calf pain. Improvement occurred in 2–3 days in 17/19 patients. Very good and good results occurred in 19/24 (79.2 percent). One subject had fair results. Four subjects experienced no improvement. Very good results were classified as greater than 80 percent relief, and good results with 70–80 percent relief. Duration of symptom improvement was 8.4 months (range 1–15 months). Seven had no relapse of symptoms. At an average follow-up of 9.6 months, 73.7 percent reported good results. The authors concluded that corticosteriod injection of the SIJ for sacroiliitis is beneficial in those who have failed medical management.

In a retrospective study, Slipman and co-workers (5) report the results of therapeutic SIJB for the treatment of SIJS. Thirty-seven patients were diagnosed with SIJS based on a minimum of 80 percent reduction in pre- and post-SIJB visual analogue scale score. Sacroiliac joint block was performed fluoroscopically utilizing a modified Hendrix technique. Each subject diagnosed with SIJS received at least one SIJB and continued with physical therapy. Each subject completed a visual analogue scale prior to undergoing a therapeutic SIJB. Thirty-four patients were then contacted at a mean follow-up of 22.9 months. An independent interviewer telephonically obtained a verbal analogue scale and Oswestry disability score. Oswestry disability scores were also completed at initial presentation. VAS was reduced by 50 percent, and Oswestry rating improved in 20 subjects, which was statistically significant. These 20 subjects upgraded their work status or maintained full duty.

The potential benefits of SIJB need to be weighed against potential risks and cost of the procedure. Prospective studies concerning complications from SIJB have not been performed in the English literature. The possibility of allergic reactions to substances injected or intravascular injection of anesthetic agent with cardiac or CNS complications requires the presence of equipment and personnel for resuscitation. Potential for viscous or vascular perforation exists, particularly in those inexperienced or unfamiliar with pelvic anatomy. Side effects from corticosteroid medication are usually dose-dependent, with injection dosages considerably less than oral corticosteroid dose packets.

Nevertheless, individuals may experience temporary increased pain, facial flushing, low-grade fever, fluid retention, insomnia, headache, and epigastric distress within the first week after injection. Cushing's syndrome has been reported after epidural injection and may be a theoretical complication with corticosteroid SIJB (96,97). At the Penn Spine Center, University of Pennsylvania Medical Center, we performed a prospective study of 29 consecutive patients presenting for SIJB utilizing an independent interviewer. Preliminary data from this study revealed no major complications. Further study with a larger sample size is required to determine the incidence of side effects and complications. The cost of SIJB including hospital and physician charges is approximately $250–$600 dollars. Individuals may require one to four injections.

The successful management of sacroiliitis in seronegative spondyloarthropathy with corticosteroid SIJB cannot be translated to SIJS. While the study by Slipman and co-workers (5) supports the use of SIJB in the management of SIJS, further prospective studies are needed. Studies concerning the use of nonfluoroscopically guided SIJ injections were not included. Blinded SIJ injections are most likely periarticular injections and nonspecific.

## BRACING

Various investigators have advocated the use of bracing in the treatment of SIJS (36,40). No prospective studies have been performed to evaluate the effectiveness of bracing in SIJS. Vleeming and co-workers (99) evaluated the biomechanical effects of pelvic belts in 12 sacroiliac joints in six cadavers. The specimens were placed into a frame and 150 Newton force was applied to produce nutation and counternutation of the SIJ. Movement of the SIJ was recorded with and without the use of a pelvic belt. Without a belt, 0.12 to 4.54 degrees of nutation and counternutation were produced. With use of a 50 Newton belt, 7/12 sacroiliac joints had an average motion decrease of 29.3 percent. All 12 had motion reduction of 18.8 percent. With a 100 Newton belt, motion decrease was similar to the 50 Newton belt. The authors concluded that movement is reduced with a 50 Newton pelvic belt, resulting in increased pelvic stability. There is no advantage to use of increased force over 50 Newtons. The belt should be located just above the greater trochanter.

This study offers some support for the use of pelvic belts to reduce SIJ motion. However, biomechanical assessment in vivo in different age groups needs to be performed. SIJ belt is in the low cost category.

## EXERCISE

There are no prospective trials that have evaluated the effect of aerobic exercise, stabilization exercises, or restoration of range of motion in SIJS. Empirically, exercise has been an important aspect in the treatment of SIJS. Corrective exercises may be utilized to position the innominates in proper position relative to the sacrum (100). General principles of rehabilitation, but specific for SIJ, should be utilized. Stretching exercises should focus on the trunk and lower extremity. In particular, the hamstrings, gluteus

maximus, and piriformis should be evaluated because of their attachment to the sacrotuberous ligament and potential influence on the SIJ (35). The erector spinae, latissimus dorsi via the thoracodorsal fascia, iliacus, quadratus lumborum, and gluteus minimus should also be addressed because of potential influence on the SIJ (17). Evaluation of antagonistic muscle groups and the lower extremity kinetic chain needs to be included. Exercises should progress to strengthening and stabilization. Postural correction and correction of compensatory movement need to be addressed. Aerobic conditioning is incorporated in the patient's rehabilitation. As symptoms are controlled, flexibility returns, and the patient is able to do basic stabilization, activity-specific stabilization exercises are incorporated. These need to be specific for the patient's occupation, sport, or avocational activities. Early in treatment, exercises such as straight leg raises, which contract hip flexors and may cause anterior rotation of the ilia on the sacrum, should be avoided (100).

## MANUAL THERAPY

Manual therapy is discussed in more detail in another chapter. Hence, manual therapy regarding SIJS is only briefly discussed here. Only two prospective studies were identified in the English medical literature.

Osterbauer and co-workers (101) performed a prospective, descriptive study of 10 patients presenting to a chiropractic office for treatment. Diagnosis of SIJ pain was based on history and physical examination. Patients received a course of three-times-weekly manipulation with short lever arm and manually assisted instrument adjustments to indicated spinal and pelvic segments. Visual analogue scores decreased an average of 25 to 12 in 7 patients. Oswestry decreased from a mean score of 28 to 13 in six patients. Only six patients responded to one-year follow-up. Five were improved, with three of the six having frequent recurrences.

Kirkaldy-Willis and Cassidy (102), in a prospective study on 69 patients with constant severe low back pain and leg pain, were clinically diagnosed with SIJS. Patients received daily manipulation for 2–3 weeks. At an average follow-up of 10.3 months, 71 percent of patients were symptom-free, 22 percent experienced mild intermittent pain, 3 percent reported improved but restricted activity, and 3 percent had constant severe pain.

While suggesting benefit, the two prospective studies cited here are indeterminate. The study of Osterbauer and co-workers (101) had a small sample, non-blinded study, with 40 percent lost to one-year follow-up. In the study by Kirkaldy-Willis and Cassidy (102), diagnosis of SIJS was based on history and physical examination. Based on recent studies, outcomes of interventions with

SIJS diagnosed by history and physical examination is suspect (47,63,64). Further studies with one-year outcome are needed to evaluate the effectiveness of manual therapy in those with fluoroscopically guided SIJB-confirmed SIJS. If one chooses to utilize manual therapy, treatment should be in conjunction with an active exercise program (20,100).

## SURGERY

Surgery is not indicated for acute sacroiliac joint pain. Results of surgery are discussed for the clinician faced with patients who become chronic SIJ pain sufferers. Gaenslen (103) reported results of sacroiliac joint fusion in nine patients—four with tuberculosis of the SIJ and five with SIJ strain. Very good to good results were obtained in eight patients. Seven patients returned to work; one patient with tuberculosis and one with SIJ did not return.

Miltner and Lowendorf (40) retrospectively report their experience of 525 cases of SIJ sprain, of which 326 had only SIJ joint sprain. The other 199 had combined disorders. Of 153 SIJ sprains followed for at least one year, nine went to surgery. Good results were obtained in eight patients and fair results in one.

Waisbrod and co-workers (104) retrospectively report their results in 21 patient who underwent 22 SIJ fusions. Subjects had positive SIJB, plain films, CT, bone scan, and physical examination. Later in the study, individuals with positive psychological testing were excluded. At least 50 percent decrease in pain occurred in 11 patients, all of whom fused. These 11 did not require analgesics and resumed their preoperative occupation. Follow-up ranged from 12 to 65 months, with a mean of 30 months. Five subjects previously underwent lumbar spine fusion, with relief of symptoms after SIJ fusion in three patients. Six other subjects underwent various surgeries prior to sacroiliac joint fusion. Two subjects were improved. The authors conclude that if strict criteria are followed, success from sacroiliac arthodesis should be 70 percent. In their study, if the seven psychosomatic patients were identified, their results would improve from 50 percent to 73 percent.

The studies of Gaenslen (103) and Miltner (40) are mainly of historical interest. The study of Waisbrod and co-workers (104) may be criticized as a retrospective study with a small sample size and alteration of exclusion criteria during the study, i.e., addition of psychologic testing. The strength of the study was the selection criteria. A prospective study with a blinded independent observer, objective outcome measures, and randomized into two groups—with and without surgery—needs to be performed. Ethical considerations may render use of a control group difficult.

*S*ummary

The sacroiliac joint may be a source of acute low back pain. The incidence of sacroiliac joint syndrome is unknown. A recent study suggests that history and physical examination are unable to differentiate acute sacroiliac joint syndrome from other causes of low back pain (47). Prior to this study, pain over the sacral sulcus with or without radiation into the lower extremity and groin pain was suggestive of SIJS. Provocative maneuvers may be helpful in raising the suspicion of SIJS. However, recent studies question the usefulness of these tests (47,64,66). Mobility tests are probably not useful in the diagnosis of SIJS. Imaging studies are not diagnostic of SIJS and are only utilized to rule out other causes of SIJ pain. In the acute SIJS patient without risk factors for neoplasia, infection, fracture, metabolic disorder, or seronegative spondyloarthropathy, imaging studies are probably not indicated. The diagnosis of SIJS is confirmed with fluoroscopically guided sacroiliac joint block with anesthetic agent. Sacroiliac joint block without fluoroscopic guidance is not recommended, as these injections are nonspecific injections into soft tissue around the SIJ and not diagnostic. However, justification of a diagnostic SIJB in the acute low back pain patient is questionable given that the majority of acute low back pain patients have resolution of symptoms in 2 months (105).

Those who are unable to perform light duty and patients with moderate to severe pain not responding to general treatment for idiopathic mechanical low back pain and lumbar stabilization rehabilitation programs after 4 weeks may be considered for diagnostic fluoroscopically guided SIJB when SIJS is suspected. Additionally, patients who have not responded to care after 2 months with clinical suspicion of SIJS are candidates for diagnostic SIJB. With confirmation of the diagnosis of SIJS by a diagnostic SIJB, specific therapy for SIJ may then be initiated. Unfortunately, no prospective studies with fluoroscopically guided SIJB-confirmed SIJS utilizing mobilization, manipulation, or bracing have been performed. Kirkaldy-Willis and Cassidy (102) demonstrated benefit of SIJ manipulation in a prospective study with SIJS diagnosed by history and physical examination. Slipman and co-workers (5) performed a retrospective study in which 59 percent were successfully treated with therapeutic fluoroscopically guided SIJB and a dynamic lumbar stabilization program. Until further research is performed, other treatment for SIJS needs to be balanced against potential medical risks to the patient and financial costs.

*Acknowledgment:* Ms. Robin Westler for illustration of Figures 13–5 to 13–9.

## References

1. Miron SD, Khan MA, Wiesen EJ, Kushner I, et al. The value of quantitative sacroiliac scintigraphy in detection of sacroiliitis. *Clin Rheum* 1983; 2:407–414.
2. Esdaile JM, Rosentall L, Terkeltaub R, Kloeiber R. Prospective evaluation of sacroiliac scintigraphy in chronic inflammatory back pain. *Arthritis Rheum* 1980; 23:998–1003.
3. Fortin JD, Apill CN, Ponthieux B, Pier J. Sacroiliac joint: Pain referral maps upon applying a new injection/arthrography technique. Part II: Clinical evaluation. *Spine* 1994; 19:1483–1489.
4. Schwarzer AC, April CN, Bogduk N. The sacroiliac joint in chronic low back pain. *Spine* 1995; 20:31–37.
5. Slipman CW, Plastaras CT, Yang ST, Huston CW, et al. Outcomes of therapeutic fluoroscopically guided sacroiliac joint injections for definitive SIJS. *Arch Phys Med Rehabil* 1996; 77:937.
6. Mierau DR, Cassidy JD, Hamin T, Milne RA. Sacroiliac joint dysfunction and low back pain in school aged children. *J Manipulative Physiol Ther* 1984; 7:81–84.
7. Potter NA, Rothstein JM. Intertester reliability for selected clinical tests of the sacroiliac joint. *Phys Ther* 1985; 65:1671–1675.
8. Bowen V, Cassidy JD. Macroscopic and microscopic anatomy of the sacroiliac joint from embryonic life until the eighth decade. *Spine* 1981; 6:620–628.
9. Albee FH. A study of the anatomy and the clinical importance of the sacroiliac joint. *JAMA* 1909; LIII:1273–1276.
10. MacDonald GR, Hunt TE. Sacro-iliac joints. Observations on the gross and histological changes in the various age groups. *Canad M A J* 1952; 66:157–163.
11. Walker JM. Age-related differences in the human sacroiliac joint: a histological study; implications for therapy. *J Orthop* 1986; 7:325–334.
12. Weisel H. The ligaments of the sacro-iliac joint examined with particular reference to their function. *Acta Anat* 1954; 20:201–213.
13. Sashin D. A critical analysis of the anatomy and the pathologic changes of the sacro-iliac joints. *J Bone Joint Surg* 1930; 12A:891–910.
14. Gardner E, Gray DJ, O'Rahilly R. Muscles, vessels, nerves, and joints of back. In: *Anatomy. A regional study of human structure.* 4th ed. Philadelphia: WB Saunders, 1975:525–545.
15. Vleeming A, Pool-Goudzwaard AL, Hammudoghlu D, Stoeckart R, et al. The function of the long dorsal sacroiliac ligament. Its implication for understanding low back pain. *Spine* 1996; 21:556–562.
16. Vleeming A, Stoeckart R, Snijders CJ. The sacrotuberous ligament: a conceptual approach to its dynamic role in stabilizing the sacroiliac joint. *Clin Biomech* 1989; 4:210–203.
17. Walker JM. The sacroiliac joint: A critical review. *Phys Ther* 1992; 7:903–916.
18. Steindler A, Luck JV. Differential diagnosis of pain low in the back. Allocation of the source of pain by the procaine hydrochloride method. *JAMA* 1938; 110:106–113.
19. Solonen KA. The sacroiliac joint in the light of anatomical, roentgenological and clinical studies. *Acta Orthop Scand* 1957; 27 (Suppl):1–127.
20. Bernard TN, Jr, Cassidy JD. The sacroiliac joint syndrome. Pathophysiology, diagnosis, and management. In: Frymoyer JW, Ducker TB, Hadler NM, Kostuik JP, et al. (eds.). *The adult spine: Principles and practice.* New York: Raven Press, 1991:2107–2130
21. Ebraheim NA, Padanilam TG, Waldrop JT, Yeasting RA. Anatomic consideration in the anterior approach to the sacro-iliac joint. *Spine* 1994; 19:721–725.
22. Hershey CD. The sacro-iliac joint and pain of sciatic radiation. *JAMA* 1943; 122:983–986.
23. Trotter M. Accessory sacro-iliac articulations. *Am J Phys Anthrop* 1937; 22:247–261.
24. Ehara S, El-Khoury GY, Bergman RA. The accessory sacroiliac joint: A common anatomic variant. *Am J Radiol* 1988; 150:857–859.
25. Stewart TD. Pathologic changes in aging sacroiliac joints. A study of dissecting-room skeletons. *Clin Orthop Rel Res* 1984; 183:188–196
26. Hollinshead WH, Jenkins DB. The bony pelvis, femur, and hip joint. In: *Functional anatomy of the limbs and back.* 5th ed. Philadelphia: WB Saunders 1981:231–240.
27. Egund N, Olsson TH, Schmid H, Selvik G. Movements in the sacroiliac joint demonstrated with roentgen stereophotogrammetry. *Acta Radiologica Diagnosis* 1978; 19:833–846.
28. Sturesson B, Selvik G, Uden A. Movements of the sacroiliac joints. A roentgen stereophotogrammetric analysis. *Spine* 1989; 14:162–165.
29. Frigereio NA, Stowe RR, Howe JW. Movement of the sacroiliac joint. *Clin Orthop Rel Res* 1974; 100:370–377.
30. Grieve EFM. Mechanical dysfunction of the sacro-iliac joint. *Int Rehabil Med* 1983; 5:46–52.
31. Miller JAA, Schultz AB, Andersson GBJ. Load-displacement behavior of sacroiliac joints. *J Orthop Res* 1987; 5:92–101.
32. Rothkotter HJ, Berner W. Failure load and displacement of the human sacroiliac joint under in vitro loading. *Arch Orthop Trauma Surg* 1988; 107:283–287.
33. Weisl H. The movements of the sacro-iliac joint. *Acta Anat* 1955; 23:80–91.
34. Lavignolle B, Vital JM, Destandau J, Toson B, et al. An approach to the functional anatomy of the sacroiliac joints in vivo. *Anat Clin* 1983; 5:169–176.
35. Vleeming A, Van Wingerden JP, Snijders CJ, Stoeckart R, et al. Load application to the sacrotuberous ligament: Influences on sacroiliac joint mechanics. *Clin Biomech* 1989; 4:204–209.
36. Fitch RR. Mechanical lesions of the sacroiliac joints. *Am J Orthop Surg* 1908; 6:693–698.
37. Martin ED. Sacro-iliac sprain. *Southern Med J* 1922; 15:135–139.
38. Kirkaldy-Willis WH. A more precise diagnosis for low back pain. *Spine* 1979; 4:102–109.
39. Fortin JD. Sacroiliac joints dysfunction. A new perspective. *J Back Musculoskel Rehabil* 1993; 3:31–43.
40. Miltner LJ, Lowendorf CS. Low back pain. A study of

525 cases of sacro-iliac and sacrolumbar sprain. *J Bone Joint Surg* (Am) 1931; 13:16–28.

41. Fortin JD, Dwyer AP, West S, Pier J. Sacroiliac joint : Pain referral maps upon applying a new injection/arthrography technique. Part I: Asymptomatic volunteers. *Spine* 1994; 19:1475–1482.

42. Smith-Petersen MN. Clinical diagnosis of common sacroiliac conditions. *Am J Roent Radium Ther* 1924; 12:546–550.

43. LeBlanc KE. Sacroiliac sprain: an overlooked cause of back pain. *Am Family Physician* 1992; 46:1459–1463.

44. Norman GF. Sacroiliac disease and its relationship to lower abdominal pain. *Am J Surg* 1968; 116:54–56.

45. Schuchmann JA, Cannon CL. Sacroiliac strain syndrome: diagnosis and treatment. *Texas Med* 1986; 82:33–36.

46. Cox HH. Sacro-iliac subluxation as a cause of backache. *Surg Gynecol Obstet* 1927; 45:637–649.

47. Dreyfuss P, Michaelsen M, Pauza K, McLarty J, et al. The value of medical history and physical examination in diagnosing sacroiliac joint pain. *Spine* 1996; 21:2594–2602.

48. Chisin R, Milgrom C, Margulies J, Giladi M, et al. Unilateral sacroiliac overuse syndrome in military recruits. *Br Med J* 1984; 289:590–591.

49. Marymont JV, Lynch MA, Henning CE. Exercise-related stress reaction of the sacroiliac joint. An unusual cause of low back pain in athletes. *Amer J Sports Med* 1986; 14:320–323.

50. Malawista SE, Seegmiller JE, Hathaway BE, Sokoloff L. Sacroiliac gout. *JAMA* 1965; 194:106–108.

51. Kerr R. Sacroiliac joint involvement by gout and hyperparathyroidism. *Orthop* 1988; 11:187–190.

52. Lehman TJA, Hanson V, Kornreich H, Peters RS, et al. HLA-B27–negative sacroiliitis: a manifestation of familial Mediterranean fever in childhood. *Pediatrics* 1978; 61:423–426.

53. Miskew DB, Block RA, Witt PF. Aspiration of infected sacro-iliac joints. *J Bone Joint Surg* 1979; 61A:1071–1072.

54. Dunn EJ, Bryan DM, Nugent JT, Robinson RA. Pyogenic infections of the sacro-iliac joint. *Clin Orthop Rel Res* 1976; 118:113–117.

55. Pouchot J, Vinceneux P, Barge J, Boussougant Y, et al. Tuberculosis of the sacroiliac joint: Clinical features, outcome, and evaluation of closed needle biopsy in 11 consecutive cases. *Am J Med* 1988; 84:622–628.

56. Reginato AJ, Ferreiro-Seoane JL, Falasca G. Unilateral sacroiliitis in secondary syphilis. *J Rheum* 1988; 15: 717–719.

57. Brand C, Warren R, Luxton M, Barraclough D. Cryptococcal sacroiliitis. Case report. *Ann Rheum Dis* 1985; 44:126–127.

58. Engelsbel S, Swartjes JM, Schutte MF. Case report. Pyogenic sacro-iliitis, a rare cause of peripartum pelvic pain. *Eur J Obstet Gyn Reproductive Bio* 1995; 62:125–126.

59. Humphrey SM, Inman RD. Metastatic adenocarinoma mimicking unilateral sacroiliitis. *J Rheum* 1995; 22:970–972.

60. Abdelwahab IF, Miller TT, et al. Transarticular invasion of joints by bone tumors: hypothesis. *Skeletal Radiol* 1991; 20:279–283.

61. Sarma NHHN. Pigmented villonodular synovitis of sacral joints by bone tumor. *Central African J Med* 1985; 31:156–157.

62. Gaucher A, Thomas JL, Netter P, Faure G. Osteomalacia, pseudosacroiliitis and necrosis of the femoral heads in Fanconi syndrome in an adult. *J Rheum* 1981; 8:512–515.

63. Dreyfuss P, Dreyer S, Griffin J, Hoffman J, Walsh N. Positive sacroiliac screening tests in asymptomatic adults. *Spine* 1994; 19:1138–1143.

64. Slipman CW, Sterenfeld EB, Chou LH, Vreslovic EJ, Jr. The predictive value of provocative sacroiliac joint stress maneuvers in defining sacroiliac joint syndrome. North American Spine Society, 10th Annual Proceedings. Washington, DC 1995:321.

65. Slipman CW. Verbal communication 1997.

66. Maigne JY, Aivaliklis A, Pfefer F. Results of sacroiliac joint double block and value of sacroiliac pain provocation tests in 54 patients with low back pain. *Spine* 1996; 21:1889–1892.

67. Cohen AS, McNeill JM, Calkins E, Sharp JT, Schubart A. The normal sacroiliac joint. An analysis of 88 sacroiliac roentgenograms. *Am J Roent Radium Ther* 1967; 100: 559–563.

68. Jajic I, Jajic Z. The prevalence of osteoarthrosis of the sacroiliac joints in an urban population. *Clin Rheum* 1987; 6:39–41.

69. Chamberlain MA, Robertson RJH. A controlled study of sacroiliitis in Behcet's disease. *Brit J Rheum* 1993; 32:693–698.

70. Yazici H, Turunc M, Ozdogan H, Yurdakul S, Akinci A, Barnes CG. Observer variation in grading sacroiliac radiographs might be a cause of sacroiliitis reported in certain disease states. *Ann Rheum Dis* 1987; 46:139–145.

71. Ryan LM, Carrera GF, Lightfoot RW Jr, et al. The radiographic diagnosis of sacroiliitis. A comparison of different view with computed tomograms of the sacroiliac joint. *Arthritis Rheum* 1983; 26:760–763.

72. LaBan MM, Meershaert JR, Taylor RS, Tabor HD. Symphyseal and sacroiliac joint pain associated with pubic symphysis instability. *Arch Phys Med Rehabil* 1978; 59:470–472.

73. Resnik CS, Resnick D. Radiology of disorders of the sacroiliac joints. *JAMA* 1985; 253:2863–2866.

74. Dodig D, Domljan Z, Popovic S, Simonovic I. Effect of imaging time on the values of the sacroiliac index. *Eur J Nucl Med* 1988; 14:504–506.

75. Lantto T. The scintigraphy of sacroiliac joints. A comparison of 99mTc DPD and 99mTc-MDP. *Eur J Nucl Med* 1990; 16:677–681.

76. Russell AS, Lentle BC, Percy JS. Investigation of sacroiliac disease: Comparative evaluation of radiological and radionuclide techniques. *J Rheum* 1975; 2:45–51.

77. Battafarano DF, West SG, Rak KM, Fortenbery EJ, Chantelois AE. Comparison of bone scan, computed tomography, and magnetic resonance imaging in the diagnosis of active sacroiliitis. *Sem Arthritis Rheum* 1993; 23:101–176.

78. Hanly JG, Mitchell MJ, Barnes DC, MacMillan L. Early recognition of sacroiliitis by magnetic resonance imaging and single photon emission computed tomography. *J Rheum* 1994; 21:2088–2095.

79. Chalmers IM, Lentle BC, Percy JS, Russell AS. Sacroiliitis detected by bone scintiscanning: a clinical, radiological, and scintigraphic follow-up study. *Ann Rheumatic Dis* 1979; 38:112–117.

80. Goldberg RP, Genant HK, Shimshak R, Shames D. Radiology 1978; 128:68

81. Verlooy H, Mortelmans L, Vleugels S, DeRoo M. Quantitative scintigraphy of the sacroiliac joints. *Clin Imaging* 1992; 16:230–233.

82. Slipman CW, Sterenfeld EB, Chou LH, Herzog R, Vresilovic E. The value of radionuclide imaging in the diagnosis of sacroiliac joint syndrome. *Spine* 1996; 19:2251–2254.

83. Horgan JG, Walker M, Newman JH, Watt I. Scintigraphy in the diagnosis and management of septic sacro-iliitis. *Clin Radiol* 1983; 34:337–346.

84. Kumar R, Balachandran S. Unilateral septic sacro-iliitis importance of the anterior view of the bone scan. *Clin Nucl Med* 1983; 8:413–415.

85. Salomon CG, Ali A, Fordham EW. Bone scintigraphy in tuberculous sacroiliitis. *Clin Nucl Med* 1986; 11:407–408.

86. Lawson TL, Foley WD, Carrera GF, Berland LL. The sacroiliac joints: anatomic, plain roentgenographic, and computed tomographic analysis. *J Comput Assist Tomogr* 1982; 6:307–314.

87. Taggart AJ, Desai SM, Iveson JM, Verow PW. Computerized tomography of the sacro-iliac joints in the diagnosis of sacro-iliitis. *Brit J Rheum* 1984; 23:258–266.

88. Durback MA, Edelstein G, Schumacher RH, Jr. Abnormalities of the sacroiliac joints in diffuse idiopathic skeletal hyperostosis: Demonstration by computed tomography. *J Rheum* 1988; 15:1506–1511.

89. Olivieri I, Gemignani G, Camerini E, Semeria R, et al. Computed tomography of the sacroiliac joints in four patients with Behcet's syndrome on by computed tomography. *Brit J Rheum* 1990; 29:264–267.

90. Hooge WA, Li D. CT of sacroiliac joints in secondary hyperparathyroidism. *J de L'Assoc Canadienne Des Radiologistes* 1981; 31:42–44.

91. Vogel JB, III, Brown WH, Helms CA, Genant HK. The normal sacroiliac joint: A CT study of asymptomatic patients. *Radiol* 1984; 151:433–437.

92. Vogel JB, III, Brown WH, Helms CA, Genant HK. The normal sacroiliac joint: A CT study of asymptomatic patients. *Radiol* 1984; 151:433–437.

93. Haldeman KO, Soto-Hall R. The diagnosis and treatment of sacro-iliac conditions by the injections of procaine (novocain). *J Bone Jt Surg* 1938; 20:675–685.

94. Norman GF, May A. Sacroiliac conditions simulating intervertebral disc syndrome. *West J Surg* 1956; 64:461–462.

95. Hendrix RW, Lin PJP, Kane WJ. Brief note. Simplified aspiration or injection technique for the sacro-iliac joint. *J Bone Joint Surg* 1982; 64A:1249–1252.

96. Maugars Y, Mathis C, Vilon P, Prost A. Corticosteroid injection of the sacroiliac joint in patients with seronegative spondylarthropathy. *Arthritis Rheum* 1992; 35:564568.

97. Derby R Jr. Point of View. *Spine* 1994; 19:1489.

98. Schwarzer AC, Derby R, Aprill CN, Fortin J, et al. The value of the provocation response in lumbar zygapophyseal joint injections. *Clin J Pain* 1994; 10:309–313.

99. Vleeming A, Buyruk HM, Stoeckart R, Karamursel S, Snijders CJ. An integrated therapy from peripartum pelvic instability: A study of the biomechanical effects of pelvic belts. *Am J Obstet Gynecol* 1992; 166:1243–1247.

100. DonTigny RL. Function and pathomechanics of the sacroiliac joint. A review. *Phys Ther* 1985; 65:35–44.

101. Osterbauer PJ, DeBoer KF, Widmaier R, Petermann E, Fuhr AW. Treatment and biomechanical assessment of patients with chronic sacroiliac syndrome. *J Manipulative Physiol Ther* 1993; 16:82–90.

102. Kirkaldy-Willis WH, Cassidy JD. Spinal manipulation in the treatment of low-back pain. *Can Fam Physician* 1985; 31:535–540.

103. Gaenslen FJ. Sacro-iliac arthordesis. Indications, author's technic and end-results. *JAMA* 1927; 89:.63–682031–2035.

104. Waisbrod H, Krainick JU, Gerbershagen HU. Sacroiliac joint arthodesis for chronic lower back pain. *Arch Orthop Trauma Surg* 1987; 106:238–240.

105. Spitzer WO, LeBlanc FE, Dupuis M, et al. Scientific approach to the assessment and management of activity-related spinal disorders. A monograph for clinicians. Report of the Quebec task force on spinal disorders. *Spine* 1987; 12 (Suppl):S1–S59.

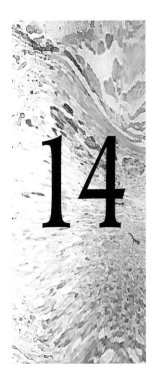

# 14 Trigger Point Management

*Edward S. Rachlin, M.D., F.A.C.S.*

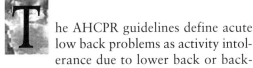he AHCPR guidelines define acute low back problems as activity intolerance due to lower back or back-related leg symptoms of less than 3 months' duration. The panel has made specific recommendations concerning trigger point injections in the management of acute low back pain.

The AHCPR panel findings and recommendations noted, "trigger point injections are invasive and not recommended in the treatment of patients with acute low back problems (strength of evidence = C)." This statement is not clinically valid. Injection of trigger points in acute low back pain depends on the clinical circumstances.

*The panel describes trigger point injection as involving the injection of local anesthetic into soft tissue (muscles) near localized tender points in the paravertebral area.*

This statement ignores the equally important muscles to be treated in the management of back pain, e.g., gluteal, piriformis, and tensor fasciae latae.

This chapter includes a discussion of trigger point management in addition to the panel recommendations, and a discussion of the research articles on which these recommendations were made. The instructional content will enable the physician to achieve better results in the management of myofascial trigger points associated with back pain, in addition to the ability to evaluate the AHCPR guideline recommendations.

Therapeutic results in the management of regional myofascial pain due to trigger point pathology depend on an accurate diagnosis and total assessment of all factors related to muscle pain. Myofascial trigger points should not be evaluated as a single entity, but as one component of interrelated causes of muscle pain (muscle spasm, muscle tension, muscle deficiency, trigger points). The necessity for a thorough history and physical examination, including a muscle evaluation, cannot be overemphasized. It is rarely possible to identify trigger points in the acute stage of low back pain if spasm is present (1). Injection into an area of muscle spasm is often confused with trigger point injection. Trigger points are best identified after spasm has been relieved. Uncertainty also exists in the diagnosis of trigger points when differentiating the tender points found in fibromyalgia with findings typical of trigger points in myofascial pain syndromes. Tender points found in fibromyalgia are typically characterized as areas of local tenderness, multiple in nature, symmetrically located, and not associated with referred pain patterns. A small subgroup of fibromyalgia patients are diffusely tender all over. Skinfold tenderness is present in many fibromyalgia patients (2). In contrast to tender points, the classical characteristics of trigger points include not only local tenderness but also the palpation of a taut band, which causes a local twitch response when stimulated. Trigger points may be singular or multiple. They may occur in any skeletal muscle. Specific referred pain patterns are typical of myofascial trigger points (3). Trigger points may also cause autonomic and proprioceptive symptoms. Tenderness and trigger points can occur simultaneously in fibromyalgia patients. The findings of a trigger point on physical examination should not lead one to the conclusion that therapy by injection is necessarily indicated. One must distinguish between acute low back pain, which may be due to the activation of a pre-existing asymptomatic latent trigger point found in the chronic stage (dystropic stage) or the early stages of a developing trigger point (neuromuscular dysfunctional stage) prior to the development of fibrotic pathologic changes (4). Trigger points in the early stage of development usually respond to physical therapy and may not require injections (5). The definition of acute low back pain, pain of less than 3 months, does not necessarily relate to the acute or chronic nature of a trigger point that may be present.

## DEFINITION AND TYPES OF TRIGGER POINTS

Myofascial trigger points are small, circumscribed, hyperirritable foci in muscles and fascia, often found within a firm or taut band of skeletal muscle. Nonmyofascial trigger points may also occur in ligaments, tendons, joint capsule, skin, and periosteum (6,7). Myofascial trigger points have been described as tender nodes of degenerated muscle tissue that can cause local and radiating pain. Historically, they have been referred to as *muskelharten* (muscle hardening) or *mygelosen* (myogelosis) by Lange (8), as myalgic spots by Gutstein (9), and were later described as trigger points by Steindler (10). Travell and Simons have published extensively on trigger points and referred pain patterns (11). In regional myofascial pain syndromes, trigger points may be limited to a single muscle or to several muscle groups. Palpating the trigger point may elicit a local or referred pain pattern, or both. Several pain patterns are consistent and characteristic of the primary muscles involved.

Regional myofascial pain syndromes, defined as local and referred muscular pain arising from trigger points, are a major cause of disability and chronic pain and play a factor in most worker's compensation cases involving pain (12). Most studies concerning myofascial pain patients refer to chronic pain rather than the acute myofascial pain syndrome. In view of the fact that an untreated myofascial pain syndrome can become a chronic pain condition, it is important that the acute stage of low back pain be properly treated. Of 283 consecutive chronic pain patients who were examined independently by a neurosurgeon and physiatrist, 85 percent were found to have a diagnosis of primary myofascial pain (13). Muscles become vulnerable when they are under acute or chronic stress (14). Trigger points may occur in any skeletal muscle and arise from multiple causes. They may develop after prolonged periods of spasm, tension, stress, fatigue, and chill. Stress and tension are among the most common causes of trigger points. They are most frequently found in axial muscles used to maintain posture. Occupational or recreational activities that require repeated stress on specific muscle groups may lead to symptomatic trigger points. Acute as well as chronic trauma may give rise to symptomatic trigger points that manifest themselves as acute low back pain. Postlaminectomy pain may be due to trigger points that were present prior to surgery or developed afterward (15,16).

One must distinguish between active and latent trigger points. Active trigger points are symptomatic, tender, and painful and may cause a referred pain pattern, local twitch response, and autonomic phenomenon. A more common reaction to trigger point palpation is the "jump response" (17). The patient tends to jump or suddenly move away from the examiner's palpating hand. Referred pain patterns are often specific for primary trigger points. Specific knowledge and understanding of referred pain patterns are necessary to avoid the mistake of treating trigger points (satellite) in the referred pain areas and overlooking the primary trigger point that is the cause of the pain. A satellite myofascial trigger point is a trigger point that has developed or become active within the referred pain area (zone of reference) of another trigger point. The most common trigger point locations are listed in Table 14–1. Table 14–1 also identifies the pain patterns frequently misdiagnosed or confused with other common muscular skeletal conditions.

Latent trigger points are asymptomatic but may cause muscle shortening and weakness. They are tender on palpation but are asymptomatic. Local twitch response is also sometimes elicited to palpation. Latent trigger points are most frequently found in the shoulder girdle muscles, the trapezius and levator scapula being the most common (18,19). Satellite trigger points develop in the area of referred pain as the result of persistent motor unit activity in the referred pain area (zone of reference) (20). Trigger points may be considered primary or secondary. Primary trigger points develop independently, not as the result of trigger point activity elsewhere. Secondary trigger points develop in neighboring and antagonistic

**TABLE 14–1**
*Trigger point pain patterns*

| LOCATION OF MUSCULAR TRIGGER POINTS | PAIN PATTERN | COMMONLY CONFUSED WITH TRIGGER POINT PAIN |
|---|---|---|
| Temporal, masseter, and occipital muscles | Radiation to head, headache, and neck pain | Cervical arthritis |
| Sternocleidomastoid | Neck pain | Meniere's disease Intracranial pathology |
| Scaleni Posterior neck muscles | Dizziness, numbness in 4th and 5th fingers, and headaches | Peripheral nerve entrapment Cervical syndrome |
| Trapezius (upper) | Neck and shoulder | Cervical arthritis |
| Supraspinatus | Arm pain | Cervical disc Bicipital tendinitis |
| Infraspinatus | Arm pain | Cervical disc Bursitis of shoulder Bicipital tendinitis |
| Rhomboid (upper and lower) | Interscapula, scapula, and dorsal pain | Arthritis dorsal spine Glenohumeral arthritis |
| Pectoral | Arm pain | Bursitis (shoulder) Cardiac pain Left cervical radiculopathy |
| Deltoid | Upper back, neck, and arm pain | Cervical radiculopathy Bursitis (shoulder) |
| Forearm muscle group | Pain in forearm and elbow | Epicondylitis |
| Sacrospinalis | Pain radiates downward to buttock | Sciatica Herniated disc |
| Tensor fascia Gluteus medius | Radiation to lateral aspect of thigh and leg | Herniated disc Bursitis |
| Piriformis | Sciatic radiation | Herniated disc |
| Adductor longus | Groin pain | Arthritis of hip Adductor muscle strain |
| Gastrocnemius | Pain in calf and leg | Tennis leg Plantaris tendon Gastrocnemius rupture |
| Soleus | Heel pain | Calcaneal bursitis Achilles' tendinitis |
| Abductor hallucis | Pain metacarpal phalangeal joint of big toe | Gout Arthritis M-P joint big toe |
| Tibialis anterior | Pain in front of leg and big toe | Herniated disc Anterior compartment syndrome |
| Vastus medialis Semimembranosus Sartorius | Pain in the knee | Chondromalacia Arthritis of knee |
| Peroneus longus | Ankle pain | Arthritis of ankle |
| Interossei of foot | Pain in foot, radiates to toes | Morton's neuroma Metatarsalgia |

From Rachlin ES: "Musculofascial pain syndromes," *Medical Times: The Journal of Family Medicine* January 1984, p. 40.

muscles as the result of stress and muscle spasm. Primary trigger points as well as secondary trigger points may become latent if they are asymptomatic. A satellite trigger point is a trigger point that develops in the referred pain area, which may be symptomatic or become a latent trigger point when it is asymptomatic.

The findings of only local tenderness may be sufficient to diagnose a trigger point if there is appropriate clinical correlation for the diagnosis. One cannot always rely on the findings of a taut band, twitch response, and referred pain pattern to diagnose a myofascial trigger point. The significance of tender areas in muscle must be judged within the clinical context.

Although histopathologic abnormalities are reported, they are nonspecific and inconsistent (21). Golgowsky and Wallraff (22) described biopsy findings in palpable hardenings of hip and back muscles. They found waxy degeneration of muscle fibers, destruction of fibrils, agglomeration of nuclei, and fatty infiltration. No control groups were included for comparisons. The findings were nonspecific. In a study conducted by Bengtsson and co-workers, 77 biopsies from 57 patients showed, "motheaten" fibers in 35 of 57 patients and "ragged red fibers" in 15 of the 41 trapezius muscles biopsied. Fassbender and Wegner looked at biopsies of patients with probable myofascial pain syndromes of fibrositis. The majority of the biopsies were abnormal, initially showing swollen mitochondria and moth-eaten myofilaments, progressing to necrosis of myofilaments, irregularity of sarcomeres and greatly reduced glycogen stores. The final stage examined demonstrated dissolution of contractile elements.[1]

Latent trigger points may be found on examination in asymptomatic muscle areas as incidental findings when examinations are made for spinal or extremity complaints. Latent trigger points do not require treatment unless they become active and symptomatic (23). Not all patients with acute low back pain with trigger points require needling. To be considered for injection, trigger points should be reasonably limited in number. Diffuse tenderness (skinfold tenderness) indicative of fibrositis should not be confused with trigger points. Multiple tender points often seen in fibromyalgia or endocrine disturbance are not suitable for initial trigger point injection therapy. Dr. Lawrence Sonkin notes that thyroid insufficiency is probably the most common metabolic cause of muscle pain. The second most frequent metabolic cause of muscle pain is female menopause (24). Endocrinologic workup and therapy would be indicated prior to injection therapy. The finding of tenderness in itself is not an indication for trigger point injection.

Hypothyroidism may be demonstrated by low serum thyroxine (T4), free thyroxine index, and high thyroid-stimulating hormone (TSH) levels. Serum creatine kinase (CK) may be elevated (25).

Success in trigger point management depends on the ability of the patient to receive proper post-injection follow-up care. Kraus protocol for post-injection therapy included electrical stimulation, relaxation limbering, and stretching of the involved muscles using vapocoolant spray or ice as needed, combined with and followed by an exercise program (26). Trigger points must not be treated as an isolated phenomenon. If myofascial trigger points are treated as an isolated cause of back pain, ignoring the interrelated aspects of back pain (muscle spasm, muscle tension, muscle deficiency, perpetuating factors), in addition to omitting the appropriate physical therapy programs necessary for successful outcome of trigger point management, the conclusion that there is no proven benefit in the treatment of acute low back pain would probably be true. This would also apply to trigger point management as it applies to chronic low back pain.

Factors that may cause or perpetuate symptomatic trigger points should be evaluated. These may include a leg length discrepancy, postural corrections, e.g., using a buttock lift with a small hemipelvis when sitting, long second metatarsal bone (Morton's foot), psychological stress, poor posture, poorly designed workplace environment leading to muscle strains (poorly designed chair, incorrect computer placement), or endocrine disturbances (hypothyroidism) (27).

Avoid injecting many muscle areas at one time. Multiple site injections cause muscle spasm and irritation, which interfere with rehabilitation. I do not inject to more than one trigger point area at a time; for example, inject the gluteal and lumbar areas on separate visits. I do not inject trigger points while muscles are in spasm. Palpation of trigger points is best performed only after muscle relaxation is achieved.

## POTENTIAL HARMS AND COSTS

AHCPR guidelines suggest potential harms and costs to include (1) damage to nerves, (2) infection, and (3) hemorrhage.

Complications of trigger point injections may be due to the side effects and reactions to local anesthetics or to injection technique (28). The physician must take a history of any allergic condition. History should include inquiries concerning allergy to local anesthetics, drugs, asthma, and food allergies and perform a skin test if necessary. Use saline or dry needling technique if allergy is suspected. Complications include pneumothorax, abdominal puncture wounds, needle breakage, hematoma formation, and nerve injury.

---

[1]From Rachlin ES. *Myofascial pain and fibromyalgia, trigger point management*. Chicago: Mosby, 1994, p.151.

There are no studies dealing with appreciable frequency of complications, including any statistics concerning serious potential complications from trigger point injection. I am aware of three cases of pneumothorax. The physician should always aspirate prior to any injection. This is of special importance when injecting a trigger point in the area of the chest wall. Aspiration of air bubbles into the syringe indicates a puncture of the pleural cavity. The syringe used, however, must have a tight-fitting, airtight attachment between the needle and the syringe. If air bubbles are encountered, injection is not performed. Coughing or chest pain during the injections suggest that the pleura may have been punctured. An x-ray film should then be obtained. If a pneumothorax is present, it must be treated appropriately. Angle the needle tangentially to the chest wall to avoid entering the intercostal space. Anatomy and technique should be studied prior to any trigger point injection. There are no statistics dealing with the harms and costs of trigger point injections; complications are rare. When done properly, trigger point injection is a safe procedure. In my experience, the proper diagnosis of myofascial trigger points treated by means of physical therapy with or without injections has avoided the need for surgery and has returned many patients to their normal occupations. Unfortunately, at the present time, there are no statistics to demonstrate the savings in patient suffering and financial costs.

A treatment plan for acute low back pain due to myofascial pain syndrome is described in Table 14–2.

## LITERATURE REVIEW

The following is a review of the literature that determined the findings and recommendations of the AHCPR panel regarding guidelines concerning trigger point injections in acute low back pain. These studies are summarized, and comments are noted regarding the appropriateness of conclusions that were reached.

1. "A Control, Double-Blind Comparison of Mepivacaine Injection Versus Saline Injection for Myofascial Pain," by F.A. Frost, B. Jenssen, J. Siggaard-Andersen (29).

SUMMARY: In a double-blind study 28 patients with acute, localized muscle pain received four local injections of mepivacaine 0.5%, and 25 patients with the same type of pain received local injections of an equivalent volume of physiological saline. The group receiving saline tended to have more relief of pain, especially after the first injection. The results thus show that pain relief is not due merely to the local anesthetic. The study raises questions about the mechanism by which local injections into muscle relieve pain, since there is the possibility that a similar effect might also be achieved by merely inserting a needle

---

### TABLE 14–2
#### Treatment plan for myofascial pain

| AVOID BED REST | TREAT SPASM AND PAIN | EVALUATE | PREVENT RECURRENCES |
|---|---|---|---|
| Keep ambulatory if possible<br>Avoid immobility | Ice massage<br>Heat<br>Ethyl chloride spray<br>Tetanizing current for 10 min<br>Relaxation<br>Limbering exercises<br>Gentle stretching | TENSION<br>• Tranquilizers if necessary<br>• Biofeedback<br>• Psychological evaluation<br><br>MUSCLE DEFICIENCY<br>• Kraus-Weber muscle test<br>• Individual exercise program to relax, limber, stretch, and strengthen muscles<br><br>TRIGGER POINTS<br>• Treat trigger points before starting exercise program<br>• Needle with lidocaine or saline | MEDICAL EVALUATION<br>• Obtain endocrine workup<br>• Treat obesity<br><br>PSYCHOLOGICAL<br>• Neurosis<br>• Anxiety<br>• Tension states<br><br>EXERCISE PROGRAM AND POSTURAL CHANGES<br>• Change work habits<br>• Specific exercise program with appropriate "warm-up" and "cool-down" periods<br>• Weight control |

From: Rachlin ES: *Myofascial pain and fibromyalgia, trigger point management.* Chicago: Mosby, 1994, p. 175.

into the trigger point. Physiological saline is considered to be a more appropriate fluid for injection therapy than local anesthetic since it is less likely to produce side effects.

Treatment was aimed at focal tender areas in the muscles. These areas have an altered consistency and are known as trigger points.[2]

DISCUSSION: Although pain relief can generally be assumed to be associated with the local anesthetic effect of the fluid injected, the study shows that the pain relief is more likely to be due to reflex muscle relaxation produced by stimulation of a reflex arc, the afferent path of which includes the muscle spindles and the free nerve endings in the tissue.

COMMENT: The study included neck, shoulder, lumbar, and gluteal pain. It does not describe the technique for trigger point injection or the type of follow-up care given. It suggests the relief of symptoms by relief of muscle spasm.

2. "Treatment of Chronic Back Pain. Comparing Cortocosteroid-Lignocaine Injections with Lignocaine Alone," by I.H.J. Bourne, MBE, MD, FRCGP (30)

SUMMARY: A trial comparing the results of injecting 57 patients suffering from chronic back pain with corticosteroid-lignocaine mixture or lignocaine alone gave excellent results in 80 percent of 30 patients treated with the mixture and in only 16 percent of 19 patients treated with lignocaine alone. All the patients had failed to benefit from other treatments.[3]

COMMENT: The study concerns chronic back pain, not acute pain. The term *chronic* is not defined. The article has no muscle relevance to the issue at hand. Steroids may cause muscle fiber damage. I do not use them for the injection of myofascial trigger points.

3. "A Prospective. Randomized, Double-Blind Evaluation of Trigger-Point Injection Therapy for Low-Back Pain," by Timothy A. Garvey, M.D., Michael R. Marks, M.D., and Sam W. Weisel, M.D. (31)

SUMMARY: The efficacy of trigger point injection therapy in treatment of low back strain was evaluated in a prospective, randomized, double-blind study. The patient population consisted of 63 individuals with low back strain. Patients with this diagnosis and nonradiating low back pain, normal neurologic examination, absence of ten-

sion signs, and lumbosacral roentgenograms interpreted as being within normal limits. They were treated conservatively for 4 weeks before entering the study. Injection therapy was of four different types: lidocaine, lidocaine combined with a steroid, acupuncture, and vapocoolant spray with acupressure. Results indicated that therapy without injected medication (63 percent improvement rate) was at least as effective as therapy with drug injection (42 percent improvement rate), at a p value of 0.009. Trigger point therapy seems to be a useful adjunct in treatment of low back strain. The injected substance apparently is not the critical factor, since direct mechanical stimulus to the trigger point seems to give symptomatic relief equal to that of treatment with various types of injected medication.

Topical vapocoolant, followed by acupressure or acupuncture, resulted in the greatest pain relief of the four methods used.[4]

COMMENT: The study included only 1- and 2-week post-treatment follow-up evaluations.

4. "Injection of Steroids and Local Anaesthetics as Therapy for Low Back Pain," by Michael Sonne, Kjeld Christensen, Sven Erik Hansen, and Erik Martin Jensen (32)

SUMMARY: Thirty patients with low back pain of at least 1 month's duration were included in a double-blind controlled study with third-party administration and treated with either methylprednisolone acetate mixed with lignocaine or oxotonic saline, injected at the site of the iliolumbar ligament. The treatment was evaluated by a visual analogue scale, range of spinal flexion ad modum Wright & Moll, and of the patients' self-assessments. In the methylprednisolone group, significant decreases in pain score and in patients' self-assessments were found. The range of spinal flexion did not undergo any significant change. No significant changes were found in the control group. No side effects were observed during the study. The study suggests that certain inflammatory changes in the lumbar ligaments could be the origin of pain in some patients with persistent low back pain.

The study considers chronic pain as pain persisting 4 weeks or more. The study included 2–week follow-up after treatment. It relates to the injection of ligaments rather than myofascial muscular trigger points.[5]

---

[2]From Frost FA, Jenssen B, Singgarrd-Anderson J. "A control double-blind comparison of mepivacaine injection versus saline injection for myofascial pain," *Lancet* 1980; 8167–8168.

[3]From Bourne IHJ, "Treatment of chronic back pain. Comparing corticosteroid-lignocaine injections with lignocaine alone." *The Practitioner* 1985; 228:333–338.

[4]From Garvey TA, Marks MR, Wiesel SW. "A prospective randomized, double-blind evaluation of trigger-point injection therapy for low back pain," Department of Orthopedic Surgery, The George Washington University Medical Center, Washington, D.C., and The Cleveland Clinic, Cleveland, Ohio, 1989:962–964.

[5]From Christensen K, Hansen SE, Jensen EM, Sonne M: "Injection of steroids and local anaesthetics as therapy for low back pain," Department of Rheumatology, H. Bispebjerg Hospital,1985; 14:343–345.

5. "Iliac Crest Pain Syndrome in Low Back Pain. A Double Blind, Randomized Study of Local Injection Therapy," by Gerrit Collee, Ben A.C. Dijkmans, Jan P. Vandenbroucke, and Arnold Cats (33).

SUMMARY: In a 2–week, double-blind, randomized study we compared the efficiency of a single local injection of 5 ml lignocaine, 0.5% (L) with 5 ml isotonic saline (S) in 41 patients with the iliac crest pain syndrome (ICPS) recruited from a rheumatology clinic and a general practice. For the purpose of comparing both treatments, two major outcome variables at the end of the study were defined at the outset: 1– Pain score. In the L group the mean pain score at day 14 was 30.5, in the S group, 43.8; the difference between both treatment groups was significant ($p < 0.05$). On subgroup analysis, similar results were found in the rheumatology setting ($p < 0.05$) but not in the general practice setting (NS). 2– Pain severity compared with baseline. In the L group 52 percent of patients improved and in the S group, 30 percent. In the general practice clinic there was no significant difference (44 vs. 62 percent); however, in the rheumatology setting 58 percent of those treated with L were improved compared with 8 percent in the S group ($p < 0.01$). The data demonstrate an effect of a local injection with lignocaine that is somewhat larger than an injection with saline, which also has some beneficial effect. The difference is evident in the rheumatology setting but not in the general practice setting.

The study included one group of patients with long-standing back pain (median duration of low back pain 8 years) and a group with back pain of short duration (median duration of low back pain 18 days). A single injection was used. In the rheumatology group of patients treated with lignocaine, a beneficial effect continued for at least 2 months and within 80 percent of cases. (Note: It is not well understood why an injection of a short-acting anesthetic such as lignocaine provides prolonged pain relief. Explanations include "breaking reflex mechanisms.") It is not clear if the injection was into muscle or ligamentous attachments.[6]

COMMENT: The study is confusing concerning injection technique into muscle or ligament. The study suggests that "spasm" is being treated rather than any histopathological structure.

6. "A New Approach to the Treatment of Chronic Low Back Pain," by Milne J. Ongley, Thomas A. Dorman, Robert G. Klein, Bjorn C. Eek, Lawrence J. Hubert (34).

SUMMARY: Eighty-one patients with chronic low back pain (average duration 10 years) were randomized to two treatment groups. Forty patients received an empirically devised regimen of forceful spinal manipulation and injections of a dextrose-glycerine-phenol (proliferant) solution into soft tissue structures as part of a program to decrease pain and disability. The other 41 patients received parallel treatment in which the main differences were less extensive initial local anesthesia and manipulation, and substitution of saline for proliferant. Neither patients nor assessors knew which treatment had been given. When assessed by disability scores, the experimental group had greater improvement than the control group at 1 month ($p < 0.001$), 3 months ($p < 0.004$), and 6 months ($p < 0.001$) from the end of treatments; at 6 months an improvement of more than 50 percent was recorded in 35 of the experimental group versus 16 of the control group and the numbers free from disability were 15 and 4, respectively ($p < 0.003$). Visual analogue pain scores and pain diagrams likewise showed significant advantages for the experimental regimen.[7]

COMMENT: This study in chronic pain included injection of ligaments (supraspinous, intraspinous, iliolumbar, and sacroiliac ligaments). In addition to injection, manipulation was performed. It is not an appropriate study to evaluate myofascial trigger points in acute low back pain.

*S*ummary

The AHCPR guidelines concluded that "based on limited research evidence in studies that included patients with chronic problems, the efficacy of trigger point or ligamentous injections for treating acute low back problems appears equivocal. The injections can expose patients to serious potential complications."

Trigger points do exist in the acute stage of low back pain. Sometimes they may be masked by the presence of muscle spasm. In the acute stage of low back pain, local areas may represent muscle spasm or muscle irritability.

Injection for muscle spasm may sometimes be indicated in the acute stage. A course of physical therapy can be prescribed that would include techniques involving spray and stretch, electrical stimulation, relaxation tech-

[6]From Collee G, Dijkmans B, Cats A, Vandenbroucke JP. Iliac crest pain syndrome in low back pain. A double- blind, randomized study of local injection therapy. *J Rheumatol* 1991; 18:(7):1060–1063.

[7]From Dorman TA, Eek BC, Hubert LJ, Klein RG, Ongley MJ. A new approach to the treatment of chronic low back pain. *Lancet* July 1987; 18:143–146.

niques, and limbering exercises. If localized tenderness and muscle shortening persist, trigger point injection should be performed, followed by a physical therapy program. Precipitating factors should be evaluated. The relief of acute low back pain is not the end of treatment. An understanding of perpetuating factors and a follow-up exercise program are vital in order to prevent recurrences. Trigger point injections do not expose patients to serious potential complications when done properly. They are a safe and effective procedure to be used as an adjunct in the management of acute and chronic low back pain.

# References

1. Kraus H. *Diagnosis and treatment of muscle pain.* Chicago: Quintessence, 1988:41.
2. Rachlin ES. *Musculofascial pain and fibromyalgia, trigger point management.* Chicago: Mosby, 1994:8–9.
3. Rachlin ES. Musculofascial pain syndromes. *Medical Times: The Journal of Family Medicine* January 1984; 166.
4. Travell JG, Simons DG. *Myofascial pain and dysfunction. The trigger point manual.* Baltimore: Williams & Wilkins, 1983:8.
5. Travell JG, Simons DG. *Myofascial pain and dysfunction. The trigger point manual.* Baltimore: Williams & Wilkins, 1983:35.
6. Kellgren JH. Deep pain sensibility. *Lancet* 1949; 1:943–949.
7. Travell JG, Simons DG. *Myofascial pain and dysfunction. The trigger point manual.* Baltimore: Williams & Wilkins, 1983:19.
8. Lange M. *Die Muskelharten (Myogelosen).* Munich: Lehmann, 1931.
9. Gutstein M. Diagnosis and treatment of muscular rheumatism. *Br J Phys Med* 1938; 1:302–321.
10. Sola AE, Kuitert JH. Myofascial trigger point pain in the neck and shoulder girdle. *Northwest Medicine* 1955; 54:980–984.
11. Sola AE, Rodenberger MS, Gettys BB. Incidence of hypersensitive areas in posterior shoulder muscles: A survey of two hundred young adults. *Am J Phys Med* 1955; 34:585–590.
12. Fishbain DA, Goldberg M, Dykstra D, et al. DSM-III diagnoses of patients with myofascial pain sydrome fibrositis. *Arch Phys Med Rehabil* 1989; 70:433–438.
13. Fishbain DA, Goldberg M, Dykstra D, et al. DSM-III diagnoses of patients with myofascial pain syndrome fibrositis. *Arch Phys Med Rehabil* 1989; 70:433–438.
14. Kraus H. *Clinical treatment of back and neck pain.* New York: McGraw-Hill, 1970.
15. Rachlin ES. Musculofascial pain syndromes. *Medical Times: The Journal of Family Medicine* January 1984: 34–47.
16. Rubin D. Myofascial trigger point syndromes: An approach to management. *Arch Phys Med Rehabil* 1981; 62:107–110.
17. Gutstein M. Diagnosis and treatment of muscular rheumatism. *Br J Phys Med* 1938; 1:302–321.
18. Sola AE, Kuitert JH. Myofascial triggerpoint pain in the neck and shoulder girdle. *Northwest Medicine* 1955; 54:980–984.
19. Sola AE, Rodenberger MS, Gettys BB. Incidence of hypersensitive areas in posterior shoulder muscles: A survey of two hundred young adults. *Am J Phys Med* 1955; 34:585–590.
20. Travell JG, Simons DG. *Myofascial pain and dysfunction. The trigger point manual.* Baltimore: Williams & Wilkins, 1983:25.
21. Yunus MB, Masi AT, Calabro JJ, et al. Primary fibromyalgia (fibrositis): Clinical study of 50 patients with matched normal controls. *Sem Arthritis Rheum* 1981; 11:151–171.
22. Rachlin ES. *Myofascial pain and fibromyalgia, trigger point management.* Chicago: Mosby, 1994:151.
23. Sola AE, Rodenberger MS, Gettys BB. Incidence of hypersensitive areas in posterior shoulder muscles: A survey of two hundred young adults. *Am J Phys Med* 1955; 34:585–590.
24. Kraus Hans. *Diagnosis and treatment of muscle pain.* Chicago: Quintessence, 1988:91.
25. Rachlin ES. *Myofascial pain and fibromyalgia, trigger point management.* Chicago: Mosby, 1994:48.
26. Kraus H. *Clinical treatment of back and neck pain.* New York: McGraw-Hill, 1970.
27. Travell JG, Simons DG. *Myofascial pain and dysfunction. The trigger point manual.* Baltimore: Williams & Wilkins, 1983:103.
28. Lange M. *Die Muskelharten (Myogelosen).* Munich: Lehmann, 1931.
29. Frost FA, Jessen B, Singgarrd-Andersen J. A control double-blind comparison of mepivacaine injection versus saline injection for myofascial pain. *Lancet* 1980; 8167– 8168.
30. Bourne IHJ. Treatment of chronic back pain. Comparing corticosteroid-lignocaine injections with lignocaine alone. *Practitioner* 1984; 228:333–338.
31. Garvey TA, Marks MR, Wiesel SW. A prospective, randomized, double-blind evaluation of trigger-point injection therapy for low-back pain. *Department of Orthopedic Surgery, The George Washington University Medical Center, Washington, DC and The Cleveland Clinic, Cleveland, Ohio.* 1989; 962–964.
32. Christensen K, Hansen SE, Jensen EM, Sonne M. Injection of steroids and local anaesthetics as therapy for low back pain. *Department of Rheumatology, Bispebjerg Hospital* 1985; 14.343–345.
33. Collee G, Dijkmans B, Cats A, Vandenbroucke JP. Iliac crest pain syndrome in low back pain. A double-blind, randomized study of local injection therapy. *J Rheumatol* 1991; 18:(7):1060–1063.
34. Dorman TA, Eek BC, Hubert LJ, Klein RG, Ongley MJ. A new approach to the treatment of chronic low back pain. *Lancet* July 1987; 18:143–146.

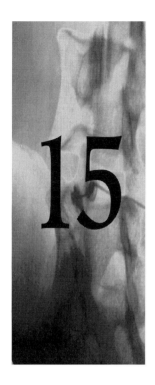

# 15 The Use of Medications

*Gerard A. Malanga, M.D.*

**P**ain is generally the chief complaint of individuals experiencing a musculoskeletal injury, and this is especially true for those presenting with disorders of the low back. Treatment of the low back pain patient often includes a progressive rehabilitation process that initially addresses local pain and inflammation before proceeding to improve range of motion, enhance strength and endurance, and ultimately a return to full activity. Successful control of pain is an essential initial goal in preparing the patient both physically and emotionally for further intervention and therapeutic exercise. Active communication with the patient is especially important during the initial treatment period as a tolerable pain level will vary in each individual.

Pain, however, should be regarded as a component of a symptom complex resulting from an underlying pathological process affecting the low back. This is similar to the cardiologist investigating a patient with congestive heart failure who seeks to determine the etiology of an underlying cardiomyopathy. The clinician caring for the back pain patient should also strive to establish a diagnosis that includes an identification of the causative dis-

order. While typically not as precise as the cardiologist in establishing a diagnosis, an understanding of functional anatomy, biomechanics, and kinesiology can help in localizing the patient's pain generators. Are the affected tissues likely bone, disc, tendon, muscle, ligament, or nerve? Is the underlying process biomechanical, inflammatory or infectious, neoplastic, or perhaps more psychological in nature? These questions are not discussed in the Agency for Health Care Policy Research (AHCPR) Guidelines for Managing Acute Low Back Pain and should be addressed prior to initiating treatment.

The answers to these questions will guide the physician toward the proper initial treatment of the low back problem, including the most appropriate choice of medications prescribed. By applying the principles of medication use in other musculoskeletal disorders, we can more strategically plan an efficacious use of pharmacological agents.

In this chapter, several classes of commonly prescribed drugs for the treatment of low back pain are considered. For each agent or group of agents considered, mechanisms of action, efficacy and current clinical research, dosing and cost, and complications and contraindications are addressed. A response to the Agency for Health Care Policy Research (AHCPR) findings and recommendations for each of the oral medications considered are included.

## ACETAMINOPHEN

Acetaminophen is the principal member of the group of drugs classified as para-aminophenol derivatives. In the late 1800s acetanilide and phenacetin were utilized for their antipyretic and analgesic properties, but significant toxicity was associated with their use. In 1949 acetaminophen became recognized as the primary active metabolite of both acetanilide and phenacetin and has now become a popular and clinically proven analgesic and antipyretic (1).

While the analgesic and antipyretic effects of acetaminophen are equal to those of aspirin, its anti-inflammatory effects are weak. Its therapeutic effects appear to be secondary to an inhibition of prostaglandin biosynthesis with a resultant increase in the pain threshold and modulation of the hypothalamic heat regulating center. The effects of acetaminophen are noted predominantly centrally and less peripherally, where it serves as only a weak inhibitor of cyclooxygenase and does not inhibit the activation of neutrophils as do other NSAIDs (1,2). The AHCPR recommends acetaminophen as a safe and acceptable medication in the treatment of acute low back pain (3).

In the setting of acute low back pain, acetaminophen can be effectively utilized as an analgesic. Several studies have shown acetaminophen to be superior to placebo in the treatment of osteoarthritis pain, and because of its efficacy it has been recommended as a first-line agent in osteoarthritis treatment (4,5,6). A 1991 study by Bradley and colleagues compared the analgesic properties of acetaminophen to ibuprofen in the treatment of pain associated with osteoarthritis of the knee. Over a four-week study period, acetaminophen was found to be as efficacious as both low dose analgesic and high dose anti-inflammatory regimens of ibuprofen in providing both pain relief and improved functional outcome (7). In a 1982 study, paracetamol, a compound similar to acetaminophen, was compared to diflunisal, an NSAID and salicylate derivative, in the treatment of chronic low back pain. Thirty patients with a six month to several year history of low back pain presumed secondary to facet pathology were treated in a randomized fashion for four weeks, and more favorable outcomes were associated with NSAID use (8).

The accepted oral dose of acetaminophen is 325–1,000 mg every four to six hours, with a 24-hour use not to exceed 4,000 mg. Peak plasma levels and analgesic effects are typically noted from 30 to 60 minutes following ingestion. Acetaminophen is generally available without prescription and is relatively inexpensive (1). While erythematous or urticarial skin rashes are occasionally observed, the most serious adverse effect of acute acetaminophen overdosage is hepatotoxicity. In adults hepatotoxicity may result from a single dose of 10 to 15 grams. More chronic abuse of acetaminophen has been associated with nephrotoxicity (1,2).

The analgesic effects of acetaminophen make it an acceptable medication in the treatment of acute low back pain. It is inexpensive and its use is typically without complications. While effective against mild to moderate pain in some acute back pain situations, it lacks other desirable effects in treating inflammation, muscle spasm, or sleep disturbance. Its efficacy as an analgesic for low back disorders associated with severe pain is questionable. This author agrees with the AHCPR recommendations that acetaminophen use is typically safe; however, its efficacy in low back pain treatment is often inadequate and has been tried by most patients prior to evaluation by a physician.

## NSAIDS

Aspirin is the prototypical member of the group of medications known as nonsteroidal anti-inflammatory drugs (NSAIDs). The glycoside salicin was first isolated in 1829 from willow bark and became recognized for its antipyretic effects. Products of salicin were converted to acetylsalicylic acid, which became recognized for its anti-inflammatory effects and was introduced as aspirin in 1899 (1). In 1984 nearly one in seven Americans was treated with an anti-inflammatory agent, and in 1986 nearly 100 million prescriptions for NSAIDs were written, resulting in worldwide annual sales estimated at $1 billion (9,10).

The primary mechanism of action of NSAIDs is a reduction of cyclooxygenase activity and a resultant decrease in prostaglandin synthesis. Prostaglandins are active mediators of the inflammatory cascade that also serve to sensitize peripheral nociceptors. A reduction in the local concentration of prostaglandins could therefore explain the combined anti-inflammatory and analgesic properties of NSAIDs (11). In single doses most of the NSAIDs are more effective analgesics than a single dose of acetaminophen or aspirin (12). Locally, NSAIDs are also thought to combat inflammation by inhibiting neutrophil function and interfering with the activity of enzymes such as phospholipase C (9). Most NSAIDs do not decrease the production of lipoxygenase-produced leukotrienes, which are also believed to significantly contribute to the inflammatory response (1). A disparity between the anti-inflammatory and analgesic potencies of these agents in clinical practice has been observed, and

**TABLE 15–1**
*Commonly prescribed nonsteroidal anti-inflammatory drugs (NSAIDs)*

| DRUG AND FAMILY | MAX DAILY DOSE (MG) | USUAL SINGLE DOSE (MG) | DOSING | HALF-LIFE (HRS) | $/MONTH |
|---|---|---|---|---|---|
| SALICYLATES | | | | | |
| Aspirin | 4,000 | 500–1,000 | q4–6h | 12 | 15 |
| Non-acetylated Salicylates | | | | | |
| Salsalate (Disalcid, others) | 4,000 | 1,000 | q8–12h | 16 | 30 |
| Diflunisal (Dolobid) | 1,500 | 1,000, 500 | q8–12h | 8–12 | 30–45 |
| Choline Mg trisalicylate (Trilisate) | 3,000 | 1,000–1500 | q8–12h | 9–17 | 40–120 |
| PROPRIONIC ACIDS | | | | | |
| Ibuprofen (Motrin, others) | 2400 | 200–400 | q4–6h | 2 | 30–80 |
| Flurbiprofen (Ansaid) | 300 | 50–100 | q6–8 | 5–7 | 50–150 |
| Fenoprofen (Nalfon) | 1,200 | 200 | q4–6 | 3 | 50–125 |
| Ketoprofen (Orudis, others) | 300 | 25–75 | q4–8h | 2–4 | 90–180 |
| Naproxen (Naprosyn) | 1,250 | 500, 250 | q6–8 | 13 | 44–80 |
| Naproxen Na (Anaprox) | 1,375 | 550, 275 | q12h | 13 | 44–80 |
| INDOLES | | | | | |
| Indomethacin (Indocin) | 150 | 25–50 | q6–8h | 4–5 | 35–100 |
| Sulindac (Clinoril) | 400 | 150–200 | q12h | 8 | 45–90 |
| Tolmetin (Tolectin) | 1,800 | 150–600 | q6–8h | 2–5 | 30–90 |
| Etodolac (Lodine) | 1,200 | 200–400 | q6–8h | 3–11 | 70–175 |
| FENAMATES | | | | | |
| Meclofenamate (Meclomen) | 400 | 100 | q6–8h | 2 | 54–162 |
| OTHERS | | | | | |
| Piroxicam (Feldene) | 40 | 20 | q24h | 50 | 80–160 |
| Nabumetone (Relafen) | 2,000 | 1,000 | q12–24h | 24 | 60–120 |
| Ketorolac (Toradol) | 40 | 10 | q6h | 4–7 | 60–120 |
| Oxaprozin (Daypro) | 1,800 | 1,200 | q24h | 24 | 70–120 |

(2, 11, 12, 63 )

recent data have suggested that pain relief from NSAIDs may in part be secondary to a more central antinociceptive component (13,14,15,16). Measurable levels of anti-inflammatory agents are appreciated in the CSF following short-term administration in the setting of a soft tissue injury (17).

NSAIDs include aspirin, which inhibits cyclooxygenase irreversibly through acetylation, and several groups of organic acids, including proprionic acid derivatives, acetic acid derivatives, and enolic acids, all of which bind to and reversibly inhibit cyclooxygenase (see Table 15–1).

Elimination half-lives of these drugs range from less than four hours for some proprionic acid derivatives to greater than 40 hours for piroxicam (11). The AHCPR recommends aspirin and NSAIDs as acceptable agents in the treatment of acute low back pain, but comments that the decision to use these drugs needs to be guided by an awareness of their potential side effects (3).

In a recent survey by McCormack and Brune of 26 studies investigating the role of NSAIDs in acute soft tissue injuries, 14 double blind placebo controlled studies were found to demonstrate a significant difference between NSAID and placebo for nine NSAIDs—clonixin, ketoprofen , naproxen , diclofenac, fenbufen, ibuprofen, indomethacin, piroxicam, and azapropazone. In those studies in which physical therapy was also administered, four NSAIDs—azapropazone, clonixin, naproxen, and ketoprofen—were demonstrated to provide unequivocal additional benefit (18). In a similar review of investigations of NSAIDs and sports-related soft tissue injuries, Weiler concluded that benefits were typically observed among treatment groups when compared with controls. These short-term studies have found that treated athletes return to practice quicker and without any apparent significant delay in the injury healing process (10). In 1987 Amlie and colleagues (19) studied the effects of seven days of oral piroxicam treatment in 278 patients with acute low back pain. Medication administration was commenced within 48 hours of symptom onset, and after three days of therapy patients in the treatment group revealed a significant amount of pain relief. After seven days the difference in pain symptoms between the treatment group and control group was no longer significant, but the treatment group demonstrated a significantly lower requirement for additional analgesics and a greater return to work rate. In a 1981 study patients with rheumatoid arthritis were found to experience little difference in symptom relief when treated with six individual NSAIDs, while in patients with ankylosing spondylitis, naproxen, indomethacin, and fenoprofen were found to be most effective (20).

The dosing and cost of each NSAID vary significantly by chemical family and agent (see Table 15–1). The choice of initial anti-inflammatory agent remains largely empirical. Aspirin is generally very inexpensive, and the newer NSAIDs often cost significantly more. In addition to cost considerations, patients have been observed to be more compliant with those agents that require less frequent dosing (20). Since steady states of plasma concentration are not typically observed until dosing has been continued for a period of three to five half-lives, plateau concentrations and maximal therapeutic effects are not realized as quickly in those agents with longer half-lives unless a loading dose is first prescribed (9). By first prescribing a loading dose, which is not often done in clinical settings, and then maintaining regular dosing as indicated for each agent, adequate plasma levels will be achieved for the anti-inflammatory abilities of these medications to be realized. Prescribing NSAIDs in lower dosages and on a less regular schedule is more likely to yield only the analgesic properties of these agents (1,9). Large variations in patient response to different NSAIDs are observed even when chemically similar drugs of a common family are prescribed (1). Over a one- to two-week period the dose may be increased to the recommended maximum, and after that time, if the results remain unsatisfactory, a different agent

should be tried (9). Side effects generally develop within the initial weeks of treatment, although gastric complications can develop at later times. Combination therapy with more than one NSAID is to be avoided as the incidence of side effects is additive and there is little evidence of added benefit to the patient (1).

Several complications are associated with NSAID use. As nonselective inhibitors of cyclooxygenase-2 (COX-2), whose activity is induced in the setting of active inflammation, and cyclooxygenase-1 (COX-1), which is responsible for thromboxane and prostaglandin synthesis and the maintenance of normal gastrointestinal mucosa, NSAIDs are commonly observed to alter gastrointestinal physiology. While dyspepsia is a very common complication, erosion, ulceration, and hemorrhage may also develop without warning symptoms (1,9). The development of NSAIDs that selectively inhibit COX-2 would theoretically provide a much safer anti-inflammatory agent. There is some evidence that nabumetone, which preferentially inhibits COX-2, is associated with a lower incidence of gastrointestinal side effects (21). Misoprostol, a synthetic prostaglandin E1 analogue, has been shown to reduce the likelihood of gastroduodenal erosion during the administration of aspirin (22). As prostaglandins also participate in the autoregulation of renal blood flow and glomerular filtration, numerous renal side effects, including acute renal failure, have been associated with NSAID use. The kidneys are most vulnerable in those individuals who might enter a hypovolemic state or in whom there is preexisting renal disease (9). While the association between NSAID use and minimal change glomerulonephropathy has been recognized, a recent study suggests that nephrotic syndrome due to membranous nephropathy should also be recognized as a possible reaction to NSAID use (23). All NSAIDs can cause central nervous system side effects such as drowsiness, dizziness, and confusion (12). Blockade of platelet aggregation, inhibition of uterine contractility, interference with antihypertensive medications, and hypersensitivity reactions are also side effects shared by many of the commonly prescribed anti-inflammatory agents (1). Some variability with regard to adverse effects has been recognized among the NSAIDs. While the non-acetylated salicylates do not prolong bleeding time and have rarely been associated with gastrointestinal complications, indomethacin has more frequently been associated with nausea, gastrointestinal bleeding, and headaches (24). NSAIDs have less potential for abuse than opioids; physical dependence on these medications has not been reported (12).

Recent studies have investigated the effects of NSAID use on the healing process of injured soft tissue, namely muscle and tendon, which they are often prescribed to treat. Almekinders investigated the *in vitro* effects of indomethacin on isolated human fibroblasts subjected to repetitive motion injury. NSAID use in this

| | TABLE 15–2 Commonly prescribed "muscle relaxants" | | |
|---|---|---|---|
| **MEDICATION** | **MECHANISM OF ACTION** | **DOSAGE** | **CONTRAINDICATIONS** |
| **MUSCLE RELAXANTS** Carisoprodol (Soma) | Blockage of interneuronal activity in reticular formation and spinal cord | 350 mg tid and hs | Acute intermittent porphyria |
| Chlorzoxazone (Parafon Forte) | Inhibition of polysynaptic reflex arcs at subcortical and spinal cord levels | 250–750 mg tid–qid | |
| Cyclobenzaprine (Flexeril) | Inhibition of alpha and gamma motor neuron activity at brainstem level | 10 mg tid | Cardiac disease, hyperthyroidism, use with MAO inhibitors |
| Methocarbamol (Robaxin) | Unknown, possible general central nervous system depression | 1,000–1,500 mg qid | |
| **BENZODIAZEPINES** Diazepam (Valium) | Depresses activity in limbic system, thalamus, hypothalamus | 2–10 mg tid–qid | Acute narrow angle glaucoma |

(2, 11)

study was associated with decreased DNA synthesis during the early proliferative healing phase but with increased protein synthesis during the later remodeling phase of healing (25). In an earlier investigation of the effects of piroxicam on the healing of rat tibialis anterior muscle subjected to strain injury, histological observation revealed a delay in the early inflammatory reactions and regeneration within the muscle tissue of the treated group. At 11 days following injury, both treated and controlled groups demonstrated similar extents of regeneration and failure loads (26). A study investigating the effects of flurbiprofen treatment on the recovery of eccentrically injured rabbit muscle revealed treated muscles to demonstrate initial histological and contractile gains but a subsequent functional loss (27). The effect of NSAIDs on chondrocyte function and the cartilage matrix has similarly been investigated (24). As these apparently timedependent effects of NSAID use on soft tissue recovery are further realized, a more scientific approach to the prescription of anti-inflammatory agents will likely arise.

This author is in agreement with the AHCPR recommendations that NSAIDs are a reasonable choice as a first-line agent for the control of acute low back pain. The patient is most likely to benefit from their combined analgesic and anti-inflammatory properties during the first week after injury onset. The anti-inflammatory properties of these agents are better attained when therapy is ini-

tiated with a loading dose and the recommended dosages are then continued at regular intervals. The prescribing physician needs to be aware of the adverse effects often associated with NSAID use. Prolonged use of anti-inflammatory medications, i.e., greater than three to four weeks, in the setting of acute low back pain is generally not indicated and should be avoided.

## MUSCLE RELAXANTS

In 1946 the discovery of mephenesin created an interest in medications that produced reversible paralysis in animals without gross sedation. With mephenesin as their prototype, muscle relaxants, which are thought to relax skeletal muscle through actions on the central nervous system (CNS) (see Table 15–2), have evolved over the past decades (29). The muscle relaxing properties of these agents arise not from direct activity at the muscular or neuromuscular junction level but rather from an inhibition of more central polysynaptic neuronal events. These agents have also been shown in some studies to demonstrate superior analgesia to either acetaminophen or aspirin, and it remains uncertain if muscle spasm is a prerequisite to their effectiveness as analgesics (11). Muscle relaxants are often prescribed in the treatment of acute low back pain in an attempt to improve the initial limitations in range of motion from muscle spasm and to interrupt the pain-spasm-pain cycle. Limiting muscle spasm and improving range of motion may prepare the patient for therapeutic exercise (29).

The AHCPR findings suggest that, in the treatment of acute low back pain, while superior to placebo, muscle relaxants do not likely provide any additional benefit when prescribed either in place of or in combination with NSAIDs. The AHCPR also cautions the prescribing physician to carefully consider the frequently observed side effects of sedation associated with their use (3).

In an attempt to determine the mechanism of action of carisoprodol in the treatment of low back pain, a double blind study was carried out comparing its effectiveness to that of a sedative control, butabarbital, and a placebo in the treatment of 48 laborers with acute lumbar pain. Carisoprodol was found to be significantly more effective in providing both subjective pain relief and objective improvements in range of motion when evaluated by finger to floor testing. The results of this study suggest that the effects of carisoprodol are not secondary to its sedative effects alone (30).

In 1989 Basmajian compared the effectiveness of cyclobenzaprine alone with diflunisal, placebo, and a combination of cylcobenzaprine and diflunisal in the treatment of acute low back pain and spasm. During the ten-day study period, the combined treatment group demonstrated significantly superior improvements in global ratings on day four, but not on days two or seven. This study suggested some effectiveness of combined analgesic and muscle relaxant therapy when utilized early in the initial week of pain onset (31). Borenstein compared the effects of combined cyclobenzaprine and naproxen with naproxen alone and also found combination therapy to be superior in reducing tenderness, spasm, and range of motion in patients presenting with ten days or less of low back pain and spasm. Adverse effects, predominantly drowsiness, were noted in 12 of 20 in the combined group and only four of 20 treated with naproxen alone (32).

Cyclobenzaprine and carisoprodol were compared in the treatment of patients with acute thoracolumbar pain and spasm rated moderate to severe and of no longer than seven days' duration. Both drugs were found to be effective, without significant differences between the treatment groups. Significant improvements were noted in physician rated mobility and in patients' visual analogue scores on follow-up days four and eight. While 60 percent of patients experienced adverse effects in the form of drowsiness or fatigue, these differences were not significantly different between groups, and only 8 percent of patients from each group discontinued treatment (29). Baratta found cyclobenzaprine, 10 mg tid, superior to placebo in a randomized, double blind study of 120 patients with acute low back pain presenting within five days of symptom onset. Significant improvement was noted in range of motion, tenderness to palpation, and pain scores on follow-up days two through nine. Sixty percent of treatment group patients reported drowsiness or dizziness compared with 25 percent of those in the placebo group (33).

In an earlier study, diazepam was found to offer no significant subjective or objective benefit, when compared to placebo, in patients treated for low back pain (34). Carisoprodol was found to be superior to diazepam in the treatment of patients with *at least moderately severe* low back pain and spasm of no longer than seven days' duration. In this study the overall incidence of adverse reactions was higher in the diazepam treated group but was not of statistical significance (35).

Muscle spasm of local origin needs to be clinically differentiated from spasticity and sustained muscle contraction in the setting of CNS and upper motor neuron injury. Baclofen and dantrolene sodium are two agents whose use is indicated in the setting of spasticity of CNS etiology. Dantrolene sodium is of particular interest as its mechanism of action is purely at the muscular level, where it serves to inhibit the release of calcium from the sarcoplasmic reticulum (2). Casale studied the effectiveness of dantrolene sodium, 25 mg daily, in the treatment of low back pain and found patients to demonstrate significant improvements in visual analogue scores, pain behavior, and EMG evaluations of *antalgic reflex motor unit firing*, when compared with the placebo group. The findings of this study are interesting in that it demonstrated improvement secondary to a pure muscle relaxant that does not possess other outside antinociceptive properties (36). Baclofen is a derivative of gamma-aminobutyric acid (GABA) and is believed to inhibit mono- and polysynaptic reflexes at the spinal level (2). Treatment with baclofen was compared to placebo in a double blind, randomized study of 200 patients with acute low back pain (37). Patients with initially severe discomfort were found to benefit from baclofen, 30–80 mg daily, on days four and ten of follow-up. Forty-nine percent of treatment patients complained of sleepiness, 38 percent of nausea, and 17 percent discontinued treatment.

Muscle relaxants (see Table 15–2) have gained wide acceptance in the treatment of acute musculoskeletal pain. Sedation is the most commonly reported adverse effect. These drugs should be used with caution in patients driving motor vehicles or operating heavy machinery. More absolute contraindications do exist to the use of carisoprodol, cyclobenzaprine, and diazepam. Rare idiosyncratic reactions have also been reported to carisoprodol and its metabolites such as meprobamate (2). Benzodiazepines have potential for abuse and their use should be avoided. By initially prescribing muscle relaxants at bedtime, the physician might take advantage of their sedative effect and minimize daytime drowsiness.

This author does not agree with the AHCPR guidelines and finds muscle relaxants to offer some additional benefits for the acute low back pain patient. These agents have been found to be effective when used in combination with an analgesic/anti-inflammatory agent within seven days of symptom onset. The prescribing physician should monitor patients receiving these medications and prescribe them for use at bedtime in an attempt to minimize daytime drowsiness and sedation often associated with their use. The use of benzodiazepines does not appear to offer any significant benefit to patients experiencing acute low back pain. Further research is needed before the role of baclofen and dantrolene sodium in the treatment of muscle spasm of local origin can be more clearly defined.

| TABLE 15–3 | |
| --- | --- |
| *Commonly prescribed opiod medications* | |
| **AGONIST DRUG** | **ORAL DOSE (MG) EQUIANALGESIC TO 20–30 MG MORPHINE** |
| Morphine | 20–30 |
| Oxycodone | 20 |
| Hydromorphone | 1.5 |
| Methadone | 10 |
| Meperidine | 75 |
| Oxymorphone | 1 |
| Levorphanol | 2 |
| ( 11 ) | |

## OPIOIDS

Opioids occupy the second rung on the World Health Organization analgesic ladder in the treatment of moderate to severe cancer pain and are commonly prescribed for postoperative pain, where they have been found to successfully treat both local and more generalized pain symptoms (11).

Opioid drugs produce analgesia by binding to multiple types of opioid receptors that are typically bound by endogenous opioid compounds. These receptors are generally classified as mu, kappa, and delta, but the opioid medications typically prescribed are morphine-like agonists that occupy the mu receptor. These receptors are located both peripherally, on sensory nerves and immune cells, and centrally, in the spinal cord and brainstem (11).

The AHCPR guidelines consider opioids as an option in the time-limited treatment of acute low back pain but suggest that they are no more effective than acetaminophen or other NSAIDSs. The AHCPR warns the prescribing physician of the potential adverse effects of opioid use, including drowsiness, impaired judgment, and the potential for physical dependence (3).

In a study by Brown and colleagues, the analgesic efficacy of diflunisal, 500 mg PO bid following a 1,000 mg loading dose, was compared to that of 300 mg of acetaminophen with 30 mg of codeine in the treatment of pain resulting from initial or recurrent low back strains. Over this 15-day trial, the analgesic efficacy of each regimen was found to be similar, but patient acceptability and tolerance were found to be superior for diflunisal. Five of 21 patients treated with acetaminophen and codeine reported adverse effects, including drowsiness, dizziness, fatigue, and nausea, compared with three of 19 patients treated with diflunisal (38). In a study of 200 patients presenting with acute

low back strain, Weisel and colleagues compared the analgesic efficacy of acetaminophen with both codeine and aspirin plus oxycodone. While all analgesic medications considered were not shown to result in a more prompt return to work, a significantly greater pain reduction, especially within the first three days of treatment, was noted for those individuals treated with codeine or aspirin plus oxycodone (39).

Additional studies have compared opioids with other analgesics in the setting of postoperative pain. Cooper found acetaminophen, 1,000 mg, in combination with oxycodone, 10 mg, to provide superior analgesia to the two combined at lower doses or either drug alone in patients experiencing postoperative dental pain (40). Acetaminophen was found to be a superior analgesic to propoxyphene in a study of 200 postpartum patients status post episiotomy (41).

For most opioids, peak drug effect occurs within one and one half to two hours following oral administration, and a second opioid dose can safely be taken two hours after the first if side effects are mild at that time. Sustained-release tablets are also available and often prove beneficial in those patients with more rapidly fluctuating pain (64). The potency of the opioid agonists are generally compared with that of morphine (see Table 15–3). Tramadol hydrochloride is a newer centrally acting analgesic that, although not chemically related to opiates, binds to mu receptors. Its mechanism of action is not completely understood, but is thought to be at least in part secondary to its inhibition of the reuptake of both serotonin and norepinephrine. Tramadol has been demonstrated to provide superior analgesia to combined acetaminophen-propoxyphene in patients experiencing severe postoperative pain, and similar analgesia, but with greater tolerability, to morphine in patients hospitalized for cancer pain (42,43). In a four-week study of 390 elderly patients with chronic pain secondary to a variety of conditions, tramadol was found to provide comparable analgesia to acetaminophen with codeine without a significant difference in associated adverse effects (44). Additional studies reveal the low abuse potential and the absence of significant respiratory depression associated with tramadol use (45,46). Individualization of tramadol dosage is recommended for those individuals either over 75 years of age, with impaired renal function, or with significant liver disease.

The goal of successful opioid prescription involves achieving a tolerable balance between analgesia and the side effects often associated with opioid use. Tolerance to adverse effects such as somnolence, nausea, and impaired thought processes typically occurs within days to weeks of initial opioid administration. Constipation is a more persistent side effect that can be managed with stool softeners and laxatives. Accumulation of normeperidine, a metabolite of meperidine, with repetitive dosing has been associated with the development of anxiety, tremors, myoclonus and generalized seizures; patients with impaired renal function are at particular risk (47). Methadone demonstrates good oral potency and a plasma half-life of 24–36 hours. Accumulation of methadone may occur with repetitive dosing, resulting in excessive sedation on days two to five (64). Physical dependence can develop after several days of administration of opioid analgesics (11).

Despite the stigmas and fears of addiction associated with their use, when properly utilized by a knowledgeable physician, opioid analgesics successfully treat otherwise intractable pain. The potential role of opioids in the treatment of nonmalignant acute low back pain is limited. While the AHCPR recommends opioids as a potential first-line agent, it is the opinion of this author that opioid use should be reserved for those patients who have either failed to obtain adequate analgesia from alternative medications, i.e., NSAIDs plus or minus a muscle relaxant, or who have contraindications to the use of other analgesics. If opioids are prescribed, a regular, rather than a PRN, dosing schedule should be prescribed, and their use should be limited to the first several days following pain onset. The prescribing physician should be aware of the possibility of dependence with more prolonged use and avoid prescribing these agents for those patients with a prior history of substance abuse.

## CORTICOSTEROIDS

The human adrenal cortex produces corticosteroids, both glucocorticoids and mineralocorticoids, and androgens. Hydrocortisone is the primary endogenous glucocorticoid, while aldosterone is the principle mineralocorticoid. The numerous effects of corticosteroids include maintenance of fluid and electrolyte balance, alterations in carbohydrate, fat, and protein metabolism, and preservation of the functions of the cardiovascular system and skeletal muscle.

Prescribed corticosteroids are typically categorized according to their relative anti-inflammatory and sodium retaining potencies (see Table 15–4). Steroid compounds that are typically prescribed for their anti-inflammatory effects often also display significant mineralocorticoid activity. Oral steroids have been found effective in the treatment of inflammatory reactions associated with allergic states, rheumatic and autoimmune diseases, and respiratory disorders. Corticosteroids interact with receptor proteins in target tissues to regulate gene expression and ultimately protein synthesis by the target tissue. As these interactions and regulatory processes occur slowly, most of the effects of corticosteroids are not immediate and become apparent hours following their introduction. Recent investigations have suggested an additional and more immediate component to corticosteroid action mediated by an interaction with membrane-bound protein receptors (1,48).

Over the past two decades, the biochemical contributions to sciatica and low back pain have been the focus of much attention (49). In the late 1970s the nuclear material of the vertebral disc was found to be antigenic and capable of producing an *in vitro* autoimmune reaction. It was hypothesized that a chemical radiculitis might explain radicular pain in the absence of a more mechanical stressor (50). Phospholipase A2 (PLA2), a potent inflammatory mediator, has been demonstrated to be released by discs following injury (51). The anti-inflammatory and immunosuppressive effects of glucocorticoids are largely secondary to their inhibition of the immune responses of lymphocytes, macrophages, and fibroblasts. Whereas NSAIDs principally inhibit prostaglandin synthesis, corticosteroids interfere earlier in the inflammatory cascade by inhibiting PLA2 actions and thereby curtailing both the leukotriene and prostaglandin mediated inflammatory response (1).

The AHCPR guidelines do not recommend the use of oral steroids in the treatment of acute low back pain. The guidelines state that severe side effects are associated with both the prolonged use of steroids and the short-term use of steroids in high dosages (3).

Studies designed to investigate the use of oral steroids in the setting of acute low back pain are limited. In 1986 Haimovic and Beresford compared oral dexamethasone with placebo in the treatment of 33 patients with lumbosacral radicular pain. Subjects receiving dexam-

**TABLE 15–4**
*Commonly prescribed oral corticosteroids*

| STEROID COMPOUND | ANTI-INFLAMMATORY POTENCY | SODIUM-RETAINING POTENCY | BIOLOGICAL HALF-LIFE (HRS) | EQUIV. DOSE (MG) |
|---|---|---|---|---|
| Cortisol | 1 | 1 | 8–12 | 20 |
| Cortisone | .8 | .8 | 8–12 | 25 |
| Prednisone | 4 | .8 | 12–36 | 5 |
| Prednisolone | 4 | .8 | 12–36 | 5 |
| 6-alpha-methyl prednisolone | 5 | .5 | 12–36 | 4 |
| Triamcinolone | 5 | 0 | 12–36 | 4 |
| Dexamethasone | 25 | 0 | 36–72 | .75 |

( 1 )

ethasone were given a tapering dose, from 64 to 8 mg over seven days. Early improvements (within seven days) were not significantly different between the two groups, occurring in 7 of 21 patients in the dexamethasone group and 4 of 12 in the placebo group. In those subjects initially found to have radicular type pain on straight leg-raising, however, 8 of 19 treated with dexamethasone, compared with only 1 of 6 in the placebo group, had diminished pain on straight leg raising repeated within 7 days. The limitations of this study include a small subject number, the use of additional analgesics that may have obscured group differences, the clinical uncertainty of a radicular process in a significant number of subjects, and the loss of several patients to follow-up after one year (52).

In the setting of acute low back pain, oral corticosteroids are typically prescribed in a quick tapering fashion over one week. The biological half-lives differ among the steroid compounds (see Table 15–4). Multiple adverse effects have been associated with prolonged steroid use, including suppression of the hypothalamic-pituitary-adrenal axis, immunosuppression, psuedotumor cerebri and psychoses, cataracts and increased intraocular pressure, osteoporosis, aseptic necrosis, gastric ulcers, fluid and electrolyte disturbances and hypertension, and impaired wound healing. The severity of these complications correlates with the dosage, duration of use, and potency of the steroid prescribed. While the incidence of steroid-induced myopathy does not appear to be directly related to the dosage of steroid prescribed or the duration of use, it appears to be more prevalent with the use of steroids containing a 9–alpha fluorine configuration, such as triamcinolone. The relationship between hypertensive side effects and duration of therapy is also not very clear;

steroids should be prescribed with greater caution in the elderly, in individuals with known hypertension, and when compounds with greater mineralocorticoid properties are prescribed. As hyperglycemia is a well-known complication of corticosteroid use, oral steroids should be avoided in the diabetic population (53).

As potent anti-inflammatory agents, oral steroids represent a theoretically useful agent in the treatment of patients with radiculopathy due to local inflammation secondary to disc injury or herniation. This author does find a use for oral steroids in the treatment of such patients who have failed a trial with oral NSAIDs. While many adverse effects are associated with oral steroid use, they are more frequently encountered in the setting of prolonged administration. The effectiveness of oral steroids in the acute low back pain population remains unproven and further research in this area is needed.

## COLCHICINE

Colchicum, a derivative of the plant *Colchicum autumnale,* was originally introduced for the treatment of gout in 1763. Benjamin Franklin, known to suffer from gout, reportedly introduced colchicum therapy in the United States. The active alkaloid, colchicine, was isolated from colchicum in 1820. By binding to tubulin, colchicine interferes with the functioning of mitotic spindles and depolymerizes fibrillar microtubules in granulocytes and other motile cells. The beneficial effects of colchicine in the treatment of gout are apparently secondary to its ability to inhibit both the metabolic and phagocytic activity and migration of granulocytes. Colchicine's inhibition of the release of histamine-containing granules from mast cells is also believed secondary to its interference with granule transportation by the microtubular system. While beneficial in the treatment of the crystal-induced inflammation observed in gout and pseudogout, colchicine is only occasionally effective in the treatment of other types of arthritides (1,54). Colchicine has been regarded by some as the most powerful anti-inflammatory agent known to man (54).

Over the past 30 years, Rask has treated thousands of patients with resistant disc disorders with oral and intravenous colchicine and has noted a 90–95 percent improvement rate. Since 1979 he has published the results of his uncontrolled studies, some involving up to 500 patients, which have suggested significant therapeutic benefits from colchicine therapy with fewer adverse effects than typically associated with the use of aspirin (54,55). In addition to the potent anti-inflammatory abilities of colchicine, other theories have been expounded in an attempt to explain its efficacy in the treatment of disc disease, including an inhibition of amyloidogenesis and an increase in endorphin production by the substantia gelatinosa (54).

The AHCPR guidelines state that the evidence of the effectiveness of colchicine in the treatment of acute low back pain is conflicting, and because of the potential for serious adverse effects, colchicine is not recommended for treating low back pain patients.

In a 1985 double blind study of 39 patients with low back pain of at least two months' duration, Meek compared combined intravenous and oral colchicine treatment with placebo. Patients in the treatment group received colchicine 0.6 mg orally bid for 14 days and 1 mg IV on days 1, 4, and 8 of the 14-day study period. While no real effect from placebo administration was observed, the treatment group demonstrated significant improvements in pain, weakness, leg raising limitations, and muscle spasm. Adverse effects from colchicine administration were documented in only one patient in the form of a burn at the IV site (54). In a double blind study of oral colchicine in the treatment of low back pain, Schnebel and Simmons compared oral colchicine with placebo in 34 patients with low back symptoms of less than three months' duration. Over the 12-week study period, both groups of patients continued in a comprehensive physical therapy program and were administered NSAIDs and muscle relaxants. No significant differences in therapeutic response were noted between the treatment and placebo groups, but an increased number of adverse effects, mainly diarrhea and vomiting, were observed in the colchicine group. This study has several limitations, including a small sample size, multiple etiologies of low back pain, poor patient compliance, and the use of concomitant treatments (55).

Colchicine use is contraindicated in patients with serious gastrointestinal, renal, hepatic, or cardiac disease. Colchicine can also harm the fetus when used during pregnancy. When administered intravenously for the treatment of an acute gouty attack, the total dosage over the first 24 hours should not exceed four milligrams, as greater cumulative dosages have been associated with multiple organ failure and death (2). Colchicine serves to inhibit the intracellular microtubules and mitotic spindles, and its adverse effects are largely secondary to its actions on the rapidly proliferating cells of the gastrointestinal epithelium. Abdominal pain, nausea, vomiting, and diarrhea are typically the earliest and most common adverse effects associated with colchicine overdosage. These gastrointestinal side effects can be almost entirely avoided with intravenous use. Colchicine has also been noted to cause a transient leukopenia, which is soon replaced with a leukocytosis. Myopathy and neuropathy have been noted in patients with impaired renal function receiving colchicine treatment (1).

The use of colchicine in the treatment of the acute low back pain patient is not common. While some practitioners have found colchicine effective in this patient population, others have not. This author is in agreement with the AHCPR recommendations on colchicine and believes further investigation in this area is needed before colchicine use can be recommended for the low back pain patient. These studies may be helpful in further defining the place of colchicine among other available anti-inflammatory and analgesic agents.

## ANTIDEPRESSANTS

The antidepressants most commonly prescribed in the United States include the tricyclic antidepressants (TCAs) and the newer selective serotonin reuptake inhibitors (SSRIs). Amitriptyline, imipramine, nortriptyline, and desipramine are representative of the TCAs, which mediate their antidepressant effects through a variable presynaptic inhibition of norepinephrine and serotonin reuptake. Fluoxetine, paroxetine, and sertraline are commonly prescribed SSRIs, which, as their name indicates, act by specifically blocking the reuptake of serotonin by the presynaptic terminal. Monoamine oxidase inhibitors (MAOIs) inhibit the activity of monoamine oxidase and thereby increase the concentrations of endogenous norepinephrine, serotonin, and epinephrine in the nervous system (56).

While several classes of antidepressants have been used successfully in the treatment of a variety of pain syndromes, the literature most strongly supports the analgesic efficacy of the tricyclics. Amitriptyline has been investigated as an analgesic more than the other antidepressant agents and appears to be the most popular anti-depressant analgesic in the clinical setting. Migraine headaches, neuropathic pain associated with diabetic neuropathy, and postherpetic neuralgia have been found to respond favorably to antidepressant administration. These agents have also been found to alleviate the pain associated with musculoskeletal conditions such as fibromyalgia, rheumatoid arthritis, and osteoarthritis (57). Antidepressants have been successfully utilized in the treatment of cancer pain. In the cancer population, when administered concurrently with an antidepressant, opioid agents may be used at a reduced dose and with a diminished incidence of side effects (58).

The analgesic abilities of antidepressants were once thought to be related to the alleviation of the depression that can often accompany persistent pain, but several antidepressants have been found to reduce pain symptoms in patients not experiencing comorbid depression (57). These agents are now believed to have primary analgesic abilities that are most likely related to their effects on monoamines in endogenous pain pathways. The efficacy of both serotonin and norepinephrine selective antidepressants would suggest that effects on pathways that involve either of these transmitters might contribute to analgesia. Other suggested mechanisms of analgesia involve the antihistamine properties of some agents, increased endorphin secretion, and an increased density of cortical calcium channels (11,56).

The AHCPR guidelines do not recommend antidepressants for the treatment of acute low back problems (3).

In a study of 44 patients admitted for low back pain, Jenkins and colleagues compared treatment with oral imipramine (Tofranil), 25 mg tid, with placebo over a four-week period. After treatment, no significant difference in improvement in straight leg raising, pain and stiffness assessments, or psychological testing was noted between the two study groups. In those individuals with apparent discogenic pain, imipramine treated patients demonstrated greater improvement in pain and stiffness, but this was not found to be statistically significant. No significant difference in side effects was noted between the two groups (59). In a study of 48 patients with chronic low back pain, treatment with imipramine was compared to placebo. Seven of the patients included were determined clinically depressed according to standard criteria. Patients completed Beck depression questionnaires at both the initial and the final visits. Depression score improvements, while not statistically significant, were noted in those patients who benefited from imipramine treatment. Individuals treated with imipramine did demonstrate a significant improvement in both limitations of work and restrictions in normal activities. Anticholinergic side effects were associated with a 10 percent dropout rate (60). In a review of the literature on antidepressants in the treatment of chronic

low back pain, Egbunike and colleagues concluded that the most consistent responses were found with doxepin and desipramine at doses above 150 mg daily. Some studies may have failed to demonstrate a response secondary to inadequate dosing. Other antidepressants were found less effective in providing analgesia. In several studies reviewed, while improvements in depression were observed, poor correlations were noted between analgesic effects and changes in the severity of depression. The relationship between pain relief and antidepressant effect remains unclear (61).

Tricyclic antidepressants produce analgesia at lower dosages than are typically prescribed for the treatment of depression. The starting dose of TCAs should be low. Initial daily dosing of amitriptyline should be 10 mg in elderly patients and 25 mg in younger individuals. An increment in dosing equal to the initial starting dose can be made every two to three days until adequate analgesia is achieved or adverse effects develop. The typical effective daily dose of amitriptyline ranges from 50 to 150 mg. As the TCA half-life is generally long and sedation is a common side effect, single nighttime dosing can be prescribed. Some patients report better pain relief and less morning drowsiness with divided daily dosing (11,56). Those studies that have investigated the analgesic efficacy of SSRIs have typically involved dosages similar to those prescribed in the management of depression, 20 to 40 mg of fluoxetine or paroxetine (57,62). Further research is needed in order to clarify the relationship between dosage and analgesia with the serotonin-specific agents (56).

The occurrence of serious adverse effects resulting from antidepressant administration is low. These complications would be rare at the generally lower dosages utilized in the treatment of pain. While cardiac side effects are uncommon, tricyclics are contraindicated in individuals with heart failure or serious cardiac conduction abnormalities. Orthostatic hypotension is the most frequent cardiovascular adverse effect, and the elderly are particularly at risk. The sedating effect often observed with antidepressant use can be beneficial as patients with pain often demonstrate diminished daytime functioning from inadequate sleep. Anticholinergic side effects such as dry mouth, blurred vision, and urinary retention are more likely with amitriptyline use than with other TCAs. These effects are also less likely at the lower dosages used for analgesia. Nortriptyline and desipramine have been found to induce fewer anticholinergic side effects and are less sedating (56,11).

While antidepressants have been demonstrated as useful adjuncts in the treatment of pain, their analgesic mechanism remains unclear. Initial dosing should be low and then slowly increased to minimize side effects. In disagreement with the AHCPR guidelines, this author does find a potential limited role for antidepressants in the treatment of the acute low back pain patient with pain and difficulty sleeping. When taken at night, the sedating properties of these agents can be beneficial in those pain patients experiencing difficulty with sleep.

# Summary

There are various agents that can be helpful in addressing the painful phase of acute low back problems. The particular medication should be chosen after consideration of the following: (1) indications; (2) contraindications; (3) goals of treatment, i.e., analgesia, reduction of inflammation, reduction of muscle spasm, etc.; and (4) the scientific and clinical evidence of their effectiveness. With the proper selection of pain medication and a positive response, the patient can be progressed through more active treatment leading to a successful outcome.

*Acknowledgment:* Special thanks to Jason Lipetz, M.D., who assisted in the research, writing, and preparation of this manuscipt in a capacity worthy of co-authorship.

# References

1. Hardman JG, Limbird LE (eds.). *Goodman and Gilman's the pharmacological basis of therapeutics,* 9th ed. New York: McGraw Hill, 1996.
2. Westley GJ, Schaefer J, Sifton DW (eds.). *Physicians' desk reference.* 49th ed. Montvale: Medical Economics, 1995.
3. Bigos SJ (chair), Acute Low Back Problems in Adults, Clinical Practice Guidelines Number 14. Rockville: U.S. Department of Health and Human Services, Public Health Service, Agency for Health Care Policy and Research, 1994.
4. Amadio P Jr, Cummings DM. Evaluation of acetaminophen in the management of osteoarthritis of the knee. *Curr Ther Res* 1983; 34:59–66.
5. Doyle DV, Lanham JG. Routine drug treatment of osteoarthritis. *Clin Rheumatol Dis* 1984; 10:277–291.
6. Calin A. Pain and inflammation. *Am J Med* 1984; 77(Suppl 3A):9–15.
7. Bradley JD, Brandt KD, Katz BP, Kalasinski LA, Ryan SI. Comparison of an antiinflammatory dose of ibuprofen, an analgesic dose of ibuprofen, and acetaminophen in the treatment of patients with osteoarthritis of the knee. *New Engl J Med* 1991; 325:87–91.
8. Hickey RFJ. Chronic low back pain: A comparison of diflunisal with paracetamol. *NZ Med J* 1982; 95: 312–314.

9. Brooks PM, Day RO. Nonsteroidal antiinflammatory drugs—differences and similarities. *New Engl J Med* 1991; 324:1716–1725.
10. Weiler JM. The use of nonsteroidal antiinflammatory drugs (NSAIDs) in sports soft-tissue injury. *Clin Sports Med* 1992; 11:625–644.
11. Portenoy RK, Kanner RM (eds.). *Pain management: Theory and practice.* Philadelphia: F.A. Davis, 1996.
12. Abramowicz M (ed.). Drugs for pain. *Medical Letter* 1993; 35:1–6.
13. McCormack K, Brune K. Dissociation between the antinociceptive and anti-inflammatory effects of the nonsteroidal anti-inflammatory drugs. *Drugs* 1991; 41: 533–547.
14. Malmerg AB, Yaksh TL. Hyperalgesia mediated by spinal glutmate or substance P receptor blocked by spinal cyclooxygenase inhibition. *Science* 1992; 257:1276–1279.
15. Gebhart GF, McCormack KJ. Neuronal plasticity. Implication for pain therapy. *Drugs* 1994; 47(Suppl 5):1–47.
16. Konttinen YT, Kemppinen P, Segerberg M, et al. Peripheral and spinal neural mechanisms in arthritis with particular reference to treatment of inflammation and pain. *Arthrit Rheum* 1994; 37:965–982.
17. Gaucher A, Netter P, Faure G, Schoeller JP, Gerardin A. Diffusion of oxyphenbutazone into synovial fluid, synovial tissue, joint cartilage and cerebrospinal fluid. *Eur J Clin Pharm* 1983; 25:107012.
18. McCormack K, Brune K. Toward defining the analgesic role of nonsteroidal anti-inflammatory drugs in the management of acute soft tissue injuries. *Clin J Sports Med* 1993; 3:106–117.
19. Amlie E, Weber H, Holme I. Treatment of acute low-back pain with piroxicam: Results of a double-blind placebo-controlled trial. *Spine* 1987; 12(5):473–476.
20. Wasner C, Britton MC, Kraines RG, Kaye RL, Bobrove AM, Fries JF. Nonsteroidal antiinflammatory agents in rheumatoid arthritis and ankylosing spondylitis. *JAMA* 1981; 246(19):2168–2172.
21. Hayllar J, Bjarnason I. NSAIDs, Cox-2 inhibitors, and the gut (commentary). *Lancet* 1995; 346:521–522.
22. Jiranek GC, Kimmey MB, Saunders DR, Willson RA, Shanahan W,
23. Silverstein FE. Misoprostol reduces gastrointestinal injury from one week of aspirin: An endoscopic study. *Gastroenter* 1989; 96:656–661.
23. Radford MG, Holley KE, Grande JP, Larson TS, Wagoner RD, Donadio J, McCarthy JT. Reversible membranous nephropathy associated with use of nonsteroidal anti-inflammatory drugs. *JAMA* 1996; 276(6):466–469.
24. Buckwalter JA. Current concepts review. Pharmacological treatment of soft-tissue injuries. *J Bone Joint Surg* 1995; 77A(12):1902–1914.
25. Almekinders LC, Baynes AJ, Bracey LW. An in vitro investigation into the effects of repetitive motion and nonsteroidal antiinflammatory medication on human tendon fibroblasts. *Am J Sports Med* 1995; 23(1): 119–123.
26. Almekinders LC, Gilbert JA. Healing of experimental muscle strains and the effects of nonsteroroidal antiinflammatory medication. *Am J Sports Med* 1986; 14(4): 303–308.
27. Mishra DK, Friden J, Schmitz MC, Lieber RL. Antiinflammatory medication after muscle injury. *J Bone Joint Surg* 1995; 77A(10):1510–1519.

28. De Lee JC, Rockwood CA. Skeletal muscle spasm and a review of muscle relaxants. *Curr Ther Res* 1980; 27(1):64–73.

29. Rollings HE, Glassman JM, Soyka JP. Management of acute musculoskeletal conditions—thoracolumbar strain or sprain: A double-blind evaluation comparing the efficacy and safety of carisoprodol with cyclobenzaprine hydrochloride. *Curr Ther Res* 1983; 34(6):917–927.

30. Hindle TH. Comparison of carisoprodol, butabarbital, and placebo in the treatment of the low back syndrome. *Calif Med* 1972; 117:7–11.

31. Basmajian JV. Acute low back pain and spasm. A controlled multicenter trial of combined analgesic and antispasm agents. *Spine* 1989; 14(4):438–439.

32. Borenstein DG, Lacks S, Wiesel SW. Cyclobenzaprine and naproxen versus naproxen alone in the treatment of acute low back pain and muscle spasm. *Clin Ther* 1990; 12(2):125–131.

33. Baratta, RR. A double-blind study of cyclobenzaprine and placebo in the treatment of acute musculoskeletal conditions of the low back. *Curr Ther Res* 1982; 32(5): 646–652.

34. Hingorani, K. Diazepam in backache. A double-blind controlled trial. *Ann Phys Med* 1965; 8:303–306.

35. Boyles WF, Glassman JM, Soyka JP. Management of acute musculoskeletal conditions: Throracolumbar strain or sprain. *Tod Ther Trends* 1983; 1:1–16.

36. Casale R. Acute low back pain. Symptomatic treatment with a muscle relaxant drug. *Clin J Pain* 1988; 4:81–88.

37. Daoas F, Hartman SE, Martinez L, Northrup BE, Nussodrf T, Silberman HM, Gross H. Baclofen for the treatment of acute low-back syndrome. A double-blind comparison with placebo. *Spine* 1985; 10(4):345–349.

38. Brown FL, Bodison S, Dixon J, Davis W, Nowoslawski J. Comparison of diflunisal and acetaminophen with codeine in the treatment of initial or recurrent low back strain. *Clin Ther* 1986; 9(Supp C).

39. Wiesel SW, Cuckler JM, Deluca F, Jones F, Zeide MS, Rothman RH. Acute low back pain. An objective analysis of conservative therapy. *Spine* 1980; 4:324–330.

40. Cooper SA, Engel J, Ladove M, Rauch D, Precheur H, Rosenheck A. An evaluation of oxycodone and acetaminophen in the treatment of postoperative dental pain. *Clin Pharm Ther* 1979; 25(2):219.

41. Hopkinson JH, Bartlett FH, Steffens AO, McGlumphy TH, Macht EL, Smith M. Acetaminophen versus propoxyphene hydrochloride for relief of pain in episiotomy patients. *J Clin Pharm* 1973; 13:251–263.

42. Wilder-Smith CH, Schimke J, Osterwalder B, Senn HJ. Oral tramadol, a mu-opiod agonist and monoamine reuptake-blocker, and morphine for strong cancer related pain. *Ann Oncol* 1994; 5(2):141–146.

43. Sunshine A, Olson NZ, Zighelboim I, DeCastro A, Minn FL. Analgesic oral efficacy of tramadol hydrochloride in postoperative pain. *Clin Pharm Ther* 1992; 51(6): 740–746.

44. Rauk RL, Ruoff GE, McMillen JI. Comparison of tramadol and acetaminophen with codeine for long-term pain management in elderly patients. *Curr Ther Res* 1994; 55(12):1417–1431.

45. Preston KL, Jasinski DR, Testa M. Abuse potential and pharmacological comparison of tramadol and morphine. *Drug Alch Dep* 1991; 27(1):7–17.

46. Houmes RJ, Voets MA, Verkaaik A, Erdmann W, Lachmann B. Efficacy and safety of tramadol versus morphine for moderate and severe postoperative pain with special regard to respiratory depression. *Anesth Analg* 1992; 74(4):510–514.

47. Kaiko RF, Foley KM, Grabinski PY, et al. Central nervous system excitatory effects of meperidine in cancer patients. *Ann Neur* 1983; 13:180–185.

48. Wehlig, M. Novel aldosterone receptors: Specificity conferring mechanism at the level of the cell membrane. *Steroids* 1994; 59:160–163.

49. Nicholas JA, Hershman EB (eds.). The lower extremity and spine in sports medicine. Vol II. St. Louis: Mosby, 1995.

50. Marshall LL, Trethewie ER, Curtain CC. Chemical radiculitis: A clinical, physiological and immunological study. *Clin Orthop* 1979; 129:61.

51. Saal JS, et al. High levels of phospholipase A2 activity in lumbar spine disc herniation. *Spine* 1990; 15:164.

52. Haimovic, IC, Beresford HR. Dexamethasone is not superior to placebo for treating lumbosacral radicular pain. *Neurology* 1986; 36:1593–1594.

53. Truhan AP, Ahmed AR. Corticosteroids: A review with emphasis on complications of prolonged systemic therapy. *Ann Allerg* 1989; 62:375–390.

54. Meek JB, Giudice VW, Mcfadden JW, Key JD, Enrick NL. Colchicine confirmed as highly effective in disk disorders. Final results of a double blind study. *J Neur Orth Med Surg* 1985; 6(3):211–218.

55. Schnebel BE, Simmons JW. The use of oral colchicine for low back pain. A double blind study. *Spine* 1988; 13(3):354–357.

56. King SA. Antidepressants: A valuable adjunct for musculoskeletal pain. *J Musculoskel Med* 1995; Oct:51–57.

57. Magni G. The use of antidepressants in the treatment of chronic pain. A review of the current evidence. *Drugs* 1991; 42:730–748.

58. Jacox A, Carr DB, Payne R, et al. Management of cancer pain. Clinical practice guideline no. 9. Rockville, Md: Agency for Health Care Policy and Research; 1994. US Dept. of Health and Human Services, Public Health Service, AHCPR publication No. 94–0592.

59. Jenkins DG, Ebbut AF, Evans CD. Tofranil in the treatment of low back pain. *J Int Med Res* 1976; 4(Supp 2):28–40.

60. Alcoff J, Jones E, Rust P, Newman R. Controlled trial of imipramine for chronic low back pain. *J Fam Pract* 1982, 14(5):841–846.

61. Egbunike IG, Chaffee BJ. Antidepressants in the management of chronic pain syndromes. *Pharmacother* 1990; 10(4):262–270.

62. Max MB, Lynch SA, Muir J, et al. Effects of desipramine, amitriptyline, and fluoxetine on pain in diabetic neuropathy. *N Engl J Med* 1992; 326:1250–56.

63. Abramowicz (ed.). Drugs for rheumatoid arthritis. *Medical Letter* 1994; 36:101–106.

64. American Pain Society. *Principles of analgesic use in the treatment of acute pain and cancer pain.* 3rd ed. Skokie: American Pain Society, 1993.

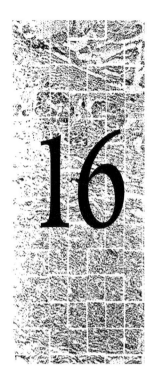

# 16 Commentary on Physical Treatments

*Myron M. LaBan, M.D., M.M.Sc., F.A.C.P.*

f you cannot catch a bird of paradise, better take a wet hen."

Nikita Khrushchev, *Time*,
January 6, 1958.

In a word, the AHCPR publication (1) was wired! Like most political documents, the conclusions were predetermined before the process was started. The 23 member panel each with their own individual agenda were eventually herded by a process of horse trading to a timely and predetermined consensus. Once again this committee reaffirmed the standard federal imperative that an elephant is really a mouse built to government specifications. As one of the predesignated reviewers, I was also "mushroomed," kept in the dark and fertilized with horse manure until the last possible minute. I was not privileged to review this document until it had already left the bindery ready for distribution. This guideline, which has sparked much controversy among those health care practitioners who treat patients with low back pain, is a sterling example of a camel built by a committee assigned the task of designing a horse. The panel in its consensus supported the guideline's beginning hypothesis that inter-

ventional treatment of low back pain is worthless. In their deliberations they charitably disregarded the tenets of the scientific process. The "authoritative" references upon which their recommendations were based were often impossibly flawed, another example of garbage in—garbage out!

The studies cited were rarely "blinded," comparison groups often had been reevaluated at different times, selection bias was flagrant, controls were infrequently available, treatment groups were statistically flawed as comparatively too small, and generic "backache" prevailed throughout as the treatment diagnosis rather than with reference to a specific etiology of the pain complaint. In some instances as many as three articles were cited as separate authorities when in fact they were the same study published in three separate journals with the lead author playing musical chairs with his co-authors. Too many of these references with all of their inherent flaws were retrospective reviews rather than prospective studies.

A critical reviewer can only conclude that, like the $25,000 Air Force toilet seats, the cost of this report to the American taxpayer was far in excess of its value. To paraphrase Tom Lehrer, like a commode, you get out that which you put in!

Unfortunately, a suit brought by Sofamor Danek Group, manufacturers of pedicle screws seeking to halt distribution of the low back guidelines, has recently been rejected by the United States Supreme Court. However, the AHCPR, apparently embarrassed by both the quality of this publication and the subsequent controversy it generated, has decided to stop developing guidelines. As a consequence they have instead shifted to developing outcome measurements. Introspective clinicians who daily treat patients with spinal pain complaints of varying etiologies have always employed outcome measures, i.e., clinical experience, as a guide to treating successive patients with similar complaints and clinical findings. In the private sector the consultant who hasn't a clue as to the diagnosis and who in turn fails to provide an appropriate, cost-effective prescription of treatment quickly finds himself without a panel of referring physicians.

"Whatever thou takest in hand, remember the end, and thou shalt never do amiss."

Apocrypha, *Ecclesiasticus 7:36*

### SPINAL MANIPULATION

At the Association of Academic Physiatrists meeting in February 1996, where "Physical Treatments" as reviewed in the guideline for Managing Acute Low Back Pain was presented, one of our assignments was to comment on the efficacy of spinal manipulation. In this publication, spinal manipulation is reviewed in depth in Chapter 18. However, as the author of a recent review on spinal manipulation (2), I cannot but help to briefly comment on the conclusions of the guideline:

* Without radiculopathy manipulation may be of value in the first month of acute low back pain.
* There is insufficient evidence to recommend manipulation in patients with a radiculopathy.
* If unsuccessful in the first couple weeks of acute back pain, continued manipulation is of no value.

All of the cited references in this section were universally flawed as none were truly "blinded," selection bias was present in almost all of the references, treatment groups were reevaluated at different times and were statistically too small to compare, the etiology of the "backache" was not delineated, and three of the references were in fact the same article cited in three different journals (3–5). Reviewing these same references we concluded:

* Spinal manipulation if useful at all should be performed within the first 2–5 days of pain complaint.

* There are insufficient statistical data to conclude that after five days of manipulation and/or conventional physical therapy (exercise and modalities) there is a difference in outcome.
* Manipulation is of no value after ten days.
* Static traction at seven days is as effective as manipulation or other physical therapy.
* Sham therapy using detuned ultrasound or short wave diathermy may be as effective as manipulation and/or physical therapy.

"The more I read, the more I meditate, and the more I acquire, the more I am enabled to affirm that I know nothing."

Voltaire, "Occult Qualities," *Philosophical Dictionary* (1764)

### PHYSICAL MODALITIES IN TREATMENT: SUPERFICIAL HEAT AND COLD, DIATHERMY

The guideline cited ten reference articles (3–12) on this subject and only two (6,8) evaluated their efficacy in patients with acute low back pain. They concluded that;

* In the treatment of acute low back pain the use of physical treatment modalities in a clinical setting is not cost-effective.
* Superficial heat and/or cold can more appropriately be recommended as a home treatment.

Reviewing the same references we concluded:

* There are relatively few reported differences between manipulation and the use of diathermy alone.
* Physical therapy modalities and manipulation are of relatively little value in treatment after the first week of low back pain.
* Placebo therapy was most effective in "treating" pain in the first seven days and less effective thereafter.
* The etiology of the back pain governs the rapidity of response to treatment.
* Back schools play no role in the acute treatment process.

In general, regardless of the physical treatment approaches during the first seven days, patients with low back pain will improve, even if sham therapy is employed. However, the reviewers do acknowledge that the speed of recovery in response to any treatment approach, physical or otherwise, is influenced by the etiology of the back pain. Unfortunately, this epiphany surfaced only briefly and is deliberately and/or otherwise disregarded in the remaining text. Also ignored is the "quality" of the recovery— that pain can be ameliorated during the acute process by employing physical modalities in treatment, each appropriately selected for a specific diagnosis. We also agree that superficial thermotherapy in the form of hot or cold packs can be successfully utilized in home treatment. On a clinical basis we would also argue that when radicular pain is a concurrent complaint, these modalities are even more effective when utilized preceding pelvic traction and/or an active exercise program in a more formal treatment setting. On the other hand, the diathermies, both ultrasound and shortwave, are preferred when facet or sacroiliac joint pain is the primary complaint (13).

"What is objectionable, what is dangerous about extremists is not that they are extreme, but that they are intolerant. The evil is not what they say about their cause, but what they say about their opponents."

Robert F Kennedy, "Extremism, Left and Right,"
*The Pursuit of Justice* (1964).

## TRANSCUTANEOUS ELECTRICAL STIMULATION (TENS)

- The guideline concluded that TENS is ineffective in the treatment of patients with acute low back pain.

Of the nine references cited as authority (12,14–21), we found only one that made reference to acute low back pain treated with TENS (17), and two references were the same study published in separate journals, *Pain* and *Archives of Physical Medicine and Rehabilitation* (20,21). TENS in one report was superior to oral anti-inflammatories (15) and in another article effective in 48 percent of cases, especially with a diagnosis of painful neuropathies and/or myofascial syndromes (16). It was also noted that in chronic pain a female sex bias with a tendency to over-report was identified. The response to TENS was attributed to a placebo effect (18). Demonstrating a cavalier license or just plain chutzpah, the reviewers "dropped the ball" on TENS as the references failed to even begin to support their preconceived conclusion that it is ineffective in acute pain management.

"It is with narrow-souled people as with narrow-necked bottles: the less they have in them, the more noise they make in pouring it out."

Alexander Pope, *Thoughts on Various Subjects*
(1727)

## INSOLES AND SHOE LIFTS

- Shoe lifts may be effective in acute low back pain, particularly in patients standing for long periods of time.

This recommendation was based on one article (22). Shoe lifts were suggested when leg length differences exceeded 2 centimeters (23). However, 51 percent of the patients reported no significant reduction in pain and 3 percent reported an increase in their discomfort. In every instance there was no proven long-term effect. Apparently, the committee agreed if for no other reason than that they were cost-effective, i.e., they were not expensive, so why not?

"Repetition does not transform a lie into truth."

Franklin D. Roosevelt, Radio Address,
October 26, 1939

## LUMBAR CORSETS AND BACK BELTS

After screening 31 articles and accepting three as authoritative, the reviewers concluded that:

- Lumbar corsets and support belts are not of proven value in patients with acute low back pain.

In two reports there was no significant difference between the controls using only exercise and the belt wearers (24,25). In another series, 58 percent discontinued wearing the belts and five of 28 subjects wearing a support were reinjured (26). All of the studies were suspect, none focused on acute low back pain only, and each could be criticized by both the limited controls and small experimental populations. The panel's insistence on drawing a conclusion—even one without any support in the literature—suggests that a preconceived conclusion far outweighed the experimental evidence.

"The great enemy of the truth is very often not the lie— deliberate, contrived and dishonest—but the myth—persistent, persuasive and unrealistic."

John F. Kennedy, Commencement Address, Yale
University, New Haven, Connecticut, June 1962

## TRACTION

- Spinal traction is not recommended in the treatment of acute low back pain.

This conclusion was based on a review of 31 articles, seven of which were selected as references (27–33).

Static, in-bed pelvic traction was reported as of no benefit with regard to pain relief, physiological status, length of hospital stay, functional outcome, or self-perception of improvement (30). Inversion traction was found to increase the incidence of hypertension and contribute to increased intraocular pressure (34). In another study, intermittent, split-table pelvic traction utilizing distraction weights of less than 30 percent of body weight was reported as ineffective in the treatment of patients with a herniated lumbar disc (27). The panel, concurring, chose either to ignore and/or in fact not recognize that the accepted initial starting distraction weight for this modality is generally that of 50 percent of gross body weight.

Split-table pelvic traction by reducing the effects of friction can be effectively employed in the management of lumbar spinal radicular syndromes associated with lumbar spinal stenosis and/or a prolapsed disc. Progressive treatments starting at 50 percent of body weight and increased successively by 5–10 pounds can successfully palliate the symptoms of pain and/or paresthesias as well as reduce weakness in the distal myotome distribution of the compromised spinal root (35). Treatment is usually preceded by superficial heat and then followed by an appropriate prescription of spinal exercises. Once again, the selected references were plagued by poor controls and with the exception of one article (33) the etiology of the low back pain was ignored.

"What people call impartiality may simply mean indifference and what people call partiality may simply mean mental activity."
G.K. Chesterton, "The Error of Impartiality,"
*All Things Considered* (1908).

## BIOFEEDBACK

- Has no role in the treatment of patients with acute low back pain?

Of the 13 articles screened, four references were used (36–39) even though two (40,41) did not meet the panel's own review criteria as there were too few subjects in each study group. All of the studies focused on patients with chronic pain. As might be expected, the results were highly variable with an identified significant placebo affect (41). With a bizarre alchemy of sleight-of-hand the panel was able to transmute lead to gold, concluding that all of these references to chronic pain could somehow be related to the treatment of acute low back pain—the raison d'etre for the guideline. Science or what?

"The best way I know to win an argument is to start by being in the right."
Lord Hailsham, *The New York Times,*
October 6, 1960.

This guideline is more of a political statement than a scientific document. Most of the references cited were suspect and could be challenged as not conforming to accepted scientific method. In reviewing this syllabus, I had the distinct impression that it had been prepared by a publication staff working without immediate "hands-on" supervision. How else could the multiple, redundant references to the same studies not be recognized? The publication staff apparently needs to reconsider that any study of outcomes as they relate to acute low back pain must address the characteristics of the review itself as well as the conclusions derived from the experimental study (42):

- Low back pain cannot be measured by "hard" outcomes. The intensity of the perceived discomfort passes through two nervous systems, that of the victim and thereafter the examiner who interprets the severity of the patient's complaint, each bringing his/her own bias to the equation.
- At best, most of the studies were confounded by poor methological outcome, i.e., an average subjective interpretation of the results with relatively small experimental populations and controls.
- If the "treaters" are also the reviewers, there can be a significant increase in bias as there is a recognized tight link to a singular treatment approach which may be important in validating the reviewer's professional identity and have a significant impact on his/her pocketbook. As a corollary, a positive outcome is more likely if the "treater" is also an author of the review.
- Any study either retrospective or prospective of acute low back pain that fails to discriminate as to the etiology of this complaint is less than valid. Studies of generic low back pain that compare apples to oranges lack science and are inherently flawed. Both metastatic cancer of the paraspinal muscle (Figure 16–1) and/or pain of vascular etiology (Figure 16–2) can produce acute low back pain. However, in both these instances the prognosis and approach to treatment are inordinately different from those that respond to two days of bed rest.
- Citing the same experimental population as multiple authority especially on repeated occasions suggests both carelessness and a "devil may care" attitude with regard to editorial accuracy. Unfortunately, it also diminishes the credibility of the well-respected and heretofore accepted Ingelfinger rule, "the under-

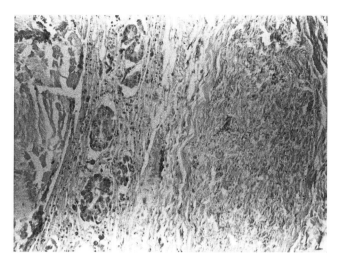

**FIGURE 16–1**

Adenocarcinoma, metastatic to paraspinal muscle adjacent to branch of posterior primary ramus.

standing is that materials submitted to the [New England] *Journal* has not been offered to any [other] book, journal or newspaper" (43).

This guideline is not the first nor will it be the last intrusion into professional practice, where political and economic rather then scientific forces unduly influence the conclusions. In 1861 Oliver Wendell Holmes (44) wrote:

"The truth is that medicine, professionally founded on observation, is as sensitive to outside influences, political, religious, philosophical, imaginative, as is the barometer to the changes of atmospheric density. Theoretically it ought to go its own straightforward inductive path, without regard to changes of government or fluctuations of public opinions. [Actually, there is] a closer relation between the medieval Sciences and the conditions of Society and the general thought of the time, than would at first be suspected."

*eferences*

1. Bigos S, Bowyer O, Braen G, et al. Acute Low Back Problems in Adults. Clinical Practice Guideline No. 14. AHCPR Publication No. 95-0642. Rockville, MD: Agency for Health Care Policy and Research, Public Health Service, U.S. Department of Health and Human Services. December 1994.

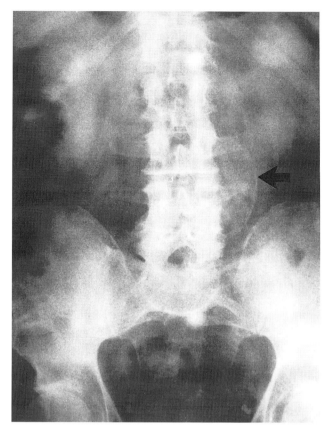

**FIGURE 16–2**

Aortic aneurysm *(arrow)* presenting as acute low back pain unresponsive to two days of bed rest.

2. LaBan MM, Taylor RS. Manipulation, An objective analysis of the literature. In: Garfin SR, Herkowitz H (eds.). The degenerative neck. *Orthop Clin North Am* 1992; 23:451–459.
3. Koes BW, Bouter LM, van Mameren H, et al. A blinded randomized clinical trial of manual therapy and physiotherapy for chronic back and neck complaints: physical outcome measures. *J Man Physical Ther* 1992; 1:16–23.
4. Koes BW, Bouter LM, van Mameren H, et al. The effectiveness of manual therapy, physiotherapy, and treatment by the general practitioner for nonspecific back and neck complaints. A randomized clinical trial. *Spine* 1992; 17:28–35.
5. Koes BW, Bouter LM, van Mameren H, et al. Randomized clinical trial of manipulative therapy and physiotherapy for persistent back and neck complaints: results of one year follow up. *Br Med J* 1992; 304:601–605.
6. Postacchini F, Facchini M, Patieri P. Efficiency of various forms of conservative treatment in low back pain. A comparative study. *Neuro-orthopedics* 1988; 6:28–35.
7. Gibson T, Grahame R, Harkness J, et al. Controlled comparison of short wave diathermy treatment with osteopathic treatment in non-specific low back pain. *Lancet* 1985; 8440:1258–1261.

8. Waterworth RF, Hunter IA. An open study of diflunisal, conservative and manipulative therapy in the management of acute mechanical low back pain. *N Z Med J* 1985; 98:372-375.

9. Klein RG, Eek BC. Low-energy laser treatment and exercise for chronic low back pain: double-blind controlled trial. *Arch Phys Med Rehabil* 1990; 71:34–37.

10. Linton SJ, Bradley LA, Jensen I, et al. The secondary prevention of low back pain: a controlled study with follow-up. *Pain* 1989; 36:197–207.

11. Manniche C, Hesselsoe G, Bentzen L, et al. Clinical trial of intensive muscle training for chronic low back pain. *Lancet* 1988; 8626-8627:1473–1476.

12. Malzack R, Vetre P, Finch L. Transcutaneous electrical nerve stimulation for low back pain. A comparison of TENS and massage for pain and range of motion. *Phys Ther* 1983; 63:489–493.

13. Falconer J, Hayes KW, Change RW. Therapeutic ultrasound in the treatment of musculoskeletal conditions. *Arthritis Care Res* 1990; 3:85–91.

14. Deyo RA, Walsh NE, Martin DC, et al. A controlled trial of transcutaneous electrical nerve stimulation (TENS) and exercise for chronic low back pain [see comments]. *N Engl J Med* 1990; 322:1627–1634.

15. Gemignani G, Olivieri I, Ruju G, et al. Transcutaneous electrical nerve stimulation in ankylosing spondylitis: a double-blind study [letter]. *Arthritis Rheum* 1991; 34:788–789.

16. Graff-Radford SB, Reeves JL, et al. Effects of transcutaneous electrical nerve stimulation on myofascial pain and trigger point sensitivity. *Pain* 1989; 37:1–5.

17. Hackett GI, Seddon D, Kaminski D. Electroacupuncture compared with paracetamol for acute low back pain. *Practitioner* 1988; 232:163–164.

18. Lehmann TR, Russell DW, Spratt KF. The impact of patients with nonorganic physical findings on a controlled trial of transcutaneous electrical nerve stimulation and electro acupuncture. *Spine* 1983; 6:625–634.

19. Lehmann TR, Russell DW, Spratt KF, et al. Efficacy of electroacupuncture and TENS in the rehabilitation of chronic low back pain patients. *Pain* 1986; 26:277–290.

20. Thorsteinsson G, Stonnington HH, Stillwell GK, et al. Transcutaneous electrical stimulation: a double-blind trial of its efficacy for pain. *Arch Phys Med Rehabil* 1977; 58:8–13.

21. Thorsteinsson G, Stonnington HH, Stillwell GK, et al. The placebo effect of transcutaneous electrical stimulation. *Pain* 1978; 5:31–41.

22. Basford JR, Smith MA. Shoe insoles in the workplace. *Orthopedics* 1988; 11:285–288.

23. Battie ML, Bigos SJ, Fisher LD, et al. The role of spinal flexibility in back pain complaints within industry. A prospective study. *Spine* 1990; 15:768–773.

24. Walsh WE, Schwartz RK. The influence of prophylactic orthosis on abdominal strength and low back injury in the work place. *Am J Phys Med Rehabil* 1990; 69:245–250.

25. Million R, Haavik Wilson K, Jayson MIV, et al. Evaluation of low back pain and assessment of lumbar corsets with and without back supports. *Ann Rheum Dis* 1981; 40:449–454.

26. Reddell CR, Congleton JJ, Hutchingson RD, et al. An evaluation of a weight lifting belt and back injury prevention training class for airline baggage handlers. *Applied Ergonomics* 1992; 23:319–329.

27. Coxhead CE, Meade TW, Inskip H, et al. Multicentre trial of physiotherapy in the management of sciatic symptoms. *Lancet* 1981; 8229:1065–1068.

28. Mathews JA, Mills SB, Jenkins VM, et al. Back pain and sciatica: controlled trials of manipulation, traction, sclerosant and epidural injections. *Br J Rheumatol* 1987; 26:416-423.

29. Mathews W, Morkel M, Mathews J. Manipulation and traction for lumbago and sciatica: physiotherapeutic techniques used in two controlled trials. *Physiother Prac* 1988; 4:201–206.

30. Larsson U, Choler U, Lidstrom A, et al. Auto-traction for treatment of lumbago-sciatica. A multicentre controlled investigation. *Acta Orthop Scand* 1980; 51:791–798.

31. Mathews JA, Hickling J. Lumbar traction: a double-blind controlled study for sciatica. *Rheumatol Rehabil* 1975; 14:222–225.

32. Pal B, Mangion P, Hossain MA, et al. A controlled trial of continuous lumbar traction in the treatment of back pain and sciatica. *Br J Rheumatol* 1986; 25:181–183.

33. Weber H, Ljunggren AE, Walker L. Traction therapy in patients with herniated lumbar intervertebral discs. *J Oslo City Hosp* 1984; 34:61–70.

34. Haskvitz EM, Hanter WP. Blood pressure response to inversion traction. *Phys Ther* 1986; 66:1361–1364.

35. Cholachis SC Jr. Traction. In: Leek JC, Gershwin ME, Fowler WM Jr (eds.). *Principles of physical medicine and rehabilitation for musculoskeletal diseases.* New York: Grune & Stratton, 1986, 121–172.

36. Asfour SS, Khalil TM, Waly SM, et al. Biofeedback in back muscle strengthening. *Spine* 1990; 15:510–513.

37. Bush C, Ditto B, Feuerstein M. A controlled evaluation of paraspinal EMG biofeedback in the treatment of chronic low back pain. *Health Psychol* 1985; 4:307–321.

38. Flor H, Haag G, Turk DC, et al. Efficacy of EMG biofeedback, pseudotherapy and conventional medical treatment for chronic rheumatic back pain. *Pain* 1983; 17:21–31.

39. Mouwen A. EMG biofeedback used to reduce standing levels of paraspinal muscle tension in chronic low back pain. *Pain* 1983; 17:353–360.

40. Flor H, Haag G, Turk DC. Long-term efficacy of EMG biofeedback for chronic rheumatic back pain. *Pain* 1986; 27:195–202.

41. Stuckey SJ, Jacobs A, Goldfarb J. EMG biofeedback training, relaxation training, and placebo for the relief of chronic low back pain. *Percept Mot Skills* 1986; 63:1023–1036.

42. Begg C, Cho M, Eastwood S, et al. Improving the quality of reporting of randomized controlled trials. *JAMA* 1996; 276:637–639.

43. Ingelfinger FJ. Definition of "sole contribution." *N Engl J Med* 1969; 281:676-677.

44. Holmes OW. *Currents and counter-currents in medical science.* Boston: Ticknor and Fields, 1861:7–8.

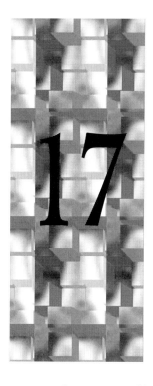

# 17 Physical Treatments for Symptom Control

*Timothy R. Dillingham, M.D., M.S., and Barbara J. deLateur, M.D., M.S.*

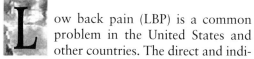ow back pain (LBP) is a common problem in the United States and other countries. The direct and indirect costs due to extended disability and time lost from work are staggering. Despite the advances in spinal imaging, the availability of many different medications for pain management, and the many rehabilitation interventions that can be used to treat patients with LBP, the problem of disability due to chronic and acute LBP continues.

The Agency for Health Care Policy and Research (AHCPR) recently published a series of guidelines for the early evaluation and care of patients with acute LBP (1,2). This document represents a formulation of relevant literature with respect to various treatments for acute LBP. An expert panel evaluated the strength and quality of the literature with respect to different treatments and made recommendations as to whether or not a particular treatment is indicated in the management of acute LBP. Many practicing clinicians found the guidelines in conflict with their established practice patterns. The economic interests of other practitioners were likewise threatened by these recommendations.

Guidelines provide valuable information for the practicing physician on the best evidence-based evaluation and management for a particular clinical problem. They become particularly important with the ever-expanding medical knowledge base that is impossible for a single individual to synthesize. However, there are many limitations to clinical guidelines. A single well-designed study cannot apply to all clinical scenarios. A body of relevant literature from different institutions is necessary to fully support definitive statements regarding optimal care. Unfortunately, this is not the case regarding many of the treatments for LBP. Guidelines are frequently rendered out-of-date when new studies are published. They may reflect the particular bias of the experts selected to produce them. The literature cited may not represent the best articles in a particular field, and these articles are frequently determined by defined literature searching strategies and selection criteria. The literature used to compile the guidelines may not be generalizable to the population targeted by the guidelines, i.e., extrapolating results from studies dealing with chronic LBP and applying them indiscriminately to patients with acute LBP. Disclaimer statements in the guidelines themselves advising readers that other diagnostic and therapeutic strategies may be appropriate and that the clinician can deviate from them and still provide competent care can be overlooked. In the current cost-conscious health care environment, third-party payors and case managers often rigidly interpret clinical guidelines as "definitive" treatment strategies.

The purpose of this chapter is to assess the literature used to generate the panel's recommendations with respect to the use of physical modalities in the treatment of acute LBP. The randomized controlled trial (RCT) provides the best assessment of efficacy. The focus of this chapter is primarily on the RCTs in the literature. The authors reviewed the literature through *Grateful Med*® back to 1991 to identify any relevant literature published after these guidelines were written.

## TRACTION

### AHCPR Conclusion

*The AHCPR panel concluded that spinal traction is not indicated in the treatment of patients with acute low back problems.*

### Relevant Literature Cited by the AHCPR Guidelines

In deriving their recommendations, the panel cited prospective randomized studies. Larsson and colleagues (3) randomly assigned 82 patients with acute LBP to auto-traction (self-administered using the arms to provide the force of traction) or corset and rest. Patients with LBP of greater than 2 weeks and less than 3.5 months and who had positive straight leg raising (SLR) test were included. The treatment group received three treatments per week for 3 weeks. Follow-up was at 1 and 3 weeks. A statistically significant benefit in terms of recovery was noted at 1 week in favor of the traction group. At 3 weeks, the differences between groups regarding who had recovered and were pain-free were still significant in favor of the traction group. The percentage of patients resolving their SLR was also significant at 3 weeks. There were no differences between the groups at 3 months. This study suggests that auto-traction may be effective for management of acute sciatica.

Mathews and colleagues (4) randomized patients with acute LBP to receive traction or infrared heat treatment. A total of 83 patients were assigned to the traction group and 60 to the control group. There were no significant differences in outcome at 2 weeks. However, a subgroup analysis revealed that for females under 45 years of age there was a significant difference favoring traction.

In a study comparing lumbar traction (5.5–8.2 kg) to sham traction (1.4–1.8 kg) for patients with acute LBP, no significant differences were found (5). This study was compromised by small sample size, with 15 subjects in the sham traction group and 24 in the traction group.

Another randomized trial (6) cited in the guidelines failed to find a significant benefit of traction but was methodologically problematic due to small sample size (13 and 14 patients in the groups) and a cross-over at 3 weeks by the control group.

Coxhead and co-workers (7) compared traction, exercises, manipulation, or elastic corset in patients with subacute LBP (average duration of symptoms was 14.3 weeks). They found no significant benefits of any treatment. After 4 weeks of treatment, 78 percent had improved, irrespective of treatment. Only for manipulation, specifically with respect to pain reduction, was the difference significant at 4 weeks. The authors concluded that there was no conclusive evidence that any of the four treatment regimens was effective.

### Additional Literature

Beurskens and colleagues (8) studied the effects of traction in reducing symptoms in patients with nonspecific LBP. Their sample consisted of patients with LBP greater than 6 weeks. Traction (n = 77) was applied with an automatic traction device producing between 35 percent and 50 percent of body weight force. Sham traction (n = 74) produced a force of less than 20 percent body weight. Approximately half the subjects in each group had pain for less than 6 months and half greater than 6 months. The researchers found no significant differences with respect to pain and disability between the two groups. This study did not specifically address acute LBP.

### Summary: Traction

We disagree with the guidelines. There is insufficient evidence to make a definitive statement. Many of the cited articles had small sample sizes or included patients with chronic LBP. Traction may be useful for acute LBP with sciatica based on findings from the study of Larsson and co-workers (3). Well-controlled trials dealing with patients with acute LBP are needed.

## TRANSCUTANEOUS ELECTRICAL NERVE STIMULATION

### AHCPR Conclusion

*TENS is not recommended in the management of acute low back pain.*

### AHCPR Literature Cited

There were several well-designed controlled trials with TENS (9,10,11,12,13,14,15). Unfortunately, these studies all addressed the use of TENS in patients with *chronic* LBP, not *acute* LBP.

In a well-designed prospective trial, Deyo and co-workers (9) found that TENS was no more effective than sham TENS in management of patients with nonspecific chronic LBP. Their sample had a median duration of pain of 4.1 years. This severely limits generalizability to patients with acute LBP. TENS did not offer any additive effect over and above the beneficial effects of exercise for these patients.

Melzack and colleagues (14), in a double blind study, compared TENS to mechanically administered massage. In this study subjects had a mean duration of pain of 36.2 weeks. TENS was found to be significantly better at pain relief and resolution of SLR than mechanical massage.

In a randomized double blind trial comparing TENS to a placebo machine, Thorsteinsson and co-workers (10) found that TENS was effective. This group of subjects had a variety of pain syndromes, postsurgical pain, neck pain, neuropathy, and so forth, which does not translate to patients with acute nonspecific LBP.

Graff-Radford and colleagues (11) looked at the effects of TENS in treatment of myofascial pain and trigger point sensitivity. Again the subjects in this study all had chronic pain syndromes and were selected from the UCLA pain center referrals. They found significant analgesic effects immediately after TENS administration for the highest intensity TENS as opposed to control TENS (placement of the unit without battery).

Lehmann and co-workers (15) pointed out the impact of patients with nonorganic signs on TENS trials. Thorsteinsson and colleagues (12) suggest that the placebo effects of TENS in patients with chronic LBP are substantial. They did not find a significant difference between TENS and control TENS (similar machine without stimulation). The patients in this trial had a variety of painful conditions. The study was similar to the same authors' study published the previous year (10). The effects of TENS were best in conditions with painful neuropathies with stimulation directly over the nerve trunk.

Lehmann and co-workers (13) compared the effects of electroacupuncture (n =17), TENS (n =18), and TENS dead-battery (placebo, n =18) in patients with chronic LBP. They found no significant benefit of TENS over placebo, but the sample size was small.

The effects of electroacupuncture (electrical stimulation over acupuncture points without needle insertion) compared with paracetamol were studied by Hackett, Seddon, and Kaminski (16). They randomized patients with acute LBP (less than 3 days). The electroacupuncture group received a placebo tablet. The paracetamol group received placebo electroacupuncture (no current). All subjects received general instructions in lifting methods and posture. Pain and mobility were significantly improved in the electroacupuncture group at week 6, but not at week 1 or week 2. The total sample size was again small—only 37 patients.

## Additional Literature

In a trial comparing TENS, placebo TENS, and no treatment in patients with chronic LBP, TENS was shown to be superior in reducing pain intensity immediately after treatment (17). TENS produced a significant additive effect over repetitive treatment sessions for pain intensity and relative pain unpleasantness, which was not found for placebo TENS. The authors concluded that TENS should be used as a short-term analgesic procedure in a multidisciplinary program for LBP rather than as an exclusive or long-term treatment.

Pope and colleagues (18) recently published the results of a study comparing the efficacy of manipulation, transcutaneous muscle stimulation, massage, and corset in the treatment of subacute (symptom duration of 3 weeks to 6 months) LBP. This was a well-designed study using massage as a control for manipulation, and clearly defined inclusion and exclusion criteria. They found no significant differences at 3 weeks for any treatment group and concluded that there were no significant differences between these treatments.

Perhaps the most relevant article to this debate was recently published by Herman and colleagues (19). They evaluated the effects of TENS in patients with LBP of 3–10 weeks in duration. TENS was randomly added to an exercise program for work-injured patients. Fifty-eight patients were randomized to exercise plus active TENS, versus placebo TENS and exercise. TENS did not significantly contribute to improved functional status, decrease in perceived pain, or earlier return to work. No additional benefits were found by adding TENS to a standard active rehabilitation program.

## Summary: TENS

We disagree with the guidelines. At this time, the scientific literature is insufficient to support any clear statement as to the effectiveness of TENS in patients with acute LBP. The results of Herman and colleagues (19) suggest that TENS is not an effective adjunctive modality for patients with acute LBP undergoing an active rehabilitation program. Pope and co-workers (18) used *muscle* stimulation, not TENS, in their well-designed RCT, limiting the generalizability of these findings. The other cited literature predominantly dealt with chronic LBP or patients with other pain syndromes.

TENS does not appear to be a clearly effective treatment for chronic LBP.

## BIOFEEDBACK

### AHCPR Conclusion

*Biofeedback is not recommended in the management of patients with acute LBP.*

### AHCPR Literature Cited

As in the case of the TENS literature, the majority of studies cited involved the use of biofeedback in management of patients with chronic back and neck symptoms.

Asfour and co-workers (20) found that EMG biofeedback could improve back muscle strengthening in patients with chronic LBP, but pain was not affected. Bush, Ditto, and Feuerstein (21) did not find any advantage of EMG biofeedback in subjects with over 2 years of LBP. Nouwen (22) arrived at a similar conclusion that for chronic LBP there is no benefit conferred by EMG biofeedback. Stuckey and colleagues (23) found that relaxation training was superior to EMG biofeedback in patients with chronic LBP.

In contrast to other studies in this area, Flor and colleagues (24) found that the short-term effects of EMG biofeedback in patients with chronic neck and back pain were significantly better than pseudotherapy at 4 weeks and 4 months. These researchers also reported the results of long-term (2.5 years) follow-up of the original sample (25). The biofeedback group maintained the significant beneficial effects from EMG biofeedback. These researchers concluded that there is long-term utility of biofeedback.

### Additional Literature

No articles that specifically deal with acute LBP could be identified via *Grateful Med®* literature searching strategies.

### Summary: Biofeedback

We disagree with the guidelines. Because of the lack of literature in this area dealing with acute LBP, no clear recommendations can be made.

## PHYSICAL AGENTS AND MODALITIES

### AHCPR Conclusions

*There is insufficiently proven benefit to justify the cost of physical agents and modalities.*

### AHCPR LITERATURE CITED

The study that clearly addressed the issue of modalities in acute pain was published by Waterworth and Hunter (26). In this trial, 112 patients with LBP that was present less than 1 month were randomized to one of three treatment regimens: diflunisal medication, physiotherapy consisting of short-wave diathermy for 15–20 minutes and ultrasound for 5–10 minutes, or manipulation of the lumbar spine. Over the 12-day assessment period, patients in all three groups showed improvement, with none of the regimens showing superior improvement. All patients were given instruction in basic spine care; the outcome raters were not blinded. This study did not show any particular benefit of heating modalities for patients with acute LBP.

Studies involving 256 patients with chronic LBP and neck pain (average symptom duration of 52 weeks) who were randomized to one of four regimens [manual therapy (manipulation), physiotherapy (heat, electrotherapy, ultrasound, short-wave diathermy, exercises, and massage), general practitioner care, or placebo (detuned diathermy)] were apparently published simultaneously in two different journals (27,28). Outcome measures were carried out at 6 and 12 months. These investigators found that the group receiving manipulation and physiotherapy had significantly better results than the other groups, but they cautioned readers about the possibility of placebo effects with both manual therapy and physiotherapy.

Laser therapy was shown to be ineffective in improving the effects of exercise (29).

Gibson and colleagues (30) studied the effects of short-wave diathermy and osteopathic manipulation versus placebo (detuned short-wave diathermy) in the management of patients with LBP of 2 to 12 months in duration. There were 109 patients randomized to one of the three groups. They found that the active treatments were no more effective than placebo and concluded that short-wave diathermy and osteopathic treatments were no more effective than placebo.

### Additional Literature

Mitchell and Carmen (31) published a study evaluating the effectiveness of an early work conditioning program for patients with acute musculoskeletal work injuries. Patients at 12 participating clinics in Ontario, Canada, with acute back and other musculoskeletal soft tissue injuries were placed in a rehabilitation program. This program consisted of ultrasound, cold packs, or interferential current for initial pain relief . This was followed by circuit training and cardiovascular exercise. These programs lasted 3 to 4 weeks with half-day or full-day programs. In this study, modalities were used as an adjunct to facilitate an active exercise program. This was a pseudo-randomization, and the treatment patients were compared to matched controls treated at other centers. The strength of this study was the large sample size (n =

1,072); they were compared to 2,172 matched controls. The initial cost of this program was more than offset by the significantly earlier return to work in the treatment group and the corresponding savings in compensation costs. This study did not specifically address ultrasound or other modalities, but it does illustrate that as part of a rehabilitation program, these modalities might be useful to facilitate active exercise and training.

### Summary: Physical Agents and Modalities

We agree with the guidelines. Although sparse, the current literature does not support the use of modalities as primary treatments in the management of acute LBP. Results of the study by Mitchell and Carmen (31) suggest that as part of a comprehensive rehabilitation program, modalities may play a role, but future studies are necessary to address this.

## LUMBAR CORSETS AND BACK BELTS

### AHCPR Conclusions

*Lumbar corsets have not been proven beneficial for treating patients with acute LBP.*

Lumbar corsets may reduce time lost from work due to LBP in individuals required to do frequent lifting at work.

### Literature Cited

Million and colleagues (32) studied chronic LBP and assessed the effectiveness of lumbar corsets with and without rigid stabilization. The sample size was quite small (n = 19). The results suggest a modest benefit of a lumbar corset with rigid support. These findings cannot be extrapolated to acute LBP sufferers.

Walsh and Schwartz (33) demonstrated in a prospective randomized trial that the use of prophylactic lumbar corsets and education for warehouse workers can reduce lost time from work.

### Additional Literature

Valle-Jones and colleagues (34) studied the effectiveness of the "Lumbotrain" back support in patients with *acute* nonspecific LBP. They randomized 111 patients with LBP (average symptom duration of 12 days) to the back support group and 105 to the control group (average 10 days of symptoms) to receive advice on rest and lifestyle. Both groups were permitted to take analgesics. The majority of patients (83%) were injured due to lifting or falling. After 3 weeks of intervention, the "Lumbotrain" back support subjects were significantly better than the control

subjects in all outcome measures: pain, duration of symptoms, and percentage returning to normal work. The authors concluded that the "Lumbotrain" back support is useful in treatment of patients with acute nonspecific LBP.

A recent summary of a large-scale study conducted by Jess F. Kraus, professor of epidemiology at the UCLA School of Public Health, supports the use of lumbar supports in the workplace (35). In this synopsis of a study yet to be published, 36,000 employees at Home Depot stores in California who logged 101 million work hours were studied. The researchers found that after implementation of mandatory back support use, the incidence of acute LBP fell from 30.6 per million hours to 20.2 per million hours.

### Summary: Lumbar Corsets and Back Belts

We disagree with the guidelines. The clinical guidelines did not cite literature dealing with acute LBP. The recent article by Valle-Jones and colleagues (34) shows a beneficial effect of lumbar support in the management of patients with acute LBP. This was a well-designed study specifically dealing with acute LBP, assessing effectiveness at pain reduction, analgesic consumption, and return to work. It is compelling evidence of efficacy and illustrates the ability of new information to render clinical guidelines obsolete. These findings should, however, be confirmed by other researchers before definitive statements are made or standards of care are developed.

We agree that for workers who do heavy lifting as part of their vocation, prophylactic lumbar support and education are useful in reducing time lost from work and reducing the incidence of acute LBP.

# *S*ummary

The AHCPR guidelines are an attempt at providing a framework for management of patients suffering from acute LBP. With respect to the interventions discussed, the guidelines frequently extrapolated findings from studies dealing with chronic LBP and applied them to patients with acute LBP. Recent literature published after the AHCPR guidelines begins to address the efficacy of specific treatments as they apply to patients with acute LBP. Considerable work remains to clarify the optimal diagnostic and therapeutic strategies for patients with acute low back pain.

*References*

1. Bigos S, Bowyer O, Braen G et al. Acute low back problems in adults. Clinical practice guideline. Quick reference Guide number 14. Rockville, MD; US Dept. of Health and Human Services, Public Health Service, Agency for Health Care Policy and Research, AHCPR Pub. No 95–0643. Dec 1994.

2. Bigos S, Bowyer O, Braen G et al. Acute low back problems in adults. Clinical practice guideline number 14. Rockville, MD; US Dept. of Health and Human Services, Public Health Service, Agency for Health Care Policy and Research, AHCPR Pub. No 95–0642. Dec 1994.

3. Larsson U, Choler U, Lidstrom A, Lind G, Nachemson A, Nilsson B, Roslund J. Auto-traction for treatment of lumbago-sciatica. A multicenter controlled investigation. *Acta Orthop Scand* 1980 Oct; 51(5):791–798.

3. Larsson U, Choler U, Lidstrom A, Lind G, Nachemson A, Nilsson B, Roslund J. Auto-traction for treatment of lumbago-sciatica. A multicenter controlled investigation. *Acta Orthop Scand* 1980 Oct; 51(5):791–798.

4. Mathews JA, Mills SB, Jenkins VM, Grimes SM, Morkel MJ, Mathews W, Scott CM, Sittampalam Y. Back pain and sciatica: controlled trials of manipulation, traction, sclerosant and epidural injections. *Br J Rheumatol* 1987 Dec; 26(6):416–423.

5. Pal B, Mangion P, Hossain MA, Diffey BL. A controlled trial of continuous lumbar traction in the treatment of back pain and sciatica. *Br J Rheumat* 1986; 25:181–183.

6. Mathews JA, Hickling J. Lumbar traction: a double-blind controlled study for sciatica. *Rheum Rehabil* 1975; 14:222–225.

7. Coxhead CE, Meade TW, Inskip H, North WRS, Troup JDG. Multicenter trial of physiotherapy in the management of sciatic symptoms. *Lancet* 1981 May; 8229:1065–1068.

8. Beurskens A, deVet HC, Koke AJ, Lindeman E, Regtop W, van der Heijden GJ, Knipschild PG. Efficacy of traction for non-specific low back pain: a randomised clinical trial. *Lancet* 1995; 346:1596–1600.

9. Deyo RA, Walsh NE, Martin DC, Schoenfeld LS, Ramamurthy S. A controlled trial of transcutaneous electrical nerve stimulation (TENS) and exercise for chronic low back pain. *New Engl J Med* 1990 Jun; 322(23):1627–1634.

10. Thorsteinsson G, Stonnington HH, Stillwell GK, Elveback LR. Transcutaneous electrical stimulation: a double-blind trial of its efficacy for pain. *Arch Phys Med Rehabil* 1977 Jan; 58:8–13.

11. Graff-Radford SB, Reeves JL, Baker RL, Chiu D. Effects of transcutaneous electrical nerve stimulation on myofascial pain and trigger point sensitivity. *Pain* 1989; 37:1–5.

12. Thorsteinsson G, Stonnington HH, Stillwell GK, Elveback LR. The placebo effect of transcutaneous electrical stimulation. *Pain* 1978; 5:31–41.

13. Lehmann TR, Russell DW, Spratt KF, Colby H, Liu YK, Fairchild ML. Christensen S. Efficacy of electro-acupuncture and TENS in the rehabilitation of chronic low back pain patients. *Pain* 1986 Sep; 26(3):277–290.

14. Melzack R, Vetere P, Finch L. Transcutaneous electrical nerve stimulation for low back pain. *Phys Ther* 1983 Apr; 63(4):489–493.

15. Lehmann TR, Russell DW, Spratt KF. The impact of patients with nonorganic physical findings on a controlled trial of transcutaneous electrical nerve stimulation and electroacupuncture, *Spine* 1983; 8(6):625–634.

16. Hackett GI, Seddon D, Kaminski D. Electroacupuncture compared with paracetamol for acute low back pain. *Practitioner* 1988 Feb; 22;232:163–164.

17. Marchand S, Charest J, Li J, Chenard JR, Lavignolle B, Laurencelle L. Is TENS purely a placebo effect? A controlled study on chronic low back pain. *Pain* 1993; 54:99–106.

18. Pope MH, Phillips RB, Haugh LD, Hsieh CY, Mac Donald L, Hadelman S. A prospective randomized three-week trial of spinal manipulation, transcutaneous muscle stimulation, massage and corset in the the treatment of sub-acute low back pain. *Spine* 1994; 19(22):2571–2577.

19. Herman E, Williams R, Stratford P, Fargas-Babjak A, Trott M. A randomized controlled trial of transcutaneous electrical nerve stimulation (CODETRON) to determine its benefits in a rehabilitation program for acute occupational low back pain. *Spine* 1994; 19(5):561–568.

20. Asfour SS, Khalil TM, Waly SM, Goldberg ML, Rosomoff RS, Rosomoff HL. Biofeedback in back muscle strengthening. *Spine* 1990 Jun;15(6):510–3.

21. Bush C, Ditto B, Feuerstein M. A controlled evaluation of paraspinal EMG biofeedback in the treatment of chronic low back pain. *Health Psychol* 1985;4(4):307–21.

22. Nouwen A. EMG biofeedback used to reduce standing levels of paraspinal muscle tension in chronic low back pain. *Pain* 1983; 17(4):353–360.

23. Stuckey SJ, Jacobs A, Goldfarb J. EMG biofeedback training, relaxation training, and placebo for the relief of chronic back pain. *Percept Motor Skills* 1986; 63:1023–1036.

24. Flor H, Haag G, Turk DC, Koehler H. Efficacy of EMG biofeedback, pseudotherapy, and conventional medical treatment for chronic rheumatic back pain. *Pain* 1983 Sep; 17(1):21–31.

25. Flor H, Haag G, Turk DC. Long-term efficacy of EMG biofeedback for chronic rheumatic back pain. *Pain* 1986 Nov; 27(2):195–202.

26. Waterworth RF, Hunter IA. An open study of diflunisal, conservative and manipulative therapy in the management of acute mechanical low back pain. *N Z Med J* 1985 May; 98(779):372–375.

27. Koes BW, Bouter LM, van Marneren H, et al. Randomized clinical trial of manipulative therapy and physiotherapy for persistent back and neck complaints: results of one year follow up. *Br Med J* 1992; 304:601–5.

28. Koes BW, Bouter LM, van Marneren H, et al. The effectiveness of manual therapy, physiotherapy, and treatment by the general practitioner for nonspecific back and neck complaints: a randomized clinical trial. *Spine* 1992; 17(1):28–35.

29. Klein RG, Eek BC. Low-energy laser treatment and exercise for chronic low back pain: double-blind controlled trial. *Arch Phys Med Rehabil* 1990 Jan; 71(1):34–37.

30. Gibson T, Grahame R, Harkness J, Woo P, Blagrave P, Hills R. Controlled comparison of short-wave diathermy treatment with osteopathic treatment in non-specific low back pain. *Lancet* 1985 Jun 1; 1(8440):1258–1261.

31. Mitchell RI, Carmen GM. Results of a multicenter trial using an intensive active exercise program for the treatment of acute soft tissue and back injuries. *Spine* 1990; 15(6):514–521.

32. Million R, Haavik Nilson K, Jayson MTV, Baker RD. Evaluation of low back pain and assessment of lumbar corsets with and without back supports. *Ann Rheum Dis* 1981; 40:449–454.

33. Walsh NE, Schwartz RK. The influence of prophylactic orthoses on abdominal strength and low back injury in the workplace. *Am J Phys Med Rehab* 1990 Oct; 69(5):245–250.

34. Valle-Jones JC, Walsh H, O'Hara J, O'Hara H, Davey NB, Hopkin-Richards H. Controlled trial of a back support ('Lumbotrain') in patients with non-specific low back pain. *Current Med Res Opinion* 1992; 12(9):604–613.

35. McIntyre DR, Bolte KM, Pope MH. Study provides new evidence of back belts' effectiveness. *Occup Health Saf* 1996 Dec; 65(12):39–41.

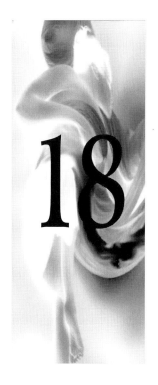

# 18 Manipulation

*James W. Atchison, D.O.*

Spinal manipulation was recommended by the AHCPR committee as one of the "physical treatments for symptom control" for the management of acute low back problems. Manipulation is defined in the AHCPR guidelines as "manual therapy in which loads are applied to the spine using short or long lever methods. The selected joint is moved to its end range of voluntary motion, followed by application of an impulse loading. The therapeutic objectives of manipulation include symptomatic relief and functional improvement."

A total of 112 articles were screened to provide 13 articles (1–13) that met inclusion for the AHCPR Guideline criteria. Additionally, five articles (14–18) that did not meet the inclusion criteria and four meta-analysis/cost-analysis (19–22) were included. Sixteen different clinical trials were accepted (1–11,13–16,18). Of the "physical treatment" options listed, manipulation was the only one with clear support by the AHCPR committee.

In the supporting literature, the AHCPR committee included two (19,21) of four (19,21,23,24) recent review articles that rated studies for scientific quality. The review articles with the highest rated manipulation studies were of average scientific merit but showed positive benefits from manipulation. Some commonly referenced articles (25–28) on manipulation were included in the review papers but not individually cited by the committee. Many of the manipulation studies with equivocal or negative results were of very low scientific merit.

The vocabulary associated with manipulation is not universal. In some countries the term *manipulation* refers only to thrusting techniques, while articulatory or oscillating treatments are classified as mobilization techniques. However, in the United States the term *manipulation* refers to any therapy in which manual loads are applied using long or short lever methods. The manipulation techniques utilized in the clinical trials referenced by the AHCPR committee included chiropractic (10), osteopathic (4,6), Maitland (1,5,16), Maigne (2), Cyriax (8,15), thrusting (3,7,9,18), oscillatory (articulatory) (14), muscle energy (11), and therapist's choice (1,13). To identify what type of treatment a patient received, techniques were classified as thrusting/high-velocity, low-amplitude (HVLA) techniques or non-thrusting techniques (see Table 18–1) (29). The non-thrusting techniques were further classified into oscillatory/articulatory (30–32),

---

**TABLE 18–1**
*Manual Medicine Techniques*

---

THRUSTING

Mobilization with Impulse or High-Velocity,
  Low-Amplitude (HVLA)

NON-THRUSTING

Mobilization without Impulse/Articulatory

Muscle Energy

Counterstrain

Functional Techniques

Myofascial Release

Soft Tissue

Craniosacral

---

From Atchison JW, Stoll ST, and Gilliar WG: Manipulation, Traction and Massage. In: Braddom RL (ed). *Physical medicine and rehabilitation*. Philadelphia: W. B. Saunders Company, 1995, p. 428.

---

myofascial (33,34), muscle energy (30,35), or functional indirect techniques such as Jones's counterstrain (36).

Within the literature referenced by the AHCPR committee, 11 of the 16 clinical trials involved some form of thrusting or HVLA manipulation (see Figure 18–1). The papers referring to thrusting (3,7,9,18), chiropractic (10), and Maigne (2) had treatment groups that received HVLA/thrusting. Additionally, the study groups in the articles reporting use of osteopathic (4,6) and Maitland (1,5,16) treatment received some thrusting treatments along with non-thrusting. The subjects often received the thrust at the end of a side-lying muscle energy or mobilization technique because thrusting could be performed in a sequential protocol without changing the patient's position.

Ten clinical trials involved the use of non-thrusting manipulation techniques, but only five of these trials had no thrusting included. Two studies (1,13) allowed therapists to use any manual technique that was indicated without a structured protocol. These techniques were most likely non-thrusting. At least seven studies involved mobilization techniques, including the Maitland treat-

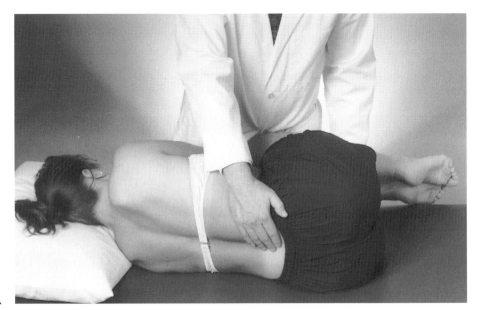

A

**FIGURE 18–1. A–D**

---

High-Velocity, Low-Amplitude treatment for the lumbar spine with rotatory thrusting. *A:* The patient is flexed to the level of the barrier from below by using the legs and hips. *B:* The lower leg is re-extended and the top knee dropped to the table which adds right sidebending and left rotation below the level of dysfunction. *C:* From above, extension, right rotation, and left sidebending are incorporated by dropping the top shoulder posteriorly and pulling the inferior arm toward the practitioner. *D:* The practitioner thrusts by dropping his/her shoulders forcing the patient's shoulder toward the table and the hip toward himself.

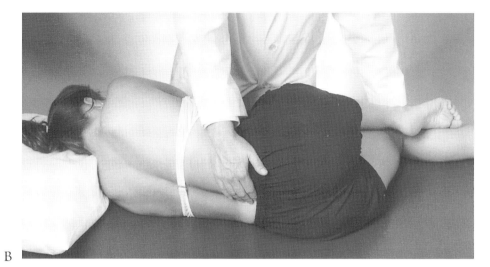

B

C

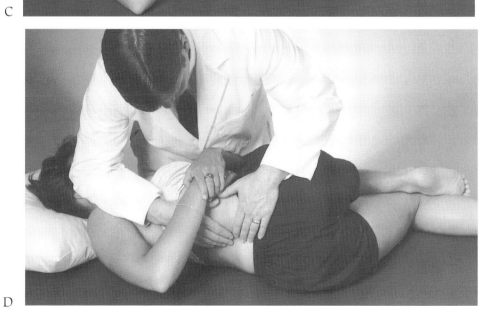

D

**FIGURE 18–1. (CONTINUED)**

ment groups (1,5,16), the osteopathic treatment groups (4,6), Nwuga's (14) study, which used oscillatory treatment (32), and the Mathews (8) study, which used Cyriax's technique (37) of distraction along with overpressure. The osteopathic combined treatment groups also received some myofascial or soft tissue techniques. Only Brodin (11) focused on a single type of osteopathic manipulation, using muscle energy techniques in his study (see Figure 18–2).

As with most treatment options for low back pain, there was no large, single population, multicenter, randomized, double-blind controlled study to indicate the absolute effectiveness or ineffectiveness of manipulation. Therefore, the committee had to use studies that encompassed a wide variety of manipulation techniques, study designs, and outcome measures to make decisions. Of the 16 clinical trials referenced by the committee, subject numbers ranged from 42 to 398 with participants distributed over two to four treatment groups. Hadler (3) reported on many of the difficulties with these studies through 1987. Unfortunately, blinded studies using therapies such as exercise and manipulation are virtually impossible to design. Additionally, the ongoing debate regarding pain control or return to function as the measurement of successful treatment has made comparing studies difficult.

Another major limitation in reviewing the literature on manipulation is that no two studies followed the same treatment regimen or included the same patient population. Many articles did not discuss the specifics of the treatment protocols. Those that did varied from a single treatment (3,7) to treatments three to five times per week for two to three weeks (1,2,4,8,10,13,14). Postacchini's study (10) is the only one to report treatment for longer than four weeks. Additionally, the patient populations were based on a variety of inclusion and exclusion criteria regarding back and/or leg pain and neurologic signs and/or symptoms. The length of symptoms was extremely variable, although several studies did limit it to less than two or three weeks. The committee had a difficult time trying to determine the most appropriate clinical pathways from the data.

## AGREEMENT OR DISAGREEMENT

*Guideline #1.* Manipulation can be helpful for patients with acute low back problems without radiculopathy when used within the first month of symptoms. (Strength of Rating = B). AGREE. As the committee pointed out with their strength of evidence ratings, the first recommendation is the only one that has literature support. All of the clinical trials reported showed some benefit to the use of manipulation, but difficulties exist in establishing

a definitive clinical regimen related to the varied outcome measures and comparison groups in the studies.

The highest scientifically rated articles (in order) according to Anderson's review (21) were by Waagen (38), Berquist-Ullman (9), Hoehler (26), Farrell (5), Glover (7), and Hadler (3). Waagen (38) is not widely quoted since there were only 19 subjects with chronic low back pain and no functional outcome measurements. Hoehler (26) reported an initially significant decrease in pain and improved dressing, reaching, sitting up in bed, and sitting in a chair after an initial rotational thrusting treatment; but after three to four weeks of treatment there was no difference in outcome measures. Berquist-Ullman (9) demonstrated "better" response to manipulation combined with other physiotherapy than placebo in persons with acute and subacute industrial injuries. Farrell (5) utilized Maitland treatment methods in patients symptomatic for less than three weeks and demonstrated significantly shorter duration of symptoms. Additionally, the patients achieved symptom-free status with fewer treatment sessions than a regimen of microwave diathermy, isometric abdominal exercises, and ergonomic instructions. Glover (7) demonstrated significant improvement in pain relief at 15 minutes with a single rotational thrust as compared to detuned (simulated) short-wave diathermy. The long-term benefit of this study was limited by the single treatment session, which allowed the placebo group to reach the same level of pain relief as the manipulation group at three- and seven-day follow-up evaluations.

Hadler (3) in 1987 was one of the first to use a functional measurement of outcome in evaluating the effectiveness of manipulation, and his study has been one of the most widely quoted in favor of manipulation. The study used a single thrusting treatment with the Roland-Morris (39,40) modification of the Sickness Impact Profile to demonstrate that subjects with symptoms between two and four weeks had more rapid reduction (of 50 percent) in outcome scores with manipulation. The major conclusion was that the rate of improvement was significantly increased with the use of manipulation. This was also one of the first manipulation studies to prospectively stratify the treatment groups based on length of symptoms and to assess the rate of improvement. This rate of improvement is extremely important in determining the potential benefit of manipulation since the follow-up outcome results were similar at two and three weeks . However, as the article notes, ". . . the ability to abrogate an episode of backache, even by a few days, has major ramifications."

Shekelle's review (19) lists the manipulation studies in order of the quality score as Ongley (41), Hadler (3), MacDonald (4), Meade (25), and Berquist-Ullman (9). Besides rating all the articles separately, Shekelle did a combined analysis indicating that the probability of recovery

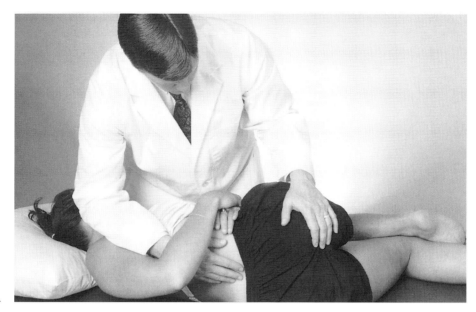

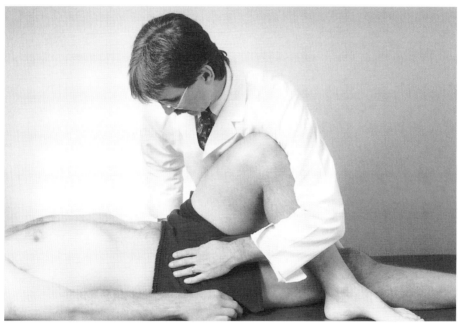

**FIGURE 18–2. A, B**

Possible muscle energy treatment techniques for the lumbar spine. There is a muscle contraction maintained for 3–5 seconds and then a relaxation phase which allows further stretching. Proper positioning allows the force of the contraction to be localized at the barrier. *A:* In the same position as for thrusting, the patient pushes up with the right shoulder and back with the right hip. During the relaxation stage, the practitioner stretches the right shoulder toward the table and the right hip toward himself. *B:* In the supine position, left hip is flexed, adducted, and internally rotated until the practitioner feels the barrier engaged with his right hand. The patient contracts the leg into the chest of the practitioner.

at three weeks is enhanced 0.17 by manipulation (if 50 percent recover, then by adding manipulation, 67 percent will recover). This is an increase of 17 percent in the number of patients who recover. The Hadler (3) and Berquist-Ullman (9) articles were previously discussed. The Ongley study (41) showed significant benefit in subjects with chronic low back pain by combining manipulation with prolotherapy. Meade's (25) study in 1990 demonstrated significant improvement in a treatment group receiving chiropractic treatment vs. therapist mobilization as determined by the Oswestry pain disability questionnaire. At two years follow-up, there was still significant improvement in the chiropractic treatment group.

MacDonald's article (4) is the other recent manipulation study that is widely quoted as it closely parallels Hadler's work (3). MacDonald used the Disability Index score as his functional measurement tool and demonstrated significant improvement in a group of patients treated with osteopathic manipulative treatment (OMT) two times per week (mean number of treatments = 5). The subgroup of patients with onset of symptoms between 14 and 28 days demonstrated the most significant improvement response between one and two weeks after beginning treatment. MacDonald reports that ". . . a larger proportion of the OMT group recovered in the first week and in the long term (eight to nine weeks)." So the rate of improvement was once again greater with manipulation.

*Guideline #1* allows for the appropriate use of manipulation as a treatment method that has been scrutinized more closely than any other therapy available for low back pain. It also emphasizes that a trial of manipulation will be most beneficial if implemented in the acute stage. As a practitioner of manual medicine, I strongly agree with both of these principles.

*Guideline #2.* When findings suggest progressive or severe neurologic deficits, an appropriate diagnostic assessment to rule out serious neurologic conditions is indicated before beginning manipulation therapy. (Strength of Rating = D). AGREE BUT DISAGREE. This guideline is unnecessary in this section because it is a true statement for all conservative treatment options, not just manipulation. This recommendation does not seem to specifically address any literature about manipulation, but seems to be an editorial comment that a good history and physical examination should be performed, and if there are objective neurologic changes further work-up may be indicated before any treatment. The guidelines address this issue in the chapters on "Initial Assessment" and "Special Studies and Diagnostic Considerations," and it seems redundant in this section. Perhaps it is mentioned in the manipulation section since manipulation is one of the few specific treatments recommended by the committee.

In my opinion, this guideline is included to emphasize the fact that there is *no* literature to support the use

of manipulation with a progressive neurologic deficit, and there are *no* studies that have looked at the use of manipulation with a nonprogressive but severe neurologic deficit. I am in agreement with the principle of this recommendation, but think the committee should say clearly that manipulation is "not recommended" in patients with progressive or severe neurologic deficits and should quantify these terms. Otherwise the "Initial Assessment" section should be relied on to emphasize the need to rule out significant neurologic deficits before any treatment.

*Guideline #3.* There is insufficient evidence to recommend manipulation for patients with radiculopathy. (Strength of Rating = C). DISAGREE. This is the most controversial area of treatment with manipulation because there may be a greater risk of the patient with radiculopathy getting worse than when treating nonradicular problems. However, at present there is no literature to suggest an increased risk. Of the 16 clinical trials accepted by the AHCPR committee, 10 specifically did not study or excluded persons with radicular signs or symptoms. The trials that addressed the question of manipulation for patients with radiculopathy were by Nwuga (14), Edwards (16), MacDonald (4), Postacchini (10), and Coxhead (1). Shekelle (19) discussed this topic specifically in his review, and in fact this guideline closely resembles one of the conclusions that Shekelle presented. The committee seems to have relied heavily on his findings.

Nwuga (14) evaluated a patient population with disc "protrusion," confirmed by myelography and electrodiagnosis, who had radiculopathy with unilateral sensory and/or reflex changes. The treatment group received oscillatory manipulation and had significant benefit compared with diathermy and isometric trunk exercises. Unfortunately, Nwuga's outcome measures were improved range of motion of the lumbar spine and improved degrees of straight leg raising maneuver instead of pain relief, return to work, or increased functional activities. Coxhead (1) studied patients with ". . . pain of sciatic distribution at least as far as the buttock crease," but did not discuss whether there were any neurologic signs present. The subgroup receiving manipulation demonstrated statistically significant improvement in the pain analogue score at four weeks while subgroups receiving traction, exercises, and corset use did not. MacDonald (4) also included subjects with signs and symptoms of radiculopathy in his treatment group who benefited from OMT. Unfortunately, he did not analyze the radiculopathy group separately to determine whether they had similar improvements in outcome to his entire group.

More than any other study, Edwards (16) demonstrated positive benefit in persons with radiculopathy using manipulation. He utilized Maitland treatment techniques compared to heat/massage/exercise in three subgroups with radicular symptoms. Subgroup II ("pain radiating into one buttock") had equal treatment benefit from the two interventions, but the manipulation subjects improved in half the time. In subgroup III ("pain radiating down the posterior aspect of the thigh to the knee" and "some subjective sensory loss or pins and needles") and subgroup IV ("pain radiating down to the posterior part of lower leg or foot" and "...neurologic changes to the extent of diminished reflexes or well marked dermatome sensory loss") there was a more pronounced benefit with manipulation. Both group III and group IV showed a statistically significant increase in ability to return to work and daily activities. Additionally, improvement occurred with fewer manipulation treatments than with the alternative treatment. The text reports that "no patients were made worse by either treatment," but Edwards emphasizes that only the mobilization techniques were utilized and did not recommend thrusting in this patient population. On the other hand, Postacchini (10) did thrusting manipulation to a subgroup of acute (symptoms less than four weeks) patients with "low back pain radiating to the buttocks and/or thighs and no neurological changes" and reported significant benefit with no adverse outcomes. Even with these findings, Postacchini does not recommend the use of thrusting manipulation with pain below the knee and/or neurologic deficit (undefined).

Although there are reports of thrusting manipulation causing cauda equina syndrome and/or progressive neurologic decline (42–46), none of the studies using patients with radiating leg symptoms and mild neurologic signs have shown any adverse outcomes or decline in neurologic status. Manipulation in the patients with radiculopathy is clearly an area where further research is needed because it is difficult to determine whether a person with slowly progressive neurologic findings has declined due to the manipulation or has simply not benefited from the treatment and is experiencing the natural progression of radiculopathy. Repeated MRI scans may help determine which patients with radiculopathy would benefit safely from manipulation and which patients would continue to decline. It is essential to identify and establish appropriate and effective treatment protocols for patients with leg pain and minimal neurologic findings because lumbar, pelvic, or sacral dysfunction can cause similar symptoms and manipulation may be an excellent choice of treatment.

If guideline #2 were revised to eliminate patients with progressive or severe neurologic deficits, then guideline #3 could clarify the use of manipulation for patients experiencing radicular symptoms (leg pain) with minimal or no neurologic deficit. In my opinion, persons with leg pain and/or mild neurologic deficits on physical examination are candidates for manipulation. However, treating this patient population with manipulation requires a great deal of experience and expertise, and the vast differences in training and skills among practitioners must

be considered when establishing guidelines. The decision of whether to initiate and/or continue manipulation treatment in a patient with radiculopathy should be based on whether or not the patient has increasing leg symptoms while positioning for the treatment technique. This guideline needs specifics that would allow treatment attempts to begin but would give the clinician some objective measures to follow as to whether to continue a particular technique. This would also allow for the appropriate use of the non-thrusting techniques that have been described as being beneficial in previous studies of this patient population (1,4,10,14,16).

*Guideline #4.* A trial of manipulation in patients without radiculopathy with symptoms longer than a month is probably safe, but efficacy is unproven. (Strength of Rating = C). DISAGREE. Five studies reviewed by the committee report the use of manipulation in a chronic low back pain population. Two of these studies showed equivocal (6) or no benefit (10). Mathews (8), however, reported a significant reduction in pain with Cyriax manipulation throughout his entire study and some of the subjects had been symptomatic for up to 13 weeks. Unfortunately, the subgroup with symptoms greater than four weeks was not analyzed separately. Coxhead (1) found improvement in pain reduction at four weeks in a group of subjects with leg pain (average 14.3 weeks) using Maitland treatment techniques daily for one week and then prn for three weeks. MacDonald (4) analyzed a subgroup of 10 subjects with symptoms greater than 28 days who showed improvement from manipulation as measured by the Disability Index.

There is additional literature to support a trial of manipulation after four weeks of low back pain. In fact, a study by Koes (47) was referenced by the AHCPR committee in the physical treatment section, but not referred to in the manipulation discussion. The study demonstrated a greater decrease in chief complaint and increase in physical functioning with manipulation/mobilization than with physiotherapy (exercises, massage, modalities) in a group of subjects with nonspecific spinal complaints for at least six weeks. Cassidy and Kirkaldy-Willis (48) also previously reported on a two to three week treatment protocol of daily thrusting manipulation in 283 patients with chronic (5.6–16.9 years) low back and leg pain. The patients were "disabled" by constant severe pain and had not responded to numerous conservative treatment regimens. They reported improvement related to pain and/or function in 54–96 percent, depending on the clinical diagnosis. This study was not analyzed by any of the review articles for quality and scientific merit, but clearly demonstrated a positive benefit for a trial of manipulation in some patients with chronic problems.

In my opinion, the literature supports the use of a trial of manipulation in persons with low back pain and/or leg pain for greater than four weeks if there are specific findings on physical examination to indicate structural or segmental abnormality. As always, if there is no specific indication for manipulation, the chances of success are limited. This patient population (symptoms greater than four weeks) may also benefit from using manipulation in combination with other treatments such as exercise (49) or specific spinal injections (41,50–53). Without question, the success of treatment should be monitored closely to limit the length of the treatment trial to an appropriate time frame.

*Guideline #5.* If manipulation has not resulted in symptomatic improvement that allows increased function after one month of treatment, manipulation therapy should be stopped and the patient reevaluated. (Strength of Rating = D). AGREE BUT DISAGREE. Of all 16 clinical trials referenced, the only study that actually addressed this guideline specifically was done by Postacchini (10). He performed chiropractic manipulation daily for one week and then two times per week for a total of six weeks (not dramatically longer than the four weeks suggested), but only in a group of subjects symptomatic for greater than two months. A combined pain and functional assessment tool was used to determine that after six months there was no difference in the group treated with manipulation. No other referenced study used a treatment trial of greater than four weeks, and several of the studies did not use functional measurements to determine the success or failure of the manipulative treatment.

This is a good general guideline that should be included in every section of the treatment guidelines. In my opinion, this guideline is included to emphasize that manipulation should be utilized for a short course of treatment and should not be continued indefinitely. This is true for any of the conservative treatment options for low back pain, but over the years manipulation has maintained a "questionable reputation" due to prolonged, unjustified treatment protocols. A limit on nonbeneficial treatment and time frames for reevaluation would be welcome additions to the guidelines by persons who practice manual medicine appropriately. In fact, a practitioner of manual medicine should reevaluate the structural diagnosis (22,30) at the start and at the end of each treatment session, and if the appropriate indications were not present manipulation would be discontinued.

It should be emphasized that this guideline indicates that manipulation should be stopped after one month if there is no increase in function. This guideline *does not say* that all manipulation has to stop at the end of one month. This means that all clinicians must monitor and document their patient's functional improvement to manipulation in order to continue treatment beyond four weeks. I am strongly in agreement with basing the need for the continuation of any treatment of low back pain on the patient's functional response.

## NEW LITERATURE

*Guideline #1.* There have been no new, well-designed, large population studies on manipulation during the first four weeks of low back pain published since the AHCPR guidelines were developed. The guidelines identified the need for evaluating specific areas related to the use of manipulation, and there are several large trials ongoing at present. Publications continue to discuss the work already done and reported. An analysis of previous work by Assendelft in *JAMA* (54) included methodologic assessment of the previous review articles and many other studies not previously reviewed. Nine of the ten highest rated articles, including studies on both acute and chronic populations, demonstrated a beneficial response to manipulation.

The guidelines have spurred many articles on the appropriate treatment of acute low back pain (55–57). Most articles have begun to include a discussion of the use of manipulation and to emphasize the point that all physicians must consider its use. The journal *Spine* has been addressing many specific treatment issues with "Contemporary Concepts" and "Spine Update" articles by experts. There have been two such articles (49,58) published supporting the use of spinal manipulation.

*Guideline #2.* There continues to be *no* study assessing the use of manipulation in a patient population with progressive or severe neurologic deficit. In my opinion, it would be unethical to do this study in a human population without several animal trials indicating potential benefit and no long-term adverse outcomes.

*Guideline #3.* There is no recent article updating the use of manipulation in patients with radiculopathy. Although there are nationally funded, large, ongoing trials of chiropractic and osteopathic manipulation, I am not aware of specific trials to address patients with minimal, stable neurologic deficits associated with radiculopathy.

*Guideline #4.* There have been two new trials since publication of the AHCPR guidelines. Triano (59) reported on the positive benefit of manipulation in 209 subjects with untreated low back pain greater than seven weeks. The treatment group received thrusting manipulation daily for two weeks and reported greater improvement in pain and activity tolerance than a manipulation "mimic" group and a back school group at the end of two and four weeks. No long-term follow-up data have been reported yet. Pope (60) found no benefit in physical outcome measures (range of motion, fatigue, strength, or pain) after three weeks of treatment with manipulation compared to massage, transcutaneous muscle stimulation, or corset use. The subjects had low back pain between three weeks and six months and received thrusting manipulation three times per week for the three weeks. Even though this study tried to specifically address criticisms of previous manipulation studies, no functional outcome measures were reported and there was no follow-up period beyond the three-week treatment period.

*Guideline #5.* There are no new studies specifically addressing time frames for appropriate treatment protocols. However, since the AHCPR published the guidelines, there have been many organizations promoting practice parameters that limit manipulative treatments to a certain number of visits and/or weeks of treatment. Much of the basis for these limitations has come from Shekelle's publications (61,62), which expressed the opinions of expert panels on treatment frequency and duration. Shekelle's recent "Spine Update" (58) reiterates the panel consensus that an appropriate trial of manipulation is about 12 treatments over a month but emphasizes that there is no scientific basis to determine that any one treatment regimen is better than another at this point.

## FUTURE RESEARCH

In my opinion, the publication of the AHCPR guidelines has identified many areas in which the literature does not provide a definite answer for the appropriate treatment of low back pain. By endorsing or not endorsing specific spinal treatments, the committee has reawakened the interest of many clinicians to research these questions and has identified many areas of potential funding opportunities for researchers and funding agencies. The publication has also brought to our attention the low scientific quality of many publications that are quoted frequently to determine clinical policy. This should make us all desire and support more rigorous clinical trials in the future. Until there is a consensus about what the key outcome measures to be used by all studies of low back pain are, further studies of manipulation will continue to raise more controversy and questions.

As identified previously in the text, the most important question regarding manipulation is in the patient population with radicular symptoms and minimal but stable neurologic deficit. In order to determine which patients with radiculopathy are candidates for manipulation, it will take MRI scans along with the initial history and physical examination on all subjects prior to manipulation, and follow-up MRI scans, physical examination, and functional outcome measurements to assess the effect on the disc and the patient. This would be an expensive study requiring a large funding agency to determine if there is a clinical presentation or specific type of disc injury that may significantly benefit safely from manipulation.

The other key questions to answer with future research include the most effective frequency and duration of treatment, the most effective type of treatment, and the type, location, and duration of symptoms in a patient that will respond the best. Although most researchers would like to isolate or limit the variables in a research study, most clinicians would like to know which treatments should be combined for the best success in treating low back pain. Of most interest at the present time is analyzing the effect of combining manipulation with active aggressive exercise programs, specific medication regimens, and/or specific spinal injections (e.g., facet, sacroiliac, lumbar sympathetic).

## CLINICAL UTILIZATION

The AHCPR guidelines were developed to introduce a more structured course of treatment for patients with acute low back pain. The use of manipulation as part of the treatment plan is approved, but it must be combined with the other components such as medications, exercise, activity modifications (including proper body mechanics), and specific spinal injections (if indicated). In order to effectively administer all of these components, physicians without training in manipulation must establish a working relationship with either a physical therapist, chiropractor, osteopathic physician, or allopathic physician who can provide manipulative treatment. Chiropractors and physical therapists should establish relationships with physicians who can manage medications and/or perform spinal injections. These referral relationships should be cultivated prior to any patient care and designed along a clinical pathway so that upon referral, treatment is clearly established and effectively coordinated. The skill of the practitioner is certainly a factor in the consideration of whether or not to refer, as well as the cost involved with having a combination of treaters.

One of the keys to clinical utilization of manipulation is the appropriate timing of the treatment. If manipulation is considered to be an option for a particular patient, treatment or referral should be done during the early stages of recovery (0–6 weeks). Manipulation should not be a consideration only after everything else has failed or it will most likely also have a high potential for failure. Unfortunately, as with most treatment approaches to low back pain, a clear picture on physical examination of who will benefit from this treatment is not available. The most important factor to consider when evaluating a patient for manipulation is the potential for decreased pain and/or improved functional ability and the rate of improvement. The physician must also combine manipulation with an active treatment program for the best long-term results. Manipulation is a passive treatment process that can initiate spinal movement, but without continued active movement this correction in the spinal biomechanics may not stabilize and symptoms will recur. The use of manual medicine within an overall treatment program of low back pain has been discussed in many review articles (55–57) over the past few years and the relationship to exercise is specifically addressed (49). It must be emphasized that even though the AHCPR guidelines discuss manipulation as a lone entity, physicians who effectively utilize manual medicine do so within a comprehensive rehabilitation treatment plan.

The AHCPR guidelines are designed specifically to reduce overall cost and to look at the long-term outcome of patients as related to large populations. This is not necessarily the best way to look at each patient who comes to your office for treatment. The patient wants pain relief as quickly as possible and often can receive it with an appropriate manual medicine technique. Reduction in pain has been demonstrated to speed recovery of functional activities by Hadler (3) and MacDonald (4). So even though most of the studies on manipulation do not show a change in long-term outcome, it is still beneficial to speed recovery in the short term. This is a very important issue to patients, employers, and third-party payors.

In today's healthcare marketplace it is employers who are paying for a large portion of the costs related to treating acute low back pain, so the rate of return to functional activities (i.e., work), is a major focus. The employer benefits significantly if a worker is pain-free and has returned to work in three weeks instead of four weeks or six weeks because it increases corporate productivity and decreases the indemnity costs related to off-work disability. Therefore, three to five visits to a practitioner of manual medicine within the first two to three weeks of treatment will demonstrate a high cost-effective ratio if indemnity costs can be reduced by two to three weeks.

When considering the use of manipulation, the physician must always consider the overall medical condition of the patient and must be aware of contraindications before treating or referring. Commonly listed medical contraindications (29,63) for thrusting and articular manipulation include spinal fracture, metabolic bone disease, bone or spinal cord tumor, rheumatoid arthritis, bleeding disorder or anticoagulant therapy, and hypermobile joints. However, none of these contraindications would prevent the use of muscle energy, indirect, or myofascial manipulation techniques. The practitioner must pay close attention to the possibility of a "red flag" during the initial history and physical examination since manipulation is recommended during the first month of treatment when imaging studies and other work-up is not recommended.

For low back pain problems that are resistant to initial conservative treatment attempts, manipulation may be effective when combined with specific spinal injections such as lumbar sympathetic blocks (52), facet injections (50,51), and sacroiliac injections (41,53). Close attention must be paid to eliminate all possible contraindications before doing any manipulation after analgesic injection.

Future considerations center around the possible use of manipulation following epidural steroid injections or selective nerve root blocks. At present, there are no specific indications for these combinations due to the fact that they most often involve patients with a known radiculopathy and they invade the neural structures. There are also no specific indications for manipulation under general anesthesia.

# Summary

In conclusion, spinal manipulation is a highly controversial treatment option for low back pain. The discussion of benefit vs. risk is often emotionally charged and lacks objectivity. It should be emphasized that the AHCPR guidelines endorse the use of manipulation as a method of treatment and do not endorse any one type of manipulation or type of practitioner.

# References

1. Coxhead CE, Meade TW, Inskip H, North WRS, Troup JDG. Multicentre trial of physiotherapy in the management of sciatic symptoms. *Lancet* 1981; 1065–1068.
2. Godfrey CM, Morgan PP, Schatzker J. A randomized trial of manipulation for low-back pain in a medical setting. *Spine* 1984; 9:301–304.
3. Hadler NM, Curtis P, Gillings DB, Stinnett S. A benefit of spinal manipulation as adjunctive therapy for acute low-back pain: a stratified controlled trial. *Spine* 1987; 12:702–706.
4. MacDonald RS, Bell CMY. An open controlled assessment of osteopathic manipulation in nonspecific low back pain. *Spine* 1990; 15:364–370.
5. Farrell JP, Twomey LT. Acute low back pain. Comparison of two conservative treatment approaches. *Med J Aust* 1982; 1:160–164.
6. Gibson T, Grahame R, Harkness J, Woo P, Blagrave P, Hills R. Controlled comparison of short-wave diathermy treatment with osteopathic treatment in non-specific low back pain. *Lancet* 1985; 1:1258–261.
7. Glover JR, Morris JG, Khosla T. Back pain: a randomized clinical trial of rotational manipulation of the trunk. *Br J Ind Med* 1974; 31:59–64.
8. Mathews JA, Mills SB, Jenkins VM, et al. Back pain and sciatica: controlled trials of manipulation, traction, sclerosant and epidural injections. *Br J Rheumatol* 1987; 26:416–423.
9. Bergquist-Ullman M, Larsson U. Acute low back pain in industry. A controlled prospective study with special

refernce to therapy and confounding factors. *Acta Orthop Scand* 1977; 170:1–117.

10. Postacchini F, Facchini M, Palieri P. Efficacy of various forms of conservative treatment in low back pain. A comparative study. *Neuro-orthopedics* 1988; 6:28–35.

11. Brodin H. Inhibition-facilitation technique for lumbar pain treatment. *Int J Rehabil Res* 1984; 7:328–329.

12. Mathews W, Morkel MJ, Mathews JA. Manipulation and traction for lumbago and sciatica: physiotherapeutic techniques used in two controlled trials. *Physiother Prac* 1988; 4:201–206.

13. Waterworth RF, Hunter IA. An open study of diflusinal, conservative and manipulative therapy in the management of acute mechanical low back pain. *N Z Med J* 1985; 98:372–375.

14. Nwuga VCB. Relative therapeutic efficacy of vertebral manipulation and conventional treatment in back pain management. *Am J Phys Med Rehabil* 1982; 6:273–278.

15. Coyer AB, Curwen IHM. Low back pain treated by manipulation. A controlled series. *Br Med J* 1955; 1:705–707.

16. Edwards BC. Low back pain and pain resulting from lumbar spine conditions. *Aust J Physiother* 1969; 15:104–110.

17. Mandell P, Lipton MH, Bernstein J, Kucera GJ, Kampner JA. *Low back pain. An historical and contemporary overview of the occupational, medical, and psychological issues of chronic back pain.* Thorofare, NJ: SLACK, Inc. 1989:219

18. Rasmussen GG. Manipulation in treatment of low-back pain (a randomized clinical trial). *Man Med* 1979; 1:8–10.

19. Shekelle PG, Adams AH, Chassin MR, Hurwitz EL, Brook RH. Spinal manipulation for low-back pain. *Ann Intern Med* 1992; 117:590–598.

20. Jarvis KB, Phillips RB, Morris EK. Cost per case comparison of back injury claims of chiropractic versus medical management for conditions with identical diagnostic codes [see comments]. *J Occup Med* 1991; 33:847–852.

21. Anderson R, Meeker WC, Wirick BE, Mootz RD, Kirk DH, Adams A. A meta-analysis of clinical trials of spinal manipulation. *J Man Physiol Ther* 1992; 15:181–194.

22. Anonymous guidelines for chiropractic quality assurance and practice parameters. Proceedings of the Mercy Center Consensus Conference. 1993. Gaitherburg, MD: Aspen Publishers, Inc., 1993:

23. Koes BW, Bowler LM, Kripschild PG. Spinal manipulation and mobilisation for back and neck pain: an indexed review. *Br Med J* 1991; 303:1298–1303.

24. Ottenbacher K, DiFabio RP. Efficacy of spinal manipulation/mobilization therapy: A meta-analysis. *Spine* 1985; 10:833–837.

25. Meade TW, Dyer S, Browne W, Townsend J, Frank AO. Low back pain of mechanical origin: randomised comparison of chiropractic and hospital outpatient treatment. *Br Med J* 1990; 300:1431–1437.

26. Hoehler FK, Tobis JS, Buerger AA. Spinal manipulation for low back pain. *JAMA* 1981; 245:1835–1838.

27. Sims-Williams H, Jayson MIV, Young SMS, Baddeley H, Collins E. Controlled trial of mobilisation and manipulation for low back pain: hospital patients. *Br Med J* 1979; 2:1318–1320.

28. Doran DML, Newell DJ. Manipulation in treatment of low back pain: a multicenter study. *Br Med J* 1975; 2:161–164.

29. Atchison JW, Stoll ST, Gilliar WG. Manipulation, trac-

tion and massage. In: Braddom RL, ed. *A textbook of physical medicine and rehabilitation.* Philadelphia: W.B. Saunders Co., 1995:421–448.

30. Greenman PE. *Principles of manual medicine.* Baltimore: Williams & Wilkins, 1989:

31. Maitland GD. *Vertebral manipulation,* 5th ed. London: Butterworths, 1986:

32. Nwuga VCB. *Manipulation of the spine.* Baltimore: Williams & Wilkins, 1976:

33. Cantu RL, Grodin AJ. *Myofascial manipulation: therory and clinical application.* Gaithersburg, MD: Aspen Publishers, Inc. 1992:

34. Ward RC. Myofascial release concepts. In: Basmajian JV, Nyberg R, eds. *Rational manual therapies.* Baltimore: Williams & Wilkins, 1993:223–241.

35. Mitchell FL, Jr., Moran PS, Pruzzo NA. *An evaluation and treatment manual of osteopathic muscle energy procedures.* Valley Park, MO: Mitchell, Moran, and Pruzzo Associates, 1979:

36. Jones LH. *Strain and counterstrain,* 13th ed. Newark, OH: American Academy of Osteopathy, 1992:

37. Cyriax J, Russell G. *Textbook of orthopaedic medicine, volume 2: treatment by manipulation, massage and injection,* 10th ed. London: Bailliere Tindall, 1980:

38. Waagen GN, Haldeman S, Cook G, Lopez D, DeBoer KF. Short term trial of chiropractic adjustments for the relief of chronic low back pain. *Man Med* 1986; 2:63–67.

39. Roland M, Morris R. A study of the natural history of low-back pain. Part II: development of guidelines for trials of treatment in primary care. *Spine* 1983; 8:145–150.

40. Roland M, Morris R. A study of the natural history of back pain. Part I: development of a reliable and sensitive measure of disability in low-back pain. *Spine* 1983; 8:141–144.

41. Ongley MJ, Klein RG, Dorman TA, Eek BC, Hubert LJ. A new approach to the treatment of chronic low back pain. *Lancet* 1987; 2:143–146.

42. Richard J. Disk rupture with cauda equina syndrome after chiropractic adjustment. *NY State J Med* 1967; 67:2496–2498.

43. Hooper J. Low back pain and manipulation: Paraparesis after treatment of low back pain by physical methods. *Med J Aust* 1973; 1:549–551.

44. Powell FC, Hanigan WC, Olivero WC. A risk/benefit analysis of spinal manipulation therapy for relief of lumbar or cervical pain. *Neurosurgery* 1992; 33:73–78.

45. Ryan MD. Massive disc sequestration after spinal manipulation [letter]. *Med J Aust* 1993; 158:718

46. Haldeman S, Rubinstein SM. Cauda equina syndrome in patients undergoing manipulation of the lumbar spine. *Spine* 1992; 17:1469–1473.

47. Koes BW, Bouter LM, van Mameren H, et al. Randomised clinical trial of manipulative therapy and physiotherapy for persistent back and neck complaints: results of one year follow up [see comments]. *BMJ* 1992; 304:601–605.

48. Cassidy JD, Kirkaldy-Willis WH. Manipulation. In: Kirkaldy-Willis WH (ed.). *Managing low back pain,* 2nd ed. New York, Edinburgh, London, Melbourne: Churchill Livingstone, 1988:287–296.

49. Twomey L, Taylor J. Exercise and spinal manipulation in the treatment of low back pain. *Spine* 1995; 20:615–619.

50. Dreyfuss PH, Dreyer SJ, Herring SA. Lumbar zygapophyseal (facet) joint injections. *Spine* 1995; 20:2040–2047.

51. Dreyfuss P, Michaelsen M, Horne M. MUJA: manipula-

tion under joint anesthesia/analgesia: a treatment approach for recalcitrant low back pain of synovial joint origin. *J Manipulative Physiol Ther* 1995; 18:537–546.

52. Atchison JW, Stoll ST, McDowell S. Manipulation under local anesthesia: lumbar sympathetic blocks followed by high velocity-low amplitude treatment. *Arch Phys Med Rehabil* 1996; 11:956.

53. Dreyfuss P, Cole AJ, Pauza K. Sacroiliac joint injection techniques. In: Weinstein SM (ed.). *Injection techniques: principles and practice.* Philadelphia: W.B. Saunders Company, 1995:785–813.

54. Assendelft WJ, Koes BW, Knipschild PG, Bouter LM. The relationship between methodological quality and conclusions in reviews of spinal manipulation [see comments]. *JAMA* 1995; 274:1942–1948.

55. Mazanec DJ. Back pain: medical evaluation and therapy. *Cleve Clin J Med* 1995; 62:163–168.

56. Reitman C, Esses SI. Conservative options in the management of spinal disorders, Part II. Exercise, education, and manual therapies. *Am J Orthop* 1995; 24:241–50.

57. Wheeler AH. Diagnosis and management of low back pain and sciatica. *Am Fam Physician* 1995; 52:1333–41:1347–1348.

58. Shekelle PG. Spinal manipulation [see comments]. *Spine* 1994; 19:858–861.

59. Triano JJ, McGregor M, Hondras MA, Brennan PC. Manipulative therapy versus education programs in chronic low back pain. *Spine* 1995; 20:948–955.

60. Pope MH, Phillips RB, Haugh LD, Hsieh CY, MacDonald L, Haldeman S. A prospective randomized three-week trial of spinal manipulation, transcutaneous muscle stimulation, massage and corset in the treatment of subacute low back pain. *Spine* 1994; 19:2571–2577.

61. Shekelle PG, Adams AH, Chassin MR, Hurwitz EL, Park RE, Phillips RB. *The appropriateness of spinal manipulation for low-back pain: indications and ratings by a multidisciplinary panel.* Santa Monica: RAND Corp., 1991.

62. Shekelle PG, Adams AH, Chassin MR, Hurwitz EL, Park RE, Phillips RB. *The appropriateness of spinal manipulation for low back pain: Indications and ratings by an all-chiropractic expert panel.* Santa Monica: RAND Corp., 1992:

63. Haldeman S. Spinal manipulative therapy in the management of low back pain. In: Finneson BE (ed.). *Low back pain,* 2nd ed. Philadelphia: J.B. Lippincott Company, 1980:245–275.

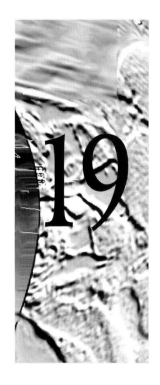

# Bed Rest and Exercise

*Jeffrey L. Young, M.D., M.A., Joel M. Press, M.D., and Stanley A. Herring, M.D.*

inety percent of people have low back pain in their lifetime, and 40 percent of these conditions can become chronic (1,2,3). When low back pain occurs acutely, the treating physician is challenged by the physical and psychoemotional needs of the patient, fiscal and work productivity needs of employers, and the constraints of a more complex and restrictive health care system. Both exercise and bed rest have been employed in the treatment of acute and subacute low back pain. The Agency for Health Care Policy Research (AHCPR) has established guidelines with respect to the utility and dosing of both bed rest and exercise in the setting of acute low back pain (4). This section reviews and critiques the guidelines and provides alternatives to these guidelines.

## AHCPR CONCLUSIONS REGARDING BED REST

The four major recommendations made regarding the use of bed rest in acute low back pain may be summarized as follows:

1. Gradual return to normal activities is more effective than prolonged bed rest.
2. Prolonged bed rest (i.e., greater than 4 days) is not recommended.
3. The majority of persons with low back pain will not require bed rest.
4. Bed rest may be an option for patients with initial symptoms of severe leg pain.

Bed rest has been traditionally prescribed to prevent worsening of pain and or dysfunction associated with acute injury. This provides the body with time to "heal itself." However, while bed rest following acute low back or any other injury initially facilitates symptomatic improvement, it does not help to restore function. Furthermore, there are a number of well-recognized deleterious effects of sustained bed rest which include but are not restricted to the following:

1. Loss of maximal aerobic capacity (5–8);
2. Elevation of resting heart rate (5–8);
3. Altered fibrinolysis/coagulation (9);
4. Reduction of oxidative enzyme enzyme levels in skeletal muscle (10,11);
5. Reduced plasticity of connective tissues (12);
6. Reduced bone mineralization (5,12);
7. Reduced cross-sectional area and strength of muscle (13–15);
8. Psychological effects such as adoption of "the sick role" (12).

A prospective, randomized study looked at the effect of bed rest in patients with and without radiating leg pain (16). The authors noted a 42 percent longer time to return to normal activity in the bed rest group. However, the methods section does not indicate if patients with back surgery were included, and they were unable to document compliance for the bed rest group. This was further complicated by members of the "not bed rest" group also trying some (unquantified) bed rest. The bed rest study often cited as a "classic" with respect to the optimum length of time for bed rest is the study by Deyo and colleagues, which was published in 1986 (17). This study purportedly compared consequences of limited (2 days) and generous (7 days) bed rest in low back pain. Although fewer days of work were lost in the 2 day group, the groups were far from pure with extensive cross-over between the non-bed rest and bed rest groups. An additional concern is that the population studied was poorly educated with many non-English speaking participants. Furthermore, the etiology of subjects' back pain was poorly described, as was existence of prior back injury, the presence of ongoing radicular symptoms, and hard neurologic findings. In general, concerns with the literature cited by the AHCPR are highly related to poor description of subjects, poor control of the length of time and number of episodes of back pain prior to intervention, poor distinction between surgerized and nonsurgerized patients, and lack of acknowledgment of the presence or absence of radiculopathy (16–20). From a philosophical standpoint, it is also curious that back pain is approached differently from other musculoskeletal injuries. There is rarely, if ever, a debate over whether 2 days or 7 days of rest is needed after a hamstring "strain"; emphasis is typically placed on early functional restoration to promote tissue healing and prepare the injured region for return to work or play.

In summary, in patients with nonradicular low back pain, there does not appear to be proven benefit of prolonged rest. The available literature is inadequate to make a definitive statement regarding the efficacy of or the appropriate amount of time of bed rest in patients with disc herniations or clear radiculopathy. Given that 70–90 percent of patients have recurrent episodes of low back pain (1,3), an argument can be made that there are anatomic changes and functional biomechanical deficits that persist following low back injury, and that these alterations need to be corrected to lessen the likelihood of further injury.

## AHCPR CONCLUSIONS REGARDING EXERCISE

1. "Low-stress aerobic exercise can prevent debilitation due to inactivity during the first month of symptoms and thereafter may help to return patients to the highest level of functioning appropriate to their circumstances" (4, p. 53).
2. "Aerobic (endurance) exercise programs, which minimally stress the back (walking, biking, or swimming), can be started during the first two weeks for most patients with acute low back problem."(4, p. 53).
3. "Back-specific exercise machines provide no apparent benefit over traditional exercise in the treatment of patients with acute low back problems"(4, p. 53).
4. Conditioning exercises for trunk muscles (especially back extensors), gradually increased, are helpful for patients with acute low back problems, especially if symptoms persist. During the first 2 weeks, these exercises may aggravate symptoms since they mechanically stress the back more than endurance exercises"(4, p. 53).
5. "Evidence does not support stretching of the back muscles in the treatment of patients with acute low back problems"(4, p. 53).
6. "Recommended exercise quotas that are gradually increased result in better outcomes than telling patients to stop exercising if pain occurs"(4, p. 54).

Overall, these recommendations are somewhat confusing and controversial. While it is true that there have been few randomized, controlled trials examining the effect of exercise in low back pain, there is an abundance of literature examining the benefits of various types of exercise in a variety of other clinical settings (5,21,22). Right or wrong, most clinicians extrapolate from this data to the low back pain population, which only adds to the confusion.

The traditional broad goals of exercise are to improve cardiovascular fitness, increase strength, increase flexibility, and increase endurance. Additional potential benefits relate to improved mood (endorphin/enkephalin effects), purported increase in pain tolerance, and "sounder" sleep (23,24). There is also evidence to suggest that spine motion improves the quality of disc nutrition and elimination of metabolic waste products of local disc metabolism (25).

Studies cited by the guidelines contribute to misconceptions about the "lack" of efficacy of exercise. It is important to recognize that absence of proof due to methodologic flaws in the available literature is not equivalent to proof of an absence of a beneficial effect of exercise. Studies by Coxhead and co-workers (1981), Gilbert and co-workers (1985), Evans and co-workers (1987), and Koes and co-workers (1991, 1995) failed to demonstrate a benefit of "exercise" over placebo treatment in acute low back pain (16,19,20,26,27). These studies were cited because they were randomized and prospective. Methodologic and statistical flaws were abundant in these reports, with absence of physical exam data, imaging data, and use of uniform exercise programs irrespective of the ill-defined underlying problem. Malmivaara and co-workers prospectively compared bed rest of 2 days, mobilizing exercises, and activity as tolerated in the treatment of patients with acute or recently exacerbated chronic low back pain (28). Patients with pain that extended down to the knee were included, but not patients with neurologic deficits. The normal-activities-as-tolerated group were utilized as the control group. Outcome and cost were assessed at 3 and 12 weeks. At both the 3 and 12 week marks, the control group fared better with respect to duration of pain, intensity of pain, lumbar flexion, ability to work as measured subjectively, Oswestry Back Disability Index, and the number of days absent from work (28). Closer examination of the study reveals that only one session of physical therapy was provided for the "intervention group," that the only patients with a prior history of spine surgery were in the exercise group, and there were twice as many subjects with chronic low back pain in the exercise group (28). Fass's work concluded that exercise therapy for patients with acute low back pain had no advantage over care from the general practitioner (18). Unfortunately, once again, exercise programs were not based on any specific diagnosis or in response to physical exam findings. It is unreasonable to expect to observe specific benefits from an exercise program if no specific diagnoses were made prior to initiation of the treatment arm of a study.

## BASIC PRINCIPLES OF AEROBIC TRAINING AND CARDIOVASCULAR CONDITIONING

Aerobic conditioning is easily lost if the back injury extends beyond one week of reduced activity levels. $VO_2$ max decreases by 25 percent from 3 weeks of bed rest (7,8). Exercise training results in a number of favorable adaptations, including improved utilization of free fatty acid metabolism; reduced body fat; increased insulin sensitivity; increased muscle blood flow; increased maximal cardiac output; increased $VO_2$ max, lower heart rate

response for any given level of exertion; reduced blood lactate accumulation for any given submaximal level of exertion; and lower minute ventilation at any submaximal level of exertion (29). Ten to 20 percent increases in $VO_2$ max with exercise training of 8 to 12 weeks' duration is common. Improvement in submaximal parameters and a subjective increase in endurance are typically observed before this. Failure to improve aerobic fitness over a 6–8 week period can result from too infrequent exercise, exercising at too low an intensity, or exercise sessions that are too short.

It is common for practitioners to advise patients that aerobic fitness confers some protective effect from development of or worsening of low back pain. Regular aerobic exercise reduces heart rate, blood pressure, and ventilatory drive for any standard intensity of work, and the assumption is that this holds for the stress encountered by the spine as well. Again, this literature is less than convincing. It is also remarkable that despite the availability of well-recognized and reliable measurement tools to assess aerobic fitness, few studies actually utilize direct or indirect metabolic measurements to quantify fitness or the cardiorespiratory response to exercise. McQuade's retrospective work indicated an association between lower cardiovascular fitness and an increased incidence of low back pain (30). It could not be determined whether the back pain preceded decreased activity and decreased fitness or vice versa (30). Brennan's comparison of aerobic fitness in patients with disc herniations versus age-matched controls presents a similar problem (31). Additionally, maximal aerobic power was derived from extrapolation of submaximal data rather than from direct respiratory gas analysis during true maximal exertion (31). The work of Cady and colleagues (1979,1985), which was predominantly observational, appeared to indicate that firefighters who were less fit had more episodes of low back injury and were more costly to take care of for work-related injuries (32,33). In the earlier study, the more fit subjects were also younger, obviously confounding the results. The work of Battie and Dehlen failed to demonstrate a beneficial effect of aerobic training (34,35). However, patient populations were not uniform in that both those with and without prior episodes of low back pain and those who did or did not have prior surgery were combined. In a prospective, randomized, controlled trial, Kellet and co-workers looked at exercise in subjects with and without prior episodes of back pain (36). No significant improvements in aerobic capacity were achieved but there were fewer sick days and less back pain reported in the treatment group. On the other hand, Lahad's work concluded that aerobic exercise may be protective against low back injury (37). A second study by Brennan and colleagues, this time using actual exercise metabolic measurement testing, demonstrated that patients post microdiscectomy provided with an aerobic training program (walking) made significantly greater gains in aerobic fitness than a matched post surgery group that was kept "sedentary" and were able to do so without enduring any increases in back pain (38). Given the available literature, the best statements about the relationship between cardiovascular fitness and the development or recurrence of low back pain are as follows:

1. Younger individuals are less likely to have low back pain.
2. More fit individuals may have less low back pain.
3. It is unclear if low back pain reduces fitness or if reduced fitness promotes low back pain.
4. Patients who already have back pain are capable of improving their aerobic fitness.

## BASIC CONCEPTS OF STRENGTHENING EXERCISES

Patients are frequently told that if they become stronger this will aid in the treatment of their low back pain. The strength literature is fraught with problems, if for no other reason than because the operational definition of the term *strength* varies from study to study. In the conventional sense, the term *strength* refers to the maximum force produced from a single effort. *Power* refers to work over a specified period of time, and *endurance* refers to the ability to sustain work at a given percentage of maximum.

Patients may have reduced strength in various muscle groups either from deconditioning or neurogenic weakness from radiculopathy. A muscle loses 1–3 percent of its strength per day and 10–15 percent per week with complete bed rest (15). There is no single best method of strengthening; all methods employ some type of overload. Increases in strength are associated with increases in cross-sectional area of skeletal muscle, or muscular hypertrophy. Strengthening exercises are more effective when muscle groups are rotated from session to session. For example, arm and chest muscles may be emphasized on days 1, 3, and 5 of the week, with emphasis on leg and back muscles on days 2, 4, and 6. Most regimens are based on how many times a percentage of the 1 RM or 10 RM is lifted. A typical beginning strength training prescription consists of 1 to 3 sets of lifting a weight 8 to 12 times, 3 times per week. If the weight can be lifted more than 12 times, it is typically too light. If it can only be lifted 6 times or fewer, the weight is too heavy. Lifting for power entails lifting somewhat lighter weights (so that they may be lifted slightly more quickly) 15–20 times. Resistance should be increased by no more than 10 percent per week. Healthy males may increase their strength by 20–40 percent over a 2–4 month period; apparent

increases in strength during the first 2 weeks of training are related to neuromuscular retraining and more efficient motor unit recruitment programs rather than due to muscular hypertrophy, which occurs at a later date (39,40). Lifting has been too strenuous if muscles remain sore beyond 24 hours post exercise. Failure to progress may relate to improper technique, too few or too many lifts per session, or continued neurogenic strength loss.

In her analysis of retrospective studies, Plowman indicated that there might be a link between trunk strength and low back pain (41). This conclusion was made with caution since assessment of maximal strength in patients with pain is almost impossible and apparent loss of strength in patients with long-term or previous episodes of low back pain could be attributed to deconditioning. Donochin's work examined hospital employees with more than three annual episodes of low back pain, enrolling participants in lumbar flexion and pelvic tilt training versus back school and a control group (42). Those who participated in the exercise arm of the study did report fewer subsequent months of back pain and demonstrated increased abdominal "strength." In a prospective, randomized, controlled trial using patients with and without back pain, Gundewall and colleagues reported fewer days of low back pain in patients given six exercise treatments a month emphasizing trunk strengthening exercises (43). Bierring-Sorensen (1994) reported trunk extension endurance testing to be predictive for development of low back pain in previously asymptomatic individuals but not in those with previous low back pain (1). In a nonrandomized trial, Troup and co-workers were unable to demonstrate a positive predictive value of trunk endurance exercises in British workers (44). Johannsen and colleagues randomized 40 consecutive chronic low back pain patients to 3 months of either "endurance" exercises or "training including coordination" exercises (45). Improvement in isokinetic back extension strength was significantly greater in the endurance group, and there was no intergroup difference with regard to disability score, although both groups improved (45). No control group was utilized and the study groups were poorly described, particularly with reference to how active the participants were on their own. Thirteen of the 40 participants dropped out of the study.

An additional problem when reviewing the literature on strength relates to whether or not isokinetic measurements are useful. An extensive review by Newton and Waddell (1993) concluded that there was inadequate evidence to support pre-employment isokinetic testing and that isokinetic tests did not help predict which initially asymptomatic individuals would be more likely to endure low back injury in the future (46). On the other hand, Reimer and colleagues suggested that the use of isokinetics to measure total work as part of a fitness test battery is a more useful tool in employee screening (47). That an endurance-type measure is more valuable intuitively makes more sense, but caution must be exercised, as this study was retrospective and an actual statistical analysis of the variables examined was omitted from the body of the paper (47).

A final area of concern with the available literature is that the lack of accurate definition of the underlying spine problems of the subject populations has led to the apparent inability to identify either flexion or extension exercises as particularly useful in the treatment of low back pain (18,19,27). This problem is exemplified by a recent paper by Dettori and co-workers (48). In this prospective study, soldiers with acute low back pain were randomized to flexion exercises and posture, to extension exercises and posture, or to no exercise for 8 weeks. Subjects were assessed at 1, 2, 4, and 8 weeks after initiation of treatment. After 1 week, both exercise groups exhibited decreased disability scores, fewer subjects with a positive straight leg raise, and a greater percentage of subjects able to return to work than the control group. A follow-up questionnaire administered 6 to 12 months after study entry did not detect a significant difference between groups for recurrence of back pain. The authors concluded that either exercise was "slightly" more effective than none, but that it made no difference if flexion or extension exercises were utilized. Unfortunately, randomization of acute low back pain patients without regard for pathology or individual position/posture preferences probably led to subjects who would have fared better with extension exercises (i.e., posterolaterally protruding disc with increased dural tension in flexion) being placed in the flexion group, and some of those who would have fared better with flexion exercise (i.e., facet synovitis) into the extension group. Both of these randomizations would lead to dilution of the potential treatment effect. Delitto and colleagues attempted to identify acute and subacute low back pain patients with or without radicular symptoms who might benefit from an extension-mobilization program (49). These patients were then randomized to either an extension motion plus sacroiliac mobilization or a flexion-type exercise program. A control group was not included. Modified Oswestry Low Back Questionnaires were administered at days 3 and 5 of treatment, with the extension group improving more rapidly. Study design did not permit distinction between the effect of the mobilizations versus the effect of the exercises (49).

In general, use of the available literature is inadequate to establish guidelines for the role of strength training in the prevention or treatment of acute low back pain. Variability in operational definitions as cited previously, lack of specificity or distinction between flexion versus extension-based exercises, the use of patients with and without back pain in the same studies, and their inclusion of industrial-based populations reveal a need for more carefully designed studies, gearing "strength" or "endurance" exercises toward the specific needs of the subject populations or the use of entirely pain-free populations followed longitudinally for the development of low back pain.

## BASIC CONCEPTS OF FLEXIBILITY EXERCISES

The literature surrounding *flexibility* is even poorer than that for cardiovascular and strength training. Definitions vary greatly from study to study and measurements are extremely hard to interpret. Stretching exercises aim to increase the available range of motion about a joint or series of joints. Their purpose is to make the patient feel less stiff, thereby making activities of daily living more comfortable, and to theoretically reduce biomechanical stresses placed on those joints. Initial application of a stretch on connective tissue straightens collagen fibers. This is an elastic stretch, which will reverse as soon as the stretching load is removed. Further load application will begin to elongate the collagen fibers. If applied for a prolonged period of time, the fibers will "deform" and retain the lengthened state. Stretches are typically applied for a prolonged period (at least 20 to 30 seconds) so that a "pulling" but not "tearing" sensation occurs and then slowly released (50,51). Proprioceptive neuromuscular facilitation (PNF) techniques (passive or static type stretches at the muscle's maximally tolerated stretch are alternated with isometric type contractions of that same muscle) are an extremely effective method of stretching that can easily be taught during the initial therapy sessions (52). Rapid, high force stretches result in tissue recoil and no persistence of stretching effect (53). Stretching exercises have been performed too vigorously if they result in muscular soreness for greater than 24 hours. Connective tissue stretching is facilitated by warming. Application of ultrasound, which can heat tissues in excess of 40° C, has been shown to be an effective method of pretreating tissues to be stretched (51). In the face of acute or chronic low back pain, this is rarely needed. Flexibility is usually improved over a 1–2 month period. If the patient does not progress and noncompliance is not an issue, persistent nerve root irritation should be considered as a cause (3,51).

As noted previously, the available literature is not particularly helpful. Cady (1985) reported that workers who had poorer flexibility cost seven times more than the most "flexible" subjects with regard to work-related low back injury (33). Battie's work was unable to demonstrate a significant difference between the flexibility of those with and without low back pain (34). Bierring-Sorrensen actually reported that those with better mobility were more likely to develop low back pain in the next year (1). Thus, the available literature is inadequate to determine guidelines and recommendations for flexibility training in acute low back pain.

## A RATIONAL APPROACH TO REHABILITATION OF ACUTE LOW BACK PAIN

Although research trials have failed to stand up to scrutiny, there is mounting clinical evidence that there is a purpose to rehabilitation and conditioning exercises in patients with low back pain, even in the face of disc herniation with radiculopathy (3,54). Exercise and physical and occupational therapy regimens can be beneficial and cost-effective when they are constructed to address specific conditions associated with accurate clinical diagnoses. A multifaceted approach appears to be more effective (3,51,54,55). Therapists who have a broad range of skills in addressing low back pain have a greater likelihood of helping patients who have different problems. Precisely prescribed rehabilitation programs tailored toward specific anatomic and biomechanical deficits are needed to optimize function following low back injury. Clinicians who are capable of modifying and upgrading regimens on the basis of changes in the patient's clinical picture rather than merely following algorithmic flow charts are needed to direct rehabilitation programs.

Goals of physical therapy include reduction of pain intensity and length of episode. This is typically accomplished by correction of abnormal skeletal shifts and posture, reduction of the associated heightened muscle tone, and establishment of comfortable body position (3,51,56). For typical discogenic pain (i.e., from a posterolaterally herniated disc), comfort incorporates an extension-based spine posture. For typical posterior element pain, a flexion-based program is typically utilized. The concept of the "neutral spine" is also utilized, as the patient is taught how to control hip, pelvic, and abdominal musculature to reduce stress on the supportive muscles and ligaments about the spine (3,51,56). The purpose of these activities is to facilitate return to work. A key to achieving a rapid progression in the exercise program is managing pain. This is accomplished via medications and/or judicious use of pain-relieving modalities. This permits the treating physician and therapist to begin actively correcting associated biomechanical flaws. Typical problem areas include tightness/inflexibility of the hamstrings, hip flexors, and hip rotators, and weakness of the hip extensors, abdominal obliques, and lower rectus abdominis. At the same time, the patient is instructed in proper ergonomics and correct lifting techniques (i.e.,

use of legs rather than flexing/extending lumbar spine emphasizing utilization of gluteal muscles and attachments of the thoracolumbar fascia) and educated to prevent reinjury.

The initial period is also critical for identification of those patients who do not benefit from exercise alone. Acute/subacute low back pain patients with persistent radicular symptoms following 6 weeks of appropriately prescribed physical therapy need to be re-evaluated to assess the need for radiologic imaging (X-ray, CT, MRI, etc.), the need for alteration of oral medication regimen, the need for diagnostic and/or therapeutic injection, or the need for surgical evaluation. Patients exhibiting persistent "centralized" low back pain following 6 weeks appropriately prescribed therapeutic exercise also require re-evaluation to assess the need for radiologic evaluation, the need for alteration of oral medication regimen, and in particular whether pharmacologic intervention is needed to restore sleep. For those exhibiting chronic nonradicular low back pain without clinical improvement following a 6-week trial therapeutic exercise, the clinician needs to be vigilant for the presence of signs of nonorganic features, and to be prepared to assess for "pain" issues rather than prescribe more therapy.

Provision of true aggressive conservative care is essential to determine if a patient falls into a surgical or nonsurgical category. The majority of spine surgeries follow failed aggressive care rather than development of cauda equina syndromes. Poorly designed physical therapy programs lead to poorer outcomes and, by default, more spine surgeries. When patients appear to have "plateaued" in their progress, the therapist and physician must re-establish goals and objectives of the program. This may lead to additional diagnostic testing (i.e., EMG, MRI) to further define pathology. Fluoroscopically guided contrast-enhanced injections can provide diagnostic and therapeutic benefit and will help patient progress in many cases.

Low back rehabilitation may be described as an orderly progression of therapeutic activities designed to reduce pain and inflammation, and facilitate healing of injured tissues, to re-establish flexibility, range of motion, strength and endurance, normal or near normal biomechanics of spine, pelvic, and hip motion and allow the individual to return to his or her activities of daily living including gainful employment, through development of work/sports specific regimens and maintenance programs.

Exercises are based on scientific evidence when available. An assumption that a complete biomechanical and neurologic evaluation will be completed prior to initiation of the program. A kinetic chain approach should be adhered to. Unless proven otherwise, all muscle strength and flexibility imbalances need to be considered relevant. Although algorithmic approaches to spine rehabilitation are attractive to many practitioners, the best programs are ultimately tailored to meet the patient's individual needs. Therapists who have a broad range of skills in addressing low back pain have a greater likelihood of helping patients who have different problems.

Therapeutic spine injections (e.g., sacroiliac joint, lumbar epidural steroid injections) can also be a valuable component of spine rehabilitation, but in most instances are performed to facilitate the therapeutic exercise program.

## EXAMPLES OF
## SPINE REHABILITATION STRATEGIES

In the 1990s, it is unusual for a team of professionals treating low back pain to use only one type of treatment program. This section describes some of the popular options available today.

In *spine stabilization exercises,* the goal is to teach the patient how to find and maintain a "neutral spine" during activities of daily living (3,51,56,57). The neutral spine position is individual-specific and is the pelvic and spine posture that places the least stress on the elements of the spine and supportive structures (56,57). In classic discogenic pain associated with a posterolateral disc herniation, neutral spine will have an extension bias (3,56). In classic posterior element pain or central spinal stenosis, neutral spine may have a mild flexion bias.

The starting position for these exercises in acute and subacute pain is frequently in the supine lie, but may also be a side-lie. Neutral spine is found by contracting abdominal and pelvic musculature to rock the pelvis anteriorly or posteriorly through the pain available range. The most functional position is in the midpoint of the range. Postural corrections incorporate the neutral spine concept. "Stabilization" is accomplished via teaching proper posture and mechanics and utilizing these potential stabilizing mechanisms:

1. Intraabdominal pressure—increases in intraabdominal pressure (utilization of a closed glottis) may transmit throughout the torso and reduce pressure placed on the spine. This does not respond to exercise training (3,56).
2. Thoracolumbar fascial (TLF) support system—the TLF has fibers that are derived from the latissimus dorsi, abdominal obliques, and gluteus maximus. Strengthening of these muscular attachments helps to stabilize the spine as the TLF spans many spine levels and is activated by flexion of the spine (3,56)
3. Hydraulic amplifier mechanism—the TLF is enhanced by the contraction of the erector spinae, which it overlies (3,56)

4. Posterior ligamentous system—the posterior ligaments engage when the spine is flexed. This reduces compressive forces placed on the other supportive structures. (3,56)
5. Muscular support mechanism—this mechanism utilizes the small intersegmental muscles between consecutive vertebrae (3,56)

Progression of treatment is a function of addressing inflexibilities and weaknesses while attempting to teach these "new" exercises. More and more dynamic challenges are added as the patient demonstrates the ability to maintain a neutral spine without worsening of lumbar spine symptoms (3,54,58).

*McKenzie exercises* are techniques that identify postures and motions that "centralize" radicular/referred low back pain (59). Although extension-based exercises are commonly utilized in classic radiculopathy associated with a posterolaterally protruding disc, these exercises are not solely extension exercises. Potential mechanisms of improvement with this type of therapy include reduction of the disc herniation and reduction of dural tension. Prior to incorporating extension-based exercises, lateral trunk shifts must be corrected. McKenzie's patient groupings include those problems due to posture, dysfunction, and derangement. Patients in the postural group develop pain from prolonged end range positioning, in the presence or absence of true pathology. Those in the dysfunctional group have shortened connective tissue and experience pain when it is stretched (i.e., scar tissue). Those in the derangement group have symptoms in response to both static loading and repeated movements. Derangement of the disc is thought to be responsible

Centralization of pain is considered to be a positive response, while persistence of radiculopathy or worsening of symptoms necessitates re-evaluating the patient. Patients with central disc herniations may not fare well with extension-based exercises

*Williams' flexion exercises* emphasize a different approach (3,51). Flexion bias exercises (i.e., posterior pelvic tilt, double knee to chest) were often prescribed with the thought that discogenic symptoms could be reduced in this manner. Flexion was theorized to decrease loading of the posterior portion of the disc (typically protruded) and to widen the neuroforamen. However, patients with acute disc herniations may have exacerbation of symptoms from increased intradiscal pressure. Alternatively, patients with posterior element pain and central spinal stenosis may benefit from this technique. Patients with presumed spinal stenosis who do not improve with flexion-based exercises should be evaluated carefully for foraminal stenosis

We have adopted an approach to treating low back pain that adheres to Kibler's model for describing musculoskeletal injuries (60,61). This model ensures that all aspects of the primary injury and any secondary sites of injury and/or dysfunction are completely diagnosed. A complete diagnosis allows a complete rehabilitation program to be developed. The components of the vicious cycle of musculotendinous overload may be described as follows.

- The *tissue injury complex* refers to the actual site of tissue disruption/ injury (60,61). It is typically the most obvious aspect of the injury.
- The *tissue overload complex* refers to the tissues subject to eccentric and tensile overloads (60,61). These structures may be local and/ or distant from the site of injury.
- The *clinical symptom complex* refers to the symptoms associated with dysfunction and injury (60,61). This is essentially what the patient complains about.
- The *functional biomechanical deficits* are those flexibility and/or strength imbalances that create abnormal/altered mechanics (60,61). These may be the cause of the pain/dysfunction, due to the pain/dysfunction or be both causes and due to the pain/dysfunction.
- The *functional adaptation complex* consists of the substitution patterns used to maintain activities of daily living (ADLs) and/ or athletic performance (60,61).

Rehabilitation may be broken into phases. During the acute phase, focus is on reducing pain from injured or inflamed tissue. This may be accomplished via medications and/or modalities (both described elsewhere in this book). Briefly, superficial cold and heat decrease spasm and pain. Deep heat (ultrasound) may decrease spasm and pain and can be used to increase collagen distensibility, which increases flexibility.

At this point, physical or occupational therapy is utilized sparingly. One to two sessions focusing on finding positions of comfort, teaching neutral spine position (see later sections), and pain-free methods of position change, i.e., lie to sit, sit to stand, and vice versa. The initial movement patterns are based on presumed pathology and pain pattern, and pain centralization (i.e., the McKenzie method). *Extension bias* is most commonly used in discogenic process with repetitive extension on motion pattern testing and centralization of pain with extension. Extension exercises may reduce intradiscal pressure and allow anterior migration of the nucleus pulposus. However, they can exacerbate the symptoms from posterior element irritation or from a central disc herniation. Flexion bias is most commonly used in posterior element pain with pain reduction in symptoms with repetitive flexion. Flexion exercises may reduce compressive forces on the facet joints. They may increase intradiscal pressure and increase radicular symptoms.

During the subacute phase, connective tissue restrictions are addressed. Manual techniques are employed to increase soft tissue distensibility along the planes of physiologic stress so to promote proper alignment of connective tissue fibers during the healing and remodeling process. Myofascial techniques are utilized to apply pressure and shear forces to the fascial layers in order to improve elasticity and produce less restricted, painful movement. The theory behind the need for these techniques assumes that fascia absorbs shock, separates and supports muscles, and helps in the transmission and attenuation of mechanical forces (3,56). It also assumes that loss of normal fascial gliding and increased cross-linking of fibers results in loss of myofascial system mobility with secondary loss of segmental bony mobility and flexibility. The purpose of mobilization is to restore optimal joint mobility by applying forces at individually targeted specific non-soft tissue motion segment levels. These are graded from I to IV, depending on the force and depth of the applied load (3,62).

Grades I and II are referred to as oscillations. Grades III and IV represent larger amplitude forces that move joint into its restricted range and provide stretch. Grade V manipulations are of a high-velocity, low-amplitude nature, taking the joint to its end range of physiologic motion (3,62).

During the recovery phase (typically the most lengthy portion of the rehabilitation program), emphasis is on restoration of function. This phase combines both supervised physical therapy and a home program, with the majority being home-based. Appropriate tissue loading is emphasized in the exercises. During this phase, resolution of tissue injury complex, restoration of the tissue overload complex, and correction of the functional biomechanical deficits occur. Goals include development of range of motion on more affected side to be within 10 percent of unaffected side and strength to be within 20 percent of unaffected side.

The maintenance phase represents the final phase and is the basis of the prevention program as well. The subclinical adaptations and biomechanical deficits are resolved. Eccentric (lengthening) muscular strengthening exercises are emphasized and work-specific training, when applicable, is incorporated. The following section outlines clinical applications of vicious overload cycle.

## ACUTE DISCOGENIC PAIN WITH RADICULOPATHY

*Clinical symptom complex*—low back and leg pain, typically worsened by flexion. If it is due to an annular tear without protrusion or extrusion of discal material, there is typically more back than leg pain. With protrusion/ extrusion of discal material, there is typically more leg than back pain. Under both circumstances, there is reduced sitting tolerance.

*Tissue injury complex*—annular fibers of disc, chemically and mechanically irritated dorsal and ventral roots, pain sensitive structures within spinal canal and vertebral foramina

*Tissue overload complex*—annulus fibrosis, nucleus pulposus, supporting muscles and ligaments of spine

*Functional biomechanical deficits*—inflexibilities and weakness of muscle and soft tissue structures. This is often manifested as inflexibility of the hamstrings and hip flexors, hypomobility of lower lumbar spine segments, and weakness of abdominal, hip abductor, and hip extensors.

*Functional adaptation complex*—increased lumbar lordosis, increased loading of posterior elements, lateral pelvic shift, and increased time spent standing

*Rehabilitation program (encapsulated)*—The initial period consists of relative rest and correction of body mechanics. Exercises to centralize pain (i.e., bring symptoms out of the legs) are then employed. Trunk shifts are corrected, as are inflexibilities. Strengthening of the abdominals, gluteal muscles is initiated, followed by dynamic conditioning exercises including inflatable gym ball exercises. Comprehensive nonsurgical spine rehabilitation programs that incorporate exercises such as the above have been shown to be highly effective in the treatment of acute and subacute discogenic pain (54,58).

## ACUTE POSTERIOR ELEMENT PAIN

*Clinical symptom complex* consists of back pain, often extending down to buttocks and posterior thigh, but rarely extending beyond the knee.

*Tissue injury complex* consists of the synovium and capsule of zygoapophyseal (z) joint.

The *tissue overload complex* acutely, consists of the synovium and capsule of the z joint. When chronic, articular cartilage is also involved.

The *functional biomechanical deficits* include posterior pelvic tilt, hamstring tightness, and weakness of the erector spinae and hamstrings

The *functional adaptation complex* includes loss of lumbar lordosis, and a preference for maintaining flexed

forward posture, side bending and rotating away from painful side

*Rehabilitation* initially consists of relative rest and teaching the patient how to "hook lie." As previously, body mechanics are corrected, but as opposed to discal injury, emphasis is placed on exercises that are flexion-based or "neutral spine"-based exercises. Once again, stretching exercises for the hamstrings and strengthening exercises for the abdominals, gluteal muscles, and spine extensors are employed.

## AQUATIC THERAPY

Although there is a limited amount of literature in the low back pain population, aquatic-based exercises are particularly useful in early phases of spine rehabilitation programs and for those whose primary sporting activity is aquatic-based (63). Advantages of aquatic-based spine exercise includes depth dependent elimination of gravitational loading and shear forces on the spine during immersion, reduced loading of injured limbs, enhanced proprioceptive feedback, and improved venous return (63). The rehabilitation team must remember that exercises learned in the water are not readily transferable to land-based exercise and vice versa. Therefore, ability to maintain a neutral based spine in the water while performing abdominal strengthening exercises does not necessarily lead to the ability to maintain a neutral spine during "crunches" on land.

"Completion" of a spine rehabilitation program is signified by the patient's demonstration of absence of signs or symptoms of the original injury, full pain-free range of motion, normal strength and flexibility, normal mechanics for work or sport, and the ability to perform job-specific skills. Under any circumstance, the philosophy adhered to is that resolution of symptoms alone is inadequate and that restoration of optimal function is the goal.

*Summary*

1. There is no proven benefit of prolonged bed rest (i.e., greater than 4 days) in acute low back pain without radiculopathy.
2. The literature does not provide adequate information to establish guidelines for the amount of rest required in the face of acute disc injury with radicular symptoms.
3. There is no conclusive proof that aerobic exercise

in or of itself prevents development of low back pain. Based on literature review, aerobic fitness may be mildly protective against low back injury and low back pain.

4. There is no conclusive evidence that aerobic exercise hastens the recovery from an episode of acute low back pain.

5. Acute low back pain results in reduction of physical activity, which leads to reduction of aerobic fitness. This problem is accentuated if low back pain occurs on a recurrent basis. This may have significant consequences with regard to physical working capacity and cardiovascular risk. On this basis alone, it is recommended that aerobic exercises be incorporated in the spine rehabilitation program as early as possible.

6. Future studies examining the role of aerobic conditioning exercises and/or the role of aerobic fitness in the prevention and treatment of low back pain should utilize direct quantification of oxygen consumption via respiratory gas analysis rather than predictive normograms or populationally based "norms."

7. Since the majority of any individual's daily activities are not performed at maximum levels, future studies examining the role of aerobic exercise should incorporate submaximal parameters such as submaximal heart rate response and rating of perceived exertion at standard workloads or relative percentages of maximal aerobic capacity.

8. Findings of reduced strength, endurance, and flexibility are common in patients with low back pain. These may be a consequence of acute deconditioning as well as a potential causative factor for dysfunction in the future.

9. Isokinetic strength testing does not appear to be helpful in the assessment of risk of development of low back pain. Isokinetic devices may prove to be useful in the quantification of work capacity.

10. Operational definitions of strength, power, and endurance are inconsistent across studies, making generalized statements about the efficacy of "strength" training or "strength" testing difficult at best. Nevertheless, there appears to be at least a mild relationship between trunk muscle "strength" and low back pain.

11. The current literature neither supports the notion that flexibility training confers protection against the development of low back pain nor that it is essential in the treatment of acute low back pain.

12. The causes of low back pain are multifactorial even when a pain generator is identified. Thus, treatment of low back pain by randomizing patients to only one method (i.e., just mobilizations, just modalities, just flexion exercises, etc.) is unrealistic. It is an error

to equate "exercise" with rehabilitation—the patient must always be taken into account.

# References

1. Biering-Soersen F. Physical measurements as risk indicators for low back trouble over a one year period. *Spine* 1994; 106–119.

2. Frymoyer JW. Back pain and sciatica. *N Engl J Med* 1988; 318:291–300.

3. Herring SA, Weinstein SM. Assessment and nonsurgical management of athletic low back injury. In: Nicholas JA, Hershman EB (eds.). *The lower extremity and spine in sports medicine.* 2nd ed. St. Louis: Mosby-Year Book, 1995:1171–1197.

4. Agency for Health Care Policy and Research. Clinical Practice Guidelines for Acute Low Back Pain, 1995.

5. Astrand PO, Rodahl K. *Textbook of work physiology.* 3rd ed. New York: McGraw-Hill, 1986.

6. Coyle EF, Hemmert MK, Coggan E. Effects of detraining on cardiovascular responses to exercise: Role of blood volume. *J Appl Physiol* 1985; 60:95–99.

7. Grimby G, Saltin B. Physiological effects of physical training. *Scand J Rehab Med* 1971; 3:6–14.

8. Saltin B, Blomqvist B, Mitchell JH, Johnson RL Jr, Wildenthal K, Chapman CB. Response to submaximal and maximal exercise after bed rest and training. *Circulation* 1968; 38(Suppl 7).

9. Bowman K, Hellsten G, Bruce A, Hallamns G, Nilsson TK. Endurance physical activity, diet and fibrinolysis. *Atherosclerosis* 1994; 196(1):65–74.

10. Henriksson J, Reitman JS. Time course of changes in human skeletal muscle succinic dehydrogenase and cytochrome oxidase activities and maximal oxygen uptake with physical activity and inactivity. *Acta Physiol Scand* 1977; 99:91–97.

11. Klaussen K, Andersen LB, Pelle I. Adaptive changes in work capacity, skeletal muscle capillarization and enzyme levels during training and detraining. *Acta Physiol Scand* 1981; 113:9–16.

12. Halar EM, Bell K. Contracture and other effects of immobility. In: DeLisa JA (ed.). *Rehabilitation medicine.* Philadelphia: JB Lippincott, 1988:448–462.

13. Booth FW, Gollnick PD. Effects of disuse on the structure and function of skeletal muscle. *Med Sci Sports Exerc* 1983; 15:415–420.

14. Eichelberger L, Roma, M, Moulder PV. Effects of immobilization on the histochemical characterization of skeletal muscle. *J Appl Physiol* 1958; 12:42–47

15. Muller EA. Influence of training and of inactivity on muscle strength. *Arch Phys Med Rehabil* 1970; 51:449–462.

16. Gilbert JR, Taylor DW, Hildebrand A, Evans C. Clinical trial of common treatments for low back pain in family practice. *Br Med J* 1985; 291:789–794.

17. Deyo RA, Diehl AK, Rosenthal M. How many days of bed rest for acute low back pain? A randomized trial. *New Engl J Med* 1986; 315:1064–1070.

18. Faas A, Chavannes AW, van Eijk JTM, Gubbels JW. A

randomized, placebo-controlled trial of exercise therapy in patients with acute low back pain. *Spine* 1993; 18:1388–1395.

19. Koes BW, Bouter LM, Beckerman H, van der Heijden GJMG, Knipschild PG. Physiotherapy exercises and back pain: a blinded review. *Br Med J* 1991; 302:1572–1576.

20. Koes BW, Bouter LM, van der Heijden GJMG. Methodological quality of randomized clinical trials on treatment efficacy in low back pain. *Spine* 1995; 20:228–235.

21. Mengshoel AM, Komnaes HB, Forre O. The effects of 20 weeks of physical fitness training in female patients with fibromyalgia. *Clin Exp Rheum* 1992; 10:345–349.

22. Scordo KA. Effects of aerobic exercise training on symptomatic women with mitral valve prolapse. *Am J Cardiol* 1991; 67:863–868.

23. O'Connor PJ, Youngstedt SD. Influence of exercise on human sleep. In: Holloszy JO (ed.). *Exercise and Sport Sciences Reviews* 1995; 23:105–134.

24. Rejeski WJ, Brawley LR, Shumaker SA. Physical activity and health related quality of life. In: Holloszy JO (ed.). *Exercise and Sport Sciences Reviews* 1996; 24:71–108.

25. Holm S, Nachemson A. Variations in the nutrition of the canine intervertebral disc induced by motion. *Spine* 1983; 8(8):867–874.

26. Coxhead CE, Meade TW, Inskip H, North WRS. Multicentre trial of physiotherapy in the management of sciatic symptoms. *Lancet* 1981; 229:1065–1068.

27. Evans C, Gilbert JR, Taylor W, Hildebrand A. A randomized controlled trial of flexion exercises, education and bed rest for patients with acute low back pain. *Physiotherapy Can* 1987; 39:96–101.

28. Milmivaara A, Hakkinen U, Aro T, et al. The treatment of acute low back pain—bed rest, exercises, or ordinary activity? *N Engl J Med* 1995; 332:351–355.

29. Young JL, Press JM. The physiologic basis of sports rehabilitation. *Phys Med Rehabil Clin N Am* 1994; 5(1):9–36.

30. McQuade KJ, Turner JA, Buchner DM. Physical fitness and chronic low back pain. *Clin Ortho Rel Res* 1988; 233:198–204.

31. Brennan GP, Ruhling RO, Hood RS, et al. Physical characteristics of patients with herniated intervertebral lumbar discs. *Spine* 1987; 12(7):699–702.

32. Cady LD, Bischoff DP, O'Connell ER, Thomas PC, Sallan JH. Strength and fitness and subsequent back injury in firefighters. *J Occup Med* 1979; 21:269–272.

33. Cady LD, Thomas PC, Karwasky RJ. Program for increasing health and physical fitness of fire fighters. *J Occup Med* 1985; 27(2):110–114.

34. Battie MC, Bigos SJ, Fisher LD, et al. A prospective study of the role of cardiovascular risk factors and fitness in industrial back pain complaints. *Spine* 1989; 14(2):141–147.

35. Dehlin O, Berg S, Hedenrud B, Andersson GBJ, Grimby. Effect of physical training and ergonomic counseling on the psychological perception of work and the subjective assessment of low back insufficiency. *Scand J Rehab Med* 1981; 13:1–9.

36. Kellett KM, Kellet DA, Nordholm LA. Effects of an exercise program on sick leave due to low back pain. *Phys Ther* 1991; 4:283–293.

37. Lahad A, Malter AD, Berg AO, Deyo RA. The effectiveness of four interventions for the prevention of low bck pain. *JAMA* 1994; 272:1286–1290.

38. Brennan GP, Shultz BB, Hood RS et al. The effects of aerobic exercise after lumbar microdiscectomy. *Spine* 1994; 19(7):735–739.

39. Basford JR. Weightlifting, weight training and injuries. *Orthopedics* 1985; 8(8):1051–1056.

40. Sale DG. Neural adaptations to resistance training. *Med Sci Sports Exerc* 1988; 20(5):S135–S145.

41. Plowman SA. Physical activity, physical fitness and low back pain. In: Holloszy JO (ed.). *Exercise and Sport Sciences Reviews* 1992; 20:221–242.

42. Donchin M. Woolf O, Kaplan L, Floman Y. Secondary prevention of low-back pain: a clinical trial. *Spine* 1990; 15:1317–1320.

43. Gundewall B, Liljeqvist M, Hansson T. Primary prevention of back symptom and absence from work. *Spine* 1993,18:587–594.

44. Troup JDG, Foreman TK, Baxter CE, Brown D. The perception of back pain and the role of physiological tests of lifting capacity. *Spine* 1987; 12:545–657.

45. Johannsen F, Remvig L, Kyger P, et al. Exercises for chronic low back pain: a clinical trial. *J Sports Phys Ther* 1995; 22(2):52–59.

46. Newton M, Waddell G. Trunk strength testing with isomachines: part I: review of a decade of scientific evidence. *Spine* 1993; 18:801–811.

47. Reimer DS, Halbrook BD, Dreyfuss PH, Tilbetti C. A novel approach to preemployment worker fitness evaluations in a material-handling industry. *Spine* 1994; 19(18):2026–2032.

48. Dettori JR, Bullock SH, Sutlive TG, Franklin RJ, Patience T. The effects of spinal flexion and extension exercises and their associated postures in patients with acute low back pain. *Spine* 1995; 20(21):2303–2312.

49. Delitto A, Cibulka MT, Erhard RE, Bowling RW, Tenhula JA. Evidence for use of an extension-mobilization category in acute low back pain syndrome: a prospective validation pilot study. *Phys Ther* 1993; 73:216–222.

50. Hallum A, Medeiros JM. Effect of duration of passive stretch on hip abduction range of motion. *J Orthop Sports Phys Ther* 1987; 18:408–415.

51. Young JL, Press JM, Cole AJ. Physical therapy options for lumbar spine pain. In: Cole AJ, Herring SA (eds.). *The low back pain handbook*. Philadelphia: Hanley & Belfus, 1996:125–140.

52. Knott M, Voss DE. *Proprioceptive neuromuscular facilitation, patterns and techniques*. New York: Harper & Row, 1965.

53. Joynt RL. Therapeutic exercise. In: DeLisa JA (ed.). *Rehabilitation medicine*. Philadelphia: JB Lippincott, 1988, pp. 346–371.

54. Saal JA, Saal JS. Nonoperative treatment of herniated lumbar intervertebral disc with radiculopathy. *Spine* 1989; 14:431–437.

55. Wiesel SW, Boden SD, Feffer HL. A quality-based protocol for management of musculoskeletal injuries. *Clin Orthop* 1994; 301:164–176.

56. Kaul MP, Herring SA. Rehabilitation of lumbar spine injuries in sports. *Phys Med Rehabil Clin N Am* 1994; 5(1):133–156.

57. DeWerd J. Stabilization exercises for the aging athlete. *J Back Musculoskel Rehabil* 1995; 5(1):75–80.

58. Saal JA. Dynamic muscular stabilization in the nonoperative treatment of lumbar pain syndromes. *Orthop Rev* 1990; 19:691–670.

59. Donelson R. The McKenzie approach in evaluating and treating low back pain. *Orthop Rev* 1990; 8:681–686.

60. Kibler WB. A framework for sports medicine: evaluation and treatment. *Phys Med Rehabil Clin N Am* 1994; 5(1):1–8.

61. Kibler WB, Chandler TJ, Pace BK. Principles of rehabilitation after chronic tendon injuries. *Clin Sports Med*1992; 11:661–671.

62. Farrell JP, Jensen GM. Manual therapy: a critical assessment of role in the profession of physical therapy. *Phys Ther* 1992; 72:843–852.

63. Cole AJ, Moschetti ML, Eagleston RE. Spine: aquatic rehabilitation strategies. *J Back Musculoskel Rehabil* 1994; 4(4):319–320.

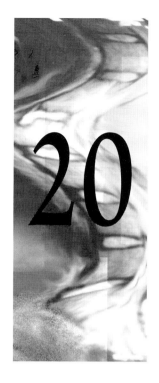

# 20 Patient Education

*Andrew J. Haig, M.D.*

What happens as the result of education? Physicians, attorneys, artists, scientists, and other "educated" persons seldom answer in terms of the information imparted to them. Rather, they are more likely to discuss the experience as a period of growth, a period of learning how to deal with more complex issues and development of relationships with peers.

While the process of educating a patient is not as time-consuming as the years of graduate training that most of the readers have experienced, the outcomes may be similar. For the patient who is in distress, educational efforts are seen as more than the simple imparting of information. As we look at efforts to educate patients—within the physician's office and within the more formal context of a back school—we need to understand the possible outcomes in a broader range than the simple imparting of information.

In this chapter we review the concept of education in back pain as outlined by the Agency for Health Care Policy and Research (AHCPR) guidelines. We begin with a discussion of the specific research that has been done to date. We then take a broader look at patient education,

especially as it may relate to low back pain. Finally, we discuss some possibilities in regard to future clinical intervention and future research into more effective educational modalities.

The AHCPR guidelines committee chose to separate patient education into two areas of study: patient education about low back symptoms in the physician's office and structured patient education such as back school. These are two prominent areas of research interest. They also encompass most of the effort directed at patient education. Before proceeding and assessing them, it is important for us to acknowledge the many other forms in which patients are educated. Long before any serious episode of back pain, patients learn about back pain through our culture. Advertisements for attorneys, chiropractors, and physicians often emphasize the catastrophic nature of back pain. Worksite education programs regarding prevention can vary highly in regard to their philosophical approach to actual injuries. In an attempt to motivate workers to pay attention to back school, educators may catastrophize regarding the prognosis for back pain once it does occur. These memories are not easily forgotten by the employee who finally has become injured. Prevention programs that emphasize body mechanics, cooperation with each other, preventive exercise, or empowerment for job redesign may have substantially different impact on the injured employee. In the early stages after injury, even before visiting with physicians, patients may have other opportunities to be educated. Co-workers, friends, family, company nurses, and others seek to impart information to the patient. The influence of these people and alternative care providers may have substantial impact on the patient.

During the course of directed treatment, there are a number of other opportunities for patient education. Videotapes, pamphlets, and books may have educational value. More individualized educational approaches combined with specific therapeutic philosophy may have different effects from a purely didactic back school (e.g., the therapist who provides a MacKenzie exercise program and teaches the patient about back pain simultaneously). While any of these may have an effect, back school and patient education within a physician's office are the most common (and most commonly studied) education efforts for patients with low back pain. We discuss each of them separately.

## PATIENT EDUCATION ABOUT LOW BACK SYMPTOMS

The AHCPR panel findings and recommendations are as follows:

Patients with acute low back problems should be given accurate information about the following: (Strength of evidence = B)

- Expectations for both rapid recovery and recurrence of symptoms based on the natural history of low back symptoms.
- Safe and effective methods of symptom control.
- Safe and reasonable activity modifications.
- The best means of limiting recurrent low back problems.
- The lack of need for specific investigations unless red flags are present.
- The effectiveness and risks of commonly available diagnostic and further treatment measures to be considered should symptoms persist.

The guidelines committee performed an important service by listing patient education among the more concrete and specific medical, diagnostic, and treatment modalities. Physicians often are oblivious to the effect of their communication on patients. Given the cultural environment surrounding low back pain, physician communication may have a profound effect on patient outcome.

Fourteen articles were screened. Two of these met the review criteria (1). Jones and colleagues studied a mixed bag of patients who presented to an emergency department. Those who received education in the emergency department or a telephone call were more likely to keep a follow-up appointment. They did not evaluate patient outcome in regard to any of the factors usually considered important in low back pain. Roland and Dixon provided an educational booklet to patients with low back pain in a primary care setting (2). At 2 weeks there was no difference in outcome, but at 1 year follow-up the patients who had received the booklet had fewer physician consultations.

These two fairly well designed studies provide a tool for physicians who wish to manage their patients. They do not appear to provide any support for the effect of education on the patients themselves. In essence, one might extrapolate that a physician who wants to follow up on patients (such as in a fee-for-service system) should provide patient education on site or with follow-up phone calls. These may provide a personal touch that results in continued seeking of attention by the patient. On the other hand, if the physician is motivated by cost cutting (as in an HMO model), a back education booklet may result in more patient independence regarding care. Studies less highly rated by AHCPR support this. Deyo and Diehl reported that patients who did not think they had received an adequate explanation about their pain wanted more tests, were less satisfied with their visit, and were less likely to follow up with the same physician. (3)

Only two of the articles directly addressed the effect of education on the patient. Neither of them directly addressed low back pain as a disease entity. Bass and colleagues found that patients with a variety of primary care complaints had earlier resolution of symptoms when they agreed with the physician (4). We might question whether this correlation implies causation. Perhaps agreement occurs more often when the physician is right regarding a final diagnosis. (Presumably physicians who are off base have less credibility with patients, but they also have worse outcomes.) Also, reasons for disagreement with the physician may be determined long before presentation to the physician. An extreme example is the patient who wants to be put on disability. The patient would disagree with any attending physician who insists on his or her return to work. The outcome in this case is poor but it is not dependent on the disagreement. It is dependent on the patient motivation. Correlation does not imply causation. Nevertheless, this article supports the common sense notion that physicians should develop consensus with their patients rather than an autocratic approach to medical problems.

Thomas performed an important interventional study (5). With a group of primary care patients who had undiagnosable syndromes including low back pain,

Thomas's physicians either said that the patient would get better and provided a specific diagnosis or did not prognosticate and provided a nonspecific diagnosis. Subsequently, patients were either given a treatment or not given a treatment. Patients who were treated positively and concretely got better faster than patients who were given nonspecific answers. This remained true whether or not the patients received the "treatment." Thomas's article provides a general framework for communication with patients who have idiopathic low back pain. It is not clear whether this framework is appropriate for patients who have specific syndromes such as disc herniation, spinal stenosis, spondylolisthesis, and the like. One would suspect that a specific and positive prognosis that underestimates the natural history of a disease would have a negative impact on patient-physician relationship. If this is true, then patients who are at risk for becoming chronic might have worsening of prognosis as a result of factors studied in Bass's paper.

The theoretical construct revolving around patient-physician interaction has been investigated in hundreds of articles and a substantial number of textbooks. This literature is largely ignored by the AHCPR guidelines. Reviews by Stewart (6) and Redelmeier (7) are readily available and prominent in the medical literature. These articles suggest that the tone of conversation has much to do with compliance, patient emotional state, and perhaps even medical outcome. The effect of (and correctness of) the facts or instructions portrayed may or may not have an actual effect on these parameters.

In the guidelines, a strength of evidence rating of "B" may be appropriate regarding the question of whether patient education has an effect on low back syndromes. The specific recommendations listed by the AHCPR, however, are unsupported in the medical literature. Indeed the recommendation that patients be taught "expectations for both rapid recovery and recurrence of symptoms based on the natural history of low back symptoms" runs contrary to the results of Thomas's study. There is no support that educating patients on "safe and effective methods of symptom control" or "safe and reasonable activity modifications" actually has any effect on patient outcome. There is substantial debate and very little literature to support any "best means of limiting recurrent low back problems." There is no evidence that teaching a patient about these has an impact on patient outcome.

Teaching patients "the lack of need for specific investigations unless red flags are present" contradicts the studies by Bass, Deyo, and Thomas. One could conclude from these studies that performing a superfluous test adds to physician-patient interaction, adds to physician credibility, and allows for more credible proclamation of a "specific" diagnosis when the physician actually views the problem as nonspecific. Most of us would concur that

special investigations (e.g., x-rays for typical acute back pain) are usually not appropriate. This is based however on our concern about patient radiation exposure, health care costs, and an overriding moral concern about truth in diagnosis. It is not based on the literature regarding patient education. Similarly one would argue from an educational standpoint that discussing diagnostic tests which are unlikely to be performed may have a contrary effect on patient outcome.

It is a major concern that the AHCPR guidelines do not consider the transition from acute to chronic pain. One could concede that 90 percent of patients who are going to get better anyhow do better when given a directed statement that they will improve. How does such a directed statement affect the 10 percent of patients who will go on to become chronic? One would suspect that these most costly and most disabled persons would only learn that they can not trust doctors. This would result in even more disability.

In summary, this reviewer can not accept the scientific validity of the panel recommendations. Many of the recommendations may be correct. There is, however, essentially no research on the effect of office education on actual recovery from back pain in terms of return to work, decreased pain, decreased medication use, decreased complications, etc. We have pointed out some controversies as well as the role of ethical and financial obligations in patient communication.

## STRUCTURED PATIENT EDUCATION: BACK SCHOOL

The AHCPR's findings are as follows:

In the workplace, back schools with worksite specific education may be effective adjuncts to individual education efforts by the clinician in the treatment of patients with acute low back problems. (Strength of evidence = C.)

The efficacy of back schools in nonoccupational settings has yet to be demonstrated. (Strength of evidence = C.)

The term *back school* is a highly variable concept. It has been used in the literature for everything from a one hour teaching session to an eight week inpatient pain program (8). Variations of the Swedish back school, a four visit program, have been studied frequently and are commonly in use throughout the world. The AHCPR definition of back school includes programs which are like the Swedish back school. In general a back school includes education regarding anatomy, diagnosis, prognosis, commonly available treatment modalities, environmental modification, and body mechanics. As spine clinicians are well aware, each of these are highly changing concepts. A therapist bias towards a manual approach, passive modalities, or exercise may greatly alter the content of back school in different communities. Therapists may not emphasize diagnostics or medications in a back school because they view it as beyond their expertise. Yet these may be key components of keeping patients out of the physicians office, as we have discussed previously. Certain concepts may be incorrect. For example, one would have a hard time finding support among biomechanics experts that "lift with your knees not with your back" is an appropriate instruction for all instances (9). Biomechanical models suggest that this approach to lifting is incorrect with large bulky objects (9). An exercise oriented therapist might be concerned that such a limitation on a patient would result in deconditioning and contracture of muscles providing long-term pain generators. Indeed Indahl has recently presented a controlled study in which persons with back pain are "untaught" body mechanics. Such patients had less pain and less work disability in the long term (10).

The effectiveness of education (i.e., did the patient actually learn what was said?) and compliance (i.e., did the patient actually do what was recommended?) are important but seldom measured components of back school. In fact there is only recent support for the concept that patients ever follow through on biomechanical advice once they leave the clinic. A newer article by Schenk and colleagues (30) seems to indicate that back school is effective in changing lifting behavior. It is possible that the entire effect of back school is the result of nonspecific patient empowerment. If this is true the style of the teacher and the group interaction may be more important than the facts presented. Certainly videotaped back school presentations might have different outcomes compared to live ones. Empathic or dynamic educators may have better results than educators who are merely effective. Cedraschi and colleagues point out that patients have a greatly distorted view of the spine anatomy and that teaching does change knowledge, but not prior notions (11). This suggests that the method of teaching in back schools must attempt to alter perceptions not just knowledge.

The AHCPR guidelines found 14 controlled studies and two meta-analyses addressing back school. They considered one other study. Certainly there have been dozens of other articles regarding back school. Many of these are uncontrolled. Others are focused primarily on the specific methodology employed rather than the outcome.

The studies selected for AHCPR consideration are interesting. While a few of these (12,13,14) include appropriate populations, the majority of studies (15,16,17,18,19, 20,21,22,23,24,25) specifically exclude acute back pain patients. It is unclear why the guidelines committee chose to accept these since there is a substantial difference in these patient populations. The patient base was not able to be determined for one article (26); others were not accessible to this writer (27,20,28). For some reason the guidelines committee violated their own premise in including studies on chronic pain. Based on a small handful of studies it is difficult to draw a consensus about effectiveness.

The study comparing back school to the MacKenzie approach is criticized by its own authors for two reasons (14). The particular back school used prohibited some exercises which may be helpful, and the back school patients only had a single group encounter with the therapist, whereas the MacKenzie group averaged 5.5 visits per patients (up to 20!). Even if the MacKenzie exercise was better, the study did not rule out the possibility that back school properly done could be a cost-effective, commonly available alternative.

It is not clear why the authors of the guidelines chose to separate occupational from nonoccupational back problems. One study in an HMO setting did not show good results (13), but nowhere else in the guideline do the authors so strongly separate occupational from nonoccupational pain. A more balanced and unbiased approach to the subject of work versus nonwork injury would have provided panel recommendations regarding surgery for patients with and without workmen's compensation issues. The guidelines should have been consistent in separating occupational from nonoccupational outcomes for all interventions.

Since publication of the AHCPR guidelines, an important study was performed by LeClaire and colleagues (29). This randomized single blind controlled trial in a private physiatric outpatient clinic randomized patients with a mean duration of low back pain of 15 days to a physical therapy routine with or without low back school. There were 168 patients. The back school provided four interventions at 0, 1, and 8 weeks after first contact. The back school was effective in accomplishing its educational goals as evidenced by statistically significant difference in patient performance on a written examination and on patient performance of an exercise program as witnessed by a research assistant. There was no statistical difference in return to work (33 days) number of recurrences (back school 14, standard care 10), duration of recurrent episodes, level of pain, spinal mobility, straight leg raise test, or functional disability as rated on two different scales.

One could raise questions as to the cultural relativity (the study was done in Quebec under the Canadian health care system) but it is really quite difficult to challenge the results of this carefully performed study.

In summary, although the AHCPR guidelines use inappropriate methodology, the very limited evidence available at the time of the guidelines in conjunction with the important study by LeClaire and colleagues do not strongly support the use of back schools. This runs contrary to many decades of medical practice, and the promotion of a number of proprietary back schools. It is possible that more intensive research on more specific populations will demonstrate effectiveness in back school. More likely the scientific trend appears to go in a different direction.

## PATIENT EDUCATION—A BROADER VIEW

It becomes apparent that the variables in patient education are many. To simply proclaim the effectiveness or ineffectiveness of patient education is simplistic. It is appropriate for the AHCPR guidelines to make comments on a specific methodology such as the Swedish Back School and its analogues. On the other hand, it is quite inappropriate to take a stand on such an amorphous and poorly understood area as physician-patient interaction.

The variables are worth understanding in detail. Table 20–1 lists information that may be imparted to patients. It is unlikely that different components of this list are equally pertinent to persons with acute, subacute, chronic, or recurrent acute back problems; to persons with work-related or litigious injuries vs. others; to those who are disabled from work vs. those who are not, to young, middle aged, or elderly patients; or to patients of different cultures, education, or sex.

Each of the areas listed in Table 20–1 is not a specific entity. Controversies in all of these areas are discussed throughout this monograph. Educators may have varying opinions or knowledge about injections, surgery, different exercise programs, the risk of recurrence, etc. Perhaps the best example of this is the work of Aage Indahl, (10) who sometimes teases his Swedish counterparts by calling his program the "Norwegian Back School." His program places great emphasis on unteaching the body mechanics and other information which patients have learned. Essentially he teaches patients to act as they would have without a back problem. Indahl's work, which received the Sofomar-Danik award at the International Society for the Study of the Lumbar Spine meeting in Burlington, Vermont, in 1996, showed substantial benefits of his "treatment" compared to usual treatment in terms of pain and disability over the three years.

Clearly the effect of "education" goes beyond the imparting of factual knowledge. Consequences of the interaction may include trust, hope, motivation, frustration, fear, anger, resignation, and a wide variety of emotional reactions. These may have profound effects on treatment compliance, the psychosocial state of the patient, secondary prevention, and the interests of the provider, payor, and society. The effects are also not easily predicted given the variations among patients, who all have differing personalities and intelligence levels. Some,

| TABLE 20–1 |
| :---: |
| *Factual information in some patient education programs* |

Anatomy

Physiology

Pathology

Diagnostics

Treatment
    Medical
    Surgical
    Physical

Rehabilitation
    Exercise and activity limitations
    Body mechanics
    Ergonomics

Prognosis

Danger signs

Treatment of recurrences

Psychological issues

Social issues

Legal issues

Consumer protection

especially in the important subgroup who are becoming chronic, may also have significant psychopathology which precludes a logical approach to education.

A discussion of the connections between the factual information imparted, the way it is imparted, the state of the student, and the actions taken by the student is quite pertinent. Space does not allow such a discussion, and indeed, to the thoughtful reader, specific issues are quite intuitive. Instead, it is worthwhile to move quickly to the end result—measurable changes in patient action.

Table 20–2 lists numerous outcomes that are possible as a result of a back pain education effect. There are scientific, economic, and ethical differences regarding the appropriateness of each of them. Each is measurable, however. In fact, there are often validated tests to determine changes in these parameters. We will not go into the specific scientific methodologies. The point is that measurement of outcome in terms of decreased pain or return to work is quite simplistic. Different programs may have intended or unintended effects in any of these areas. The design of a proper educational effort should at least involve awareness of these issues.

**TABLE 20–2**
*Potential effects of patient education*

TREATMENT EFFECTS

Improved knowledge
Decreased pain
Increased risk taking/decreased fear
Improved compliance with activity recommendations at
    home and work
Improved compliance with other treatments (drugs, etc.)
Increased neuromuscular coordination

PSYCHOSOCIAL EFFECTS

Shift to an internal locus of control
Patient belief in the provider's treatment philosophy
Decreased psychological disorders
Decreased impact on family and friends
Decreased litigation

SECONDARY PREVENTION

Decrease in recurrence of pain
Decreased work disability
Decreased progression to chronic disability

PROVIDER AND SOCIETAL EFFECTS

Bonding between the provider and the patient
More efficient use of expensive providers (P.T., group
    therapy vs. individual M.D.)
Increased profit for provider
Decreased cost to the payor
Increased satisfaction of referral sources
Decreased health care seeking with recurrences
Spread of knowledge or interest in back problems
    among co-workers and friends
Propagation or modification of societal norms regarding
    the relationship between pain and disability

## FUTURE DIRECTIONS

Measurement of the effect of patient education, whether through a back school or a physician's office, is likely to be confused by selection bias, attention bias, placebo effects, and other confounding factors. The AHCPR guidelines were appropriate in selecting, as much as possible, only randomized controlled trials. The general lack of trials devoted to LBP is a problem solvable only by additional research.

The obvious study, a large, well-controlled, randomized prospective trial of back school, crossing cultural and geographic boundaries of both the physician and patient, would solidify our understanding of back school's clinical effects. More fruitful results will come from a broader approach to patient education. A number of questions arise:

Can patient education take a different form? We have found, for instance, that patients "learn" and retain positional instructions better with audio biofeedback than with either verbal instructions and pictures or feedback from a corset (31). One wonders about the relative effectiveness of video, interactive CD ROM, education efforts with pre and post tests, or situation specific education. The cost-benefit ratio of group therapy is probably much different from one on one individual education or video/computer education..

Is back school sufficient on its own? Or is it effective as a substrate—fertile soil upon which other specific interventions, ranging from injection to counseling, will have a better effect? There is substantial literature to suggest that patients who understand their treatment are more likely to benefit.

Can the effect of back school on work readiness be measured, when the largest factor in actual return to work may be the physician's written order? Physicians have variable and highly subjective practices in this regard.

Is a more psychologically oriented back school likely to prevent long-term disability? While the anatomy and pathology of the spine are weak predictors of chronicity, psychosocial factors are paramount. It is possible that a psychological intervention regarding coping, conflict resolution, relaxation, etc., would decrease these factors, leading to less long-term disability. Unfortunately, the AHCPR chose not to address prevention of chronicity in its acute pain practice parameters. Given that chronic pain is the most costly and disabling issue in back pain management, this is a substantial oversight.

Is there a subpopulation of patients who will benefit from back school or other educational efforts? Perhaps those at risk for future disability, as we can now predict with 75 percent accuracy, using Hazard's model (32). Perhaps, as one paper suggested, back school is not effective for idiopathic back pain in an HMO (13). Perhaps there are certain medical problems or psychological mindsets which are amenable to an educational approach.

The area of physician office education is perhaps the most fruitful for future efforts. What approach to patient interaction is most effective? Is it the same for all patients? What interpersonal skills do clinicians need in order to use effective educational approaches? Are the interviewing skills of surgeons, primary care physicians, and physiatrists different? We suspect that on the average, they must be based on both personality types, clinical interests, and time commitment. What clinical biases help or interfere with patient outcome? Again, common sense and some research suggest that answers to these questions may need to be individualized. For example, if a physician simply "educates" during the physical examination, anxiety can be allayed: "I'm checking your reflexes. This is a measure of nerve messages passing the disc. Happily, they are normal."

## Summary

The AHCPR guidelines do a great service in setting the stage for debate. Unfortunately the research regarding back schools includes a large number of studies of chronic pain. This contradicts the stated methodology of the guidelines. While one more recent study casts doubt on the effectiveness of back school, any conclusions are preliminary.

Regarding education in the physician's office, the guidelines completely overstep their boundaries, making a number of specific recommendations about what to teach, when there is no research assessing the effect of education about these areas.

Patient education will always happen. Whether formally or informally, in a physician's office or on television commercials. The process is complex, and the outcomes are multifactorial. Scientifically based research on patient education in low back pain is not impossible. We look forward to the cultural changes within medicine which will support such research. Finally, we need to acknowledge that change in medical economics and technology may be the greatest factor in patient education. Physician reward for providing educational material instead of charging for an office visit depends on the insurer. In fee for service models this is an unreimbursed expense. We debate the relative effectiveness of group vs. one on one education, but internet access and interactive computer programs may prove both effective and inexpensive.

## References

1. Jones SL, Jones PK, Katz J. Compliance for low back pain patients in the emergency department. A randomized trial. *Spine* 1988 Jan; 17(1):1–8.
2. Roland M, Dixon M. Randomized controlled trial of an educational booklet for patients presenting with back pain in general practice. *J R Coll Gen Pract* 1989 Jun; 39(323):244–246.
3. Deyo RA, Diehl AK. Patient satisfaction with medical care for low back pain. *Spine* 1986 Jan-Feb; 11(1):28–30.
4. Bass MJ, Buck C, Turner L, Dickie G, Pratt G, Robinson HC. The physician's actions and the outcome of illness in family practice. *J Fam Pract* 1986 Jul; 23(1):43–47.
5. Thomas KB. General practice consultations: Is there any point in being positive? *Br Med J [Clin Res]* 1987 May 9; 294:1200–1202.
6. Stewart MA. Effective physician-patient communication and health outcomes: A review. *Can Med Assoc J* 1995; 152(9):1423–1433.
7. Redelmeier DA, Rosen P, Kahneman D. Understanding patients' decisions. Cognitive and emotional perspectives. *JAMA* 1993; 270(1):72–76.
8. Linton SJ, Kamwendo K. Low back schools. A critical review. *Phys Ther* 1987 Sep; 67(9):1375–1383.
9. Pope MH, Frymoyer JW, Andersson, G. *Occupational low back pain.* New York: Praeger Press, 1984.
10. Indahl A, Haldorson EMH, Ursin H, Reikeras O. The method, the means, or the message? An educational approach to low back pain. A three year followup of a randomized clinical trial. Sofomar Danik Award, The International Society for the Study of the Lumbar Spine Annual Meeting. June 1996, Burlington, Vermont.
11. Cedraschi C, Reust P, Roux E, Vischer TL. The role of prior knowledge on back pain education. *J Spinal Disord* 1992; 5(3):267–276.
12. Bergquist-Ullman M, Larsson U. Acute low back pain in industry. A controlled prospective study with special reference to therapy and confounding factors. *Acta Orthop Scand* 1977; (170):1–117.
13. Berwick DM, Budman S, Fieldstone M. No clinical effect of back schools in an HMO. A randomized prospective trial. *Spine* 1989 Mar; 14(3):338–344.
14. Stankovic R, Johnell O. Conservative treatment of acute low back pain. A prospective randomized trial: MacKenzie method of treatment versus patient education in "mini back school" [see comments]. *Spine* 1990 Feb; 15(2):120–123.
15. Donchin M, Woolf O, Kaplan L, Floman Y. Secondary prevention of low back pain. A clinical trial. *Spine* 1990 Dec; 15(12):1317–1320.
16. Hurri H. The Swedish back school in chronic low back pain. Part I. Benefits. *Scand J Rehab Med* 1989; 21(1):33–40.
17. Hurri H. The Swedish back school in chronic low back pain. Part II. Factors predicting the outcome. *Scand J Rehab Med* 1989; 21(1):41–44.
18. Julkunen J, Hurri H, Kankainen J. Psychological factors in the treatment of chronic low back pain. Follow-up study of a back school intervention. *Psychother Psychosom* 1988; 50(4):173–181.
19. Keijsers JF, Bouter LM, Meertens RM. Validity and comparability of studies on the effects of back schools. *Physiother Theory Pract* 1991; 7(3):177–184.
20. Keijsers JF, Groenman NH, Gerards FM, van Oudheusden E, Steenbakkers M. A back school in the Netherlands: Evaluating the results. *Patient Educ Couns* 1989 Aug; 14(1); 31–44.
21. Keijsers JF, Steenbakkers MW, Gerards FM, Meertens RM. The efficacy of the back school: An analysis of the literature. *Arthr Care Res* 1990 Dec; 3(4):210–215.
22. Klaber Moffett JA, Chase SM, Portek I, Ennis Jr. A controlled, prospective study to evaluate the effectiveness of a back school in the relief of chronic low back pain. *Spine* 1986 Mar; 11(2):120–122.
23. Lindstrom I, Ohlund C, EEk C, Wallin L, Peterson L, Fordyce WE, Nachemson AL. The effect of graded activity on patients with subacute low back pain: A random-

ized prospective clinical study with an operant conditioning behavioral approach. *Phys Ther* 1992 Apr; 72(4):279–293.

24. Lankhorst GJ, Van de Stadt RJ, Vogelaar TW, Van der Korst JK, Prevo AJ. The effect of the Swedish Back School in chronic idiopathic low back pain. A prospective controlled study. *Scand J Rehab Med* 1983; 15(3):141–145.

25. Lindquist S, Lundberg B, Wikmark R, Bergstad B, Loof B, Ottermark AC. Information and regime at low back pain. *Scand J Rehab Med* 1984; 16(3):113–116.

26. Morrison GEC, Chase W, Young V, Roberts W. Back pain: Treatment and prevention in a community hospital. *Arch Phys Med Rehabil* 1988 Aug; 69(8):605–609.

27. Evans C, Gilvert JR, Taylor W, Hildebrand A. A randomized controlled trial of flexion exercises, education, and bed rest for patients with acute low back pain. *Physiotherapy Can* 1987 Mar-Apr; 39(2):96–101.

28. Postacchini G, Facchini M, Palieri P. Efficacy of various forms of conservative treatment in low back pain. A comparative study. *Neuroorthopedics* 1988; 6(1):28–35.

29. Leclaire R, Esdaile JM, Suissa S, Rossignol M, Proulx R, Dupuis M. Back school in a first episode of compensated acute low back pain: A clinical trial to assess efficacy and prevent relapse. *Arch Phys Med Rehabil* 1996 Jul; 77:673–679.

30. Schenk RJ, Doran RL, Stachura JJ. Learning effects of a back education program. *Spine* 1996; 21(19):2183–2189.

31. Haig AJ, Grobler L, Pope MH, Haugh LD, MacDonald L, Holleran K. The relative effectiveness of lumbosacral corset and trunk inclination audio biofeedback on trunk flexion. *European J Phys Med Rehabil* 1991; 2:29–37.

32. Hazard RG, Haugh LD, Reid S, Preble JB, MacDonald L. Early prediction of chronic disability after occupational low back injury. *Spine* 1996; 21(8):945–951.

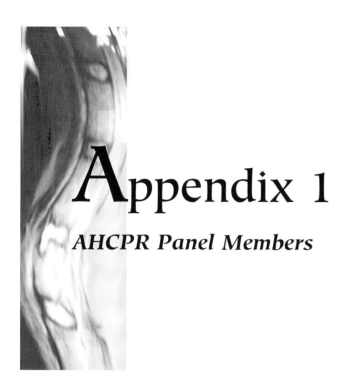

# Appendix 1

## AHCPR Panel Members

**STANLEY J. BIGOS, MD, CHAIR**
*University of Washington*
*Seattle, Washington*
*Orthopedic Surgeon*

**REVEREND O. RICHARD BOWYER**
*Fairmont State College*
*Fairmont, West Virginia*
*Consumer Representative*

**G. RICHARD BRAEN, MD**
*University of New York*
*Buffalo, New York*
*Emergency Medicine Physician*

**KATHLEEN BROWN, PHD, RN**
*University of Alabama*
*Birmingham, Alabama*
*Occupational Health Nurse*

**RICHARD DEYO, MD, MPH**
*University of Washington*
*Seattle, Washington*
*General Internist*

**SCOTT HALDEMAN, DC, MD, PHD**
*University of California at Irvine*
*Santa Ana, California*
*Neurologist/Chiropractor*

**JOHN L. HART, DO**
*Still Regional Medical Center*
*Columbia, Missouri*
*Physiatrist*

**ERNEST W. JOHNSON, MD**
*Ohio State University*
*Columbia, Ohio*
*Physiatrist*

**ROBERT KELLER, MD**
*Maine Medical Assessment Foundation*
*Belfast, Maine*
*Orthopedic Surgeon*

**DANIEL KIDO, MD, FACR**
*Washington University Medical Center*
*St Louis, Missouri*
*Radiologist*

**MATTHEW H. LIANG, MD, MPH**
*Harvard Medical School*
*Boston, Massachusetts*
*Rheumatologist*

**ROGER M. NELSON, PT, PHD**
*Thomas Jefferson University College of*
*    Allied Health Sciences*
*Philadelphia, Pennsylvania*
*Physical Therapist*

**MARGARETA NORDIN, RPT, DRSCI**
*Hospital for Joint Diseases*
*New York, New York*
*Physical Therapist/Orthopedic Researcher*

**BERNICE D. OWEN, PHD, RN**
*University of Wisconsin*
*Madison, Wisconsin*
*Community Health Nurse*

**MALCOLM H. POPE, DRMEDSC, PHD**
*University of Vermont*
*Burlington, Vermont*
*Orthopedic Researcher*

**RICHARD K. SCHWARTZ, MS, OTR, FSR**
*San Antonio, Texas*
*Occupational Therapist*

**DONALD H. STEWART, JR., MD**
*Arlington, Virginia*
*Neurosurgeon*

**JEFF SUSMAN, MD**
*University of Nebraska Medical Center*
*Omaha, Nebraska*
*Family Physician*

**JOHN J. TRIANO, MA, DC**
*Texas Back Institute*
*Piano, Texas*
*Chiropractor*

**LUCIUS C. TRIPP,MD, MPH, FACPM**
*General Motors-Henry Ford Hospital*
  *Rehabilitation Center*
*Warren, Michigan*
*Neurosurgeon/Occupational Medicine*
  *Specialist*

**DENNIS C. TURK, PHD**
*University of Pittsburgh School of Medicine*
*Pittsburgh, Pennsylvania*
*Psychologist*

**CLARK WATTS, MD, JD**
*University of Texas Health Sciences*
  *Center*
*San Antonio, Texas*
*Neurosurgeon*

**JAMES N. WEINSTEIN, DO**
*University of Iowa Hospitals*
*Iowa City, Iowa*
*Orthopedic Surgeon*

# Appendix 2

## AHCPR Acute Low Back Pain References

1. Andersson GBJ. The epidemiology of spinal disorders. In: Frymoyer JW (ed.). *The adult spine: Principles and practice.* New York: Raven Press, 1991:107–146.

2. Välfors B. Acute, subacute and chronic low back pain: Clinical symptoms, absenteeism and working environment. *Scand J Rehab Med* 1985; 11 (Suppl):1–98.

3. Sternbach RA. Survey of pain in the United States: The Nuprin pain report. *Clin J Pain* 1986; 2(1):49–53.

4. Cunningham LS, Kelsey JL. Epidemiology of musculoskeletal impairments and associated disability. *Am J Public Health* 1984; 74:574–579.

5. Cypress BK. Characteristics of physician visits for back symptoms: A national perspective. *Am J Public Health* 1983 Apr; 73(4):389–395.

6. Spengler DM, Bigos SJ, Martin NA, Zeh J, Fisher L, Nachemson A. Back injuries in industry: A retrospective study. I. Overview and cost analysis. *Spine* 1986 Apr; 11(3):241–256.

7. Kelsey JL, White AA III. Epidemiology and impact of low-back pain. *Spine* 1980 Mar–Apr; 5(2):133–142.

8. Nachemson AL. Newest knowledge of low back pain. A critical look. *Clin Orthop* 1992; 279:8–20.

9. Deyo RA, Cherkin D, Conrad D, Volinn E. Cost, controversy, crisis: Low back pain and the health of the public. *Ann Rev Public Health* 1991; 12:141–156.

10. Keller RB, Soule DN, Wennberg JE, Hanley DF. Dealing with geographic variations in the use of hospitals: The experience of the Maine medical assessment foundation orthopaedic study group. *J Bone Joint Surg* 1990 Oct; 72A(9):1286–1293.

11. Volinn E, Mayer J, Diehr P, Van Koevering D, Connell FA, Loeser JD. Small area analysis of surgery for low-back pain. *Spine* 1992; 17(5):575–581

12. Bigos SJ, Battié MC. Acute care to prevent back disability. Ten years of progress. *Clin Orthop* 1987 Aug; (221):121–130.

13. Waddell G. A new clinical model for the treatment of low-back pain. *Spine* 1987 Sep; 12(7):632–644.

14. Goertz MN. Prognostic indicators for acute low-back pain. *Spine* 1990 Dec; 15(12):1307–1310.

15. Von Korff M, Deyo RA, Cherkin D, Barlow W. Back pain in primary care: Outcomes at 1 year. *Spine* 1993 Jun; 18(7):855–862.

16. Kelsey JL. Idiopathic low back pain: Magnitude of the problem. In: White AA, Gordon SL (eds.). *American Academy of Orthopaedic Surgeons Symposium on idiopathic low back pain.* St. Louis: C.V. Mosby,1982:5–8.

17. Field MT, Lohr KN (eds.). *Guidelines for clinical practice: From development to use.* Washington, DC: National Academy Press,1992:426.

18. Woolf SH. AHCPR interim manual for clinical practice guideline development. U.S. Department of Health and Human Services: 1991 May. AHCPR Pub. No. 91-0018.

19. Quebec Task Force on Spinal Disorders. Scientific approach to the assessment and management of activity-related spinal disorders. A monograph for clinicians. Report of the Quebec Task Force on Spinal Disorders. *Spine* 1987; 12(7S):S1–S9.

20. Aejmelaeus R, Hiltunen H, Härkönen M, Silfverhuth M, Vähä-Tahlo T, Tunturi T. Myelographic versus clinical diagnostics in lumbar disc disease. *Arch Orthop Trauma Surg* 1984; 103(1):18–25.

21. Aiello I, Serra G, Migliore A, Tugnoli V, Roccella P, Cristofori MC, Manca M. Diagnostic use of H-reflex from vastus medialis muscle. *Electromyogr Clin Neurophysiol* 1983; 23:159–166.

22. Bosacco SJ, Berman AT, Garbarino JL, Teplick JG, Peyster R. A comparison of CT scanning and myelography in the diagnosis of lumbar disc herniation. *Clin Orthop* 1984 Nov; (190):124–128.

23. Cats-Baril WL, Frymoyer JW. Identifying patients at risk of becoming disabled because of low-back pain. The Vermont Rehabilitation Engineering Center predictive model. *Spine* 1991 Jun; 16(6):605–607.

24. Charnley J. Orthopaedic signs in the diagnosis of disc protrusion with special reference to the straight-leg-raising test. *Lancet* 1951 Jan 27; 1:186–192.

25. Christodoulides AN. Ipsilateral sciatica on femoral nerve stretch test is pathognomonic of an L4/5 disc protrusion. *J Bone Joint Surg [Br]* 1989 Jan; 71(1):88–89.

26. Deyo RA, Diehl AK. Cancer as a cause of back pain: Frequency, clinical presentation, and diagnostic strategies. *J Gen Intern Med* 1988 May–Jun; 3(3):230–238.

27. Giles LGF, Taylor JR. Low-back pain associated with leg length inequality. *Spine* 1981; 6:510–521.

28. Grundy PF, Roberts CJ. Does unequal leg length cause back pain? A case control study. *Lancet* 1974 Aug 4; 2(8397):256–258.

29. Gunn CC, Milbrandt WE, Little AS, Mason KE. Dry needling of muscle motor points for chronic low-back pain. A randomized clinical trial with long-term follow-up. *Spine* 1980 May/Jun; S(3):279–291.

30. Herron LD, Turner J. Patient selection for lumbar laminectomy and discectomy with a revised objective rating system. *Clin Orthop* 1985 Oct; 199:145–152.

31. Hudgins WR. The crossed straight leg raising test: A diagnostic sign of herniated disc. *J Occup Med* 1979 Jun; 21(6):407–408.

32. Jensen OH. The level-diagnosis of a lower lumbar disc herniation: The value of sensibility and motor testing. *Clin Rheumatol* 1987 Dec; 6(4):564–569.

33. Jensen OH, Schmidt-Olsen S. A new functional test in the diagnostic evaluation of neurogenic intermittent claudication. *Clin Rheumatol* 1989 Sep; 8(3):363–367.

34. Kerr RSC, Cadoux-Hudson TA, Adams CBT. The value of accurate clinical assessment in the surgical management of the lumbar disc protrusion. *J Neurol Neurosurg Psychiatry* 1988 Feb; 51(2):169–173.

35. Kortelainen P, Puranen J, Koivisto E, Läde S. Symptoms and signs of sciatica and their relation to the localization of the lumbar disc herniation. *Spine* 1985 Jan–Feb; 10(1):88–92.

36. Kosteljanetz M, Bang F, Schmidt-Olsen S. The clinical significance of straight-leg raising (Lasègue's sign) in the diagnosis of prolapsed lumbar disc. Interobserver variation and correlation with surgical finding. *Spine* 1988 Apr; 13(4):393–395.

37. Kosteljanetz M, Espersen JO, Halaburt H, Miletic T. Predictive value of clinical and surgical findings in patients with lumbago-sciatica. A prospective study (Part I). *Acta Neurochir [Wien]* 1984; 73(1–2):67–76.

38. Lacroix JM, Powell J, Lloyd GJ, Doxey NC, Mitson GL, Aldam CF. Low-back pain. Factors of value in predicting outcome. *Spine* 1990 Jun; 15(6):495–499.

39. McNeill TW, Sinkora G, Leavitt F. Psychologic classification of low-back pain patients: A prognostic tool. *Spine* 1986 Nov; 11(9):955–999.

40. Morris EW, Di Paola M, Vallance R, Waddell G. Diagnosis and decision making in lumbar disc prolapse and nerve entrapment. *Spine* 1986 Jun; 11(5):436–439.

41. Murphy KA, Cornish RD. Prediction of chronicity in acute low back pain. *Arch Phys Med Rehabil* 1984 Jun; 65(6):334–337.

42. Nehemkjs AM, Carver DW, Evanski PM. The predictive utility of the orthopedic examination in identifying the low back pain patient with hysterical personality features. *Clin Orthop* 1979 Nov–Dec; (145):158–162.

43. Nykvist F, Hurme M, Alaranta H, Miettinen ML. Social factors and outcome in a five-year follow-up study of 276 patients with sciatica. *Scand J Rehab Med* 1991; 23(1):19–26.

44. Rae PS, Waddell G, Venner RM. A simple technique for measuring lumbar spinal flexion. Its use in orthopaedic practice. *J R Coll Surg Edinb* 1984 Sep; 29(5):281–284.

45. Ransford AO, Cairns D, Mooney V. The pain drawing as an aid to the psychologic evaluation of patients with low-back pain. *Spine* 1976 Jun; 1(2):127–134.

46. Roland MO, Morrell DC, Monis RW. Can general practitioners predict the outcome of episodes of back pain? *Br Med J (Clin Res)* 1983 Feb 12; 286(6364):523–525.

47. Shiqing X, Quanthi Z, Dehao F. Significance of the straight-leg-raising test in the diagnosis and clinical evaluation of lower lumbar intervertebral-disc protrusion. *J Bone Joint Surg* 1987 Apr; 69A(4):517–522.

48. Soukka A, Alaranta H, Tallroth K, Heliövaara M. Leg-length inequality in people of working age. The association between mild inequality and low back pain is questionable. *Spine* 1991 Apr; 16(4):429–431.

49. Spengler DM, Freeman CW. Patient selection for lumbar discectomy. An objective approach. *Spine* 1979 Mar–Apr; 4(2):129–134.

50. Spengler DM, Ouellette EA, Battié M, Zeh J. Elective discectomy for herniation of a lumbar disc. Additional experience with an objective method. *J Bone Joint Surg [Am]* 1990 Feb; 72(2):230–237.

51. Takata K, Inoue SI, Takahashi K, Ohtsuka Y. Swelling of the cauda equina in patients who have herniation of a lumbar disc. A possible pathogenesis of sciatica *J Bone Joint Surg [Am]* 1988 Mar; 70(3):361–368.

52. Udén A, Landin LA. Pain drawing and myelography in sciatic pain. *Clin Orthop Rel Res* 1987 Mar; 216:124–130.

53. Von Baeyer CL, Bergstrom KT, Brodwin MG, Brodwin SK. Invalid use of pain drawings in psychological screening of back pain patients. *Pain* 1983 May; 16(l):103–107.

54. Deyo RA, Rainville J, Kent DL. What can the history and physical examination tell us about low back pain? *JAMA* 1992 Aug 12; 268(6):760–765.

55. Waddell G, Main CJ, Morris EW, Venner RM, Rae PS, Sharmy SH, Galloway H. Normality and reliability in the clinical assessment of backache. *Br Med J [Clin Res]* 1982 May 22; 284(6328):15 19–23.

56. Aronson HA, Dunsmore RH. Herniated upper lumbar discs. *J Bone Joint Surg [Am]* 1963 Mar; 45:311–317.

57. Bigos SJ, Battié MC, Fisher LD. Methodology for evaluating predictive factors for the report of back injury. *Spine* 1991 Jun; 16(6):669–670.

58. Deyo RA, Diehl AK. Psychosocial predictors of disability in patients with low back pain. *J Rheumatol* 1988 Oct; 15(10):1557–1564.

59. Deyo RA, Tsui-Wu YJ. Descriptive epidemiology of low-back pain and its related medical care in the United States. *Spine* 1987 Apr; 12(3):264–268.

60. Gran JT. An epidemiologic survey of the signs and symptoms of ankylosing spondylitis. *Clin Rheumatol* 1985 Jun; 4(2):161–169.

61. Hakelius A, Hindmarsh J. The comparative reliability of preoperative diagnostic methods in lumbar disc surgery. *Acta Orthop Scand* 1972; 43:234–238.

62. Lowery WD, Horn TJ, Boden SD, Wiesel SW. Impairment evaluation based on spinal range of motion in normal subjects. *J Spinal Disorders* 1992; 5(4):398–402.

63. Spangfort EV. The lumbar disc herniation. *Acta Orth Scand* 1972; 142 (Suppl):1–95.

64. Waldvogel FA, Vasey H. Osteomyelitis: The past decade. *N Engl J Med* 1980 Aug 14; 303(7):360–370.

65. Weber H. Lumbar disc herniation. A prospective study of prognostic factors including a controlled trial. Part I. *J Oslo City Hosp* 1978; 28:33–64.

66. Turner JA, Ersek M, Herron L, Deyo R. Surgery for lumbar spinal stenosis. Attempted meta-analysis of the literature. *Spine* 1992 Jan; 17(1):1–8.

67. Jones SL, Jones PK, Katz J. Compliance for low-back pain patients in the emergency department. A randomized trial. *Spine* 1988; 13(5):553–556.

68. Roland M, Dixon M. Randomized controlled trial of an educational booklet for patients presenting with back pain in general practice. *J R Coll Gen Pract* 1989 Jun; 39(323):244–246.

69. Bass MT, Buck C, Turner L, Dickie G, Pratt G, Robinson HC. The physician's actions and the outcome of illness in family practice. *J Fam Pract* 1986 Jul; 23(1):43–47.

70. Deyo RA, Diehl AK. Patient satisfaction with medical care for low-back pain. *Spine* 1986 Jan–Feb; 11(1):28–30.

71. Thomas KB. General practice consultations: Is there any point in being positive? *Br Med J [Clin Res]* 1987 May 9; 294:1200–1202.

72. Bergquist-Ullman M, Larsson U. Acute low back pain in industry. A controlled prospective study with special reference to therapy and confounding factors. *Acta Orthop Scand* 1977; (170):1–117.

73. erwick DM, Budman S, Feldstein M. No clinical effect of back schools in an HMO. A randomized prospective trial. *Spine* 1989 Mar; 14(3):33–44.

74. Donchin M, Woolf O, Kaplan L, Floman Y. Secondary prevention of low back pain. A clinical trial. *Spine* 1990 Dec; 15(12):1317–1320.

75. Evans C, Gilbert TR, Taylor W, Hildebrand A. A randomized controlled trial of flexion exercises, education, and bed rest for patients with acute low back pain. *Physiother Can* 1987 Mar–Apr; 39(2):96–101.

76. Hurri H. The Swedish back school in chronic low back pain. Part I. Benefits. *Scand J Rehab Med* 1989; 21(1):33–40.

77. Huni H. The Swedish back school in chronic low back pain. Part II. Factors predicting the outcome. *Scand J Rehab Med* 1989; 21(1):41–44.

78. Julkunen J, Hurri H, Kankainen J. Psychological factors in the treatment of chronic low back pain. Follow-up study of a back school intervention. *Psychother Psychosom* 1988; 50(4):173–181.

79. Keijsers JF, Groenman NH, Gerards FM, van Oudheusden E, Steenbakkers M. A back school in the Netherlands: Evaluating the results. *Patient Educ Couns* 1989 Aug; 14(1):31–44.

80. Keijsers JF, Steenbakkers MW, Gerards FM, Meertens RM. The efficacy of the back school: An analysis of the literature. *Arthr Care Res* 1990 Dec; 3(4):210–215.

81. Klaber Moffett JA, Chase SM, Portek I, Ennis JR. A controlled, prospective study to evaluate the effectiveness of a back school in the relief of chronic low back pain. *Spine* 1986 Mar; 11(2):120–122.

82. Lindequist S, Lundberg B, Wikmark R, Bergstad B, Lööf G, Otterrmark AC. Information and regime at low back pain. *Scand J Rehab Med* 1984; 16(3):113–116.

83. Lindstrtöm I, Ohlund C, Eek C, Wallin L, Peterson L, Fordyce WE, Nachemson AL. The effect of graded activity on patients with subacute low-back pain: A randomized prospective clinical study with an operant conditioning behavioral approach. *Phys Ther* 1992 Apr; 72(4):279–293.

84. Morrison GEC, Chase W, Young V, Roberts WL. Back pain: Treatment and prevention in a community hospital. *Arch Phys Med Rehabil* 1988 Aug; 69(8):605–609.

85. Postacchini F, Facchini M, Palieri P. Efficacy of various forms of conservative treatment in low back pain. A comparative study. *Neuroorthopedics* 1988; 6(1):28–35.

86. Stankovic R, Johnell O. Conservative treatment of acute low-back pain. A prospective randomized trial: McKenzie method of treatment versus patient education in "mini back school" [see comments]. *Spine* 1990 Feb; 15(2):120–123.

87. Keijsers JFEM, Bouter LM, Meertens RM. Validity and comparability of studies on the effects of back schools. *Physiother Theory Pract* 1991; 7(3):177–182.

88. Linton SJ, Kamwendo K. Low back schools. A critical review. *Phys Ther* 1987 Sep; 67(9):1375–1383.

89. Lankhorst GJ, Van de Stadt KT, Vogelaar TW, Van der Korst JK, Prevo AT. The effect of the Swedish Back School in chronic idiopathic low back pain. A prospective controlled study. *Scand J Rehab Med* 1983; 15(3):141–145.

90. Amlie E, Weber H, Holme I. Treatment of acute low-back pain with piroxicam: Results of a double-blind placebo-controlled trial. *Spine* 1987 Jun; 12(5):473–476.

91. Basmajian JV. Acute back pain and spasm. A controlled multicenter trial of combined analgesic and antispasm agents. *Spine* 1989 Apr; 14(4):438–439.

92. Berry H, Bloom B, Hamilton EBD, Swinson DR. Naproxen sodium, diflunisal, and placebo in the treatment of chronic back pain. *Ann Rheum Dis* 1982; 41:129–132.

93. Brooks PM, Day RO. Nonsteroidal antiinflammatory drugs—differences and similarities. *N Engl J Med* 1991 Jun 13; 32A:1716–1725.

94. Cooper SA, Engel J, Ladove M, Rauch D, Precheur H, Rosenheck A. An evaluation of oxycodone and acetaminophen in the treatment of postoperative dental pain. *Clin Pharmacol Ther* 1979; 23(2):219.

95. Fowler PD. Aspirin, paracetamol and non-steroidal antiinflammatory drugs: A comparative review of side effects. *Med Toxicol* 19X7; 2:338–366.

96. Gall EP, Caperton EM, McComb JE, Messner R, Murz CV, O'Hanlan M, Willkens RF. Clinical comparison of ibuprofen, fenoprofen calcium, naproxen and tolmetin sodium in rheumatoid arthritis. *J Rheumatol* 1982; 9(3):402–407.

97. Hickey RFJ. Chronic low back pain: A comparison of diflunisal with paracetamol. *N Z Med J* 1982; 95:312–314.

98. Hopkinson JH, Bartlett FH, Steffens AO, McGlumphy TH, Macht EL, Smith M. Acetaminophen versus propoxyphene hydrochloride for relief of pain in episiotomy patient. *J Clin Pharm* 1973; 13:251–263.

99. Jiranek GC, Kimmey MB, Saunders DR, Willson RA, Shanahan W, Silverstein FE. Misoprostol reduces gastroduodenal injury from one week of aspirin: An endoscopic study. *Gastroenterology* 1989; 96:656–661.

100. Lanza F, Peace K, Gustitus L, Rack MF, Dickson B. A blinded endoscopic comparative study of misoprostol versus sucralfate and placebo in the prevention of aspirin-induced gastric and duodenal ulceration. *Am J Gastroenterol* 1988; 83(2):143.

101. Scott DL, Roden S, Marshall T, Kendall MJ. Variations in responses to non-steroidal anti-inflammatory drugs. *Br J Clin Pharmacol* 1982; 14:691–694.

102. Wallenstein SL, Houde RW. Clinical comparison of the analgesic effectiveness of N-acetyl-p-aminophenol, salicylamide and aspirin [abstract]. *Fed Proc* 1954; 13:414.

103. Wasner C, Britton MC, Kraines G, Kaye RL, Bobrove AM, Fries JF. Non steroidal anti-inflammatory agents in rheumatoid arthritis and ankylosing spondylitis. *JAMA* 1981; 246:2168–2172.

104. Arbus L, Fajadet B, Aubert D, Morre M, Goldberger E. Activity of tetrazepam (Myolastan®) in low back pain. A double-blind trial v placebo. *Clin Trials J* 1990; 27(4):258–267.

105. Baratta RR. A double-blind study of cyclobenzaprine and placebo in the treatment of acute musculoskeletal conditions of the low back. *Curr Ther Res* 1982 Nov; 32(5):646–652.

106. Borenstein DG, Lacks S, Wiesel SW. Cyclobenzaprine and naproxen versus naproxen alone in the treatment of acute low back pain and muscle spasm. *Clin Ther* 1990 Mar–Apr; 12(2):125–131.

107. WF, Glassman JM, Soyka JP. Management of acute musculoskeletal conditions: Thoracolumbar strain or sprain. A double-blind evaluation comparing the efficacy and safety of carisprodol with diazepam. *Today's Ther Trends* 1983; 1(1):1–16.

108. Casale R. Acute low back pain. Symptomatic treatment with a muscle relaxant drug. *Clin J Pain* 1988; 4(2):81–88.

109. Dapas F, Hartman SF, Martinez L, Northrup BE, Nussdorf RT, Silberman HM, Gross H. Baclofen for the treatment of acute low-back syndrome. A double-blind comparison with placebo. *Spine* 1985 May; 10(4):345–349.

110. Gold RH. Orphenadrine citrate: Sedative or muscle relaxant? *Clin Ther* 1978; 1(6):451–453.

111. Hindle TH 3d. Comparison of carisoprodol, butabarbital, and placebo in treatment of the low back syndrome. *Calif Med* 1972 Aug; 117(2):7–11.

112. Hingorani K. Diazepam in backache: A double-blind controlled trial. *Ann Phys Med* 1965; 8:303–306.

113. Klinger NM, Wilson RR, Kanniainen CM, Wagenknecht KA, Re ON, Gold RH. Intravenous orphenadrine for the treatment of lumbar paravertebral muscle strain. *Curr Ther Res* 1988; 43(2):207–254.

114. Rollings HE, Glassman JM, Soyka TP. Management of acute musculoskeletal conditions—thoracolumbar strain or sprain: A double-blind evaluation comparing the efficacy and safety of carisoprodol with cyclobenzaprine hydrochloride. *Curr Ther Res* 1983 Dec; 34(6):917–928.

115. Brown FL Jr, Bodison S, Dixon J, Davis W, Nowoslawski J. Comparison of diflunisal and acetaminophen with codeine in the treatment of initial or recurrent acute low back strain. *Clin Ther* 1986; 9 (Suppl C):52–58.

116. Muncie KL Jr, King DE, DeForge B. Treatment of mild to moderate pain of acute soft tissue injury: Diflunisal vs acetaminophen with codeine. *J Fam Pract* 1986 Aug; 23(2):125–127.

117. Wiesel SW, Cuckler M, Deluca F, Jones F, Zeide MS, Rothman RH. Acute low-back pain: An objective analy-

sis of conservative therapy. *Spine* 1980 Jul/Aug; 5(4):324–330.

118. Heishman SJ, Stilzer ML, Bigelow GE, Liebson IA. Acute opioid physical dependence in humans: Effect of varying the morphine-naloxone interval. *J Pharmacol Exp Ther* 1989 Aug; 250(2):485–491.

119. Haimovic IC, Beresford HR. Dexamethasone is not superior to placebo for treating lumbosacral radicular pain. *Neurology* 1986 Dec; 36(12):1593–1594.

120. Felson DT, Anderson JJ. A cross-study evaluation of association between steroid dose and bolus steroids and avascular neurosis of bone. *Lancet* 1987 Apr 18; 1(8538):902–906.

121. Truhan AP, Ahmed AR. Corticosteroids: A review with emphasis on complications of prolonged systemic therapy. *Ann Allergy* 1989 May; 62:375–390.

122. Meek JB, Giudice VW, McFadden JW, Key JD. Colchicine confirmed as highly effective in disk disorders. Final results of a double-blind study. *J Neuro & Orthop Med & Surg* 1985 Oct; 6(3):211–218.

123. Schnebel BE, Simmons JW. The use of oral colchicine for low-back pain. A double-blind study. *Spine* 1988 Mar,13(3):354–357.

124. Simmons JW, Harris WP, Koulisis CW, Kimmich SJ. Intravenous colchicine for low-back pain: A double-blind study. *Spine* 1990 Jul; 15(7):716–717.

125. Alcoff J Jones E, Rust P, Newman R. Controlled trial of imipramine for chronic low back pain. *J Fam Pract* 1982 May; 14(5):841–846.

126. Goodkin K, Gullion CM, Agras WS. A randomized, double-blind, placebo-controlled trial of trazodone hydrochloride in chronic low back pain syndrome. *J Clin Psychopharmacol* 1990 Aug; 10(4):269–278.

127. Jenkins DG, Ebbutt AF, Evans CD. Tofranil in the treatment of low back pain. *J Int Med Res* 1976; 4(28):28–40.

128. Blackwell B. Adverse effects of antidepressant drugs. Part 1: Monoamine oxidase inhibitors and tricyclics. *Drugs* 1981; 21:201–219.

129. Blackwell B. Adverse effects of antidepressant drugs. Part 2: "Second generation" antidepressants and rational decision making in antidepressant therapy. *Drugs* 1981; 21:272–282.

130. Brodin H. Inhibition-facilitation technique for lumbar pain treatment. *Int J Rehabil Res* 1984; 7(3):328–329.

131. Coxhead CE, Meade TW, Inskip H, North WRS, Troup JDG. Multicentre trial of physiotherapy in the management of sciatic symptoms. *Lancet* 1981 May 16; 8229:1065–1068.

132. Farrell JP, Twomey LT. Acute low back pain. Comparison of two conservative treatment approaches. *Med J Aust* 1982 Feb 20; 1(4):1604.

133. Gibson T, Grahame R, Harkness J, Woo P, Blagrave P, Kills R. Controlled comparison of short-wave diathermy treatment with osteopathic treatment in non-specific low back pain. *Lancet* 1985 Jun 1; 1(8440):1258–1261.

134. Glover JR, Morris JG, Khosla T. Back pain: A randomized clinical trial of rotational manipulation of the trunk. *Br J Ind Med* 1974 Jan; 31(1):59–64.

135. Godfrey CM, Morgan PP, Schattker J. A randomized trial of manipulation for low-back pain in a medical setting. *Spine* 1984 Apr; 9(3):301–304.

136. Hadler NM, Curtis P, Gillings DB, Stinnett S. A benefit of spinal manipulation as adjunctive therapy for acute low-back pain: A stratified controlled trial. *Spine* 1987 Sep; 12(7):703–706.

137. MacDonald RS, Bell CM. An open controlled assessment of osteopathic manipulation in nonspecific low-back pain (published erratum appears in *Spine* 1991 Jan; l6(1):l04). *Spine* 1990 May; 15(5):364–370.

138. Mathews JA, Mills SB, Jenkins VM, Grimes SM, Morkel MJ, Mathews W, Scott CM, Sittampalam Y. Back pain and sciatica: Controlled trials of manipulation, traction, sclerosant and epidural injections. *Br J Rheumatol* 1987 Dec; 26(6):416–423.

139. Mathew's W, Morkel M, Mathews J. Manipulation and traction for lumbago and sciatica: Physiotherapeutic techniques used in two controlled trials. *Physiother Prac* 1988 Dec; 4(4):201–206.

140. Waterworth RF, Hunter IA. An open study of diflunisal, conservative and manipulative therapy in the management of acute mechanical low back pain. *N Z Med J* 1985 May 22; 98(779):372–375.

141. Anderson R, Meeker WC, Wirick BE, Mootz RD, Kirk DH, Adams A. A meta-analysis of clinical trials of spinal manipulation. *J Man Physiol Ther* 1992 Mar–Apr; 15(3):181–194.

142. Haldeman S, Chapman-Smith D, Petersen DM (eds.). *Guidelines for chiropractic quality assurance and practice parameters.* Proceedings of the Mercy Center Consensus Conference, 1993. Gaithersburg, MD: Aspen Publishers,1993.

143. Jarvis KB, Phillips RB, Morris EK. Cost per case comparison of back injury claims of chiropractic versus medical management for conditions with identical diagnostic codes. *J Occup Med* 1991 Aug; 33(8):847–852.

144. Shekelle PG, Adams AK, Chassin MR, Hurwitz EL, Brook RH. Spinal manipulation for low-back pain. *Ann Intern Med* 1992 Oct; 117(7):590–598.

145. Coyer AB, Curwen IHM. Low back pain treated by manipulation. A controlled series. *Br Med J* 1955 Mar 19; 1:705–707.

146. Edwards BC. Low back pain and pain resulting from lumbar spine conditions. *Aust J Physiother* 1969 Sep; 15(3):104–110.

147. Mandell P, Lipton MH, Bernstein J, Kucera GJ, Kampner JA. *Low back pain. An historical and contemporary overview of the occupational, medical, and psychosocial issues of chronic back pain.* Thorofare, NJ: SLACK, Inc., 1989:219.

148. Nwuga VCB. Relative therapeutic efficacy of vertebral manipulation and conventional treatment in back pain management. *Am J Phys Med* 1982 Dec; 61(6):273–278.

149. Rasmussen GG. Manipulation in treatment of low-back pain (a randomized clinical trial). *Man Med* 1979; 1:8–10.

150. Klein RG, Eek BC. Low-energy laser treatment and exercise for chronic low back pain: Double-blind controlled trial. *Arch Phys Med Rehabil* 1990 Jan; 71(1):34–37.

151. Koes BW, Bouter LM, van Mameren H, Essers AHM, Verstegen GMJR, Hofhuizen DM, Houben JP, Knipschild PG. A blinded randomized clinical trial of manual therapy and physiotherapy for chronic back and neck complaints: Physical outcome measures. *J Man Physiol Ther* 1992 Jan; 15(1):16–23.

152. Koes BW, Bouter LM, van Mameren H, Essers AHM, Verstegen GMJR, Hofhuizen DM, Houben P, Knipschild PG. The effectiveness of manual therapy, physiotherapy, and treatment by the general practitioner for nonspecific back and neck complaints. A randomized clinical trial. *Spine* 1992; 17(1):28–35.

153. Koes BW, Bouter LM, van Mameren H, Essers AHM, Verstegen GM, Hofhuizen DM, Houben JP, Knipschild PG. Randomised clinical trial of manipulative therapy and physiotherapy for persistent back and neck complaints: Results of one year follow up. *Br Med J* 1992; 304:601–605.

154. Linton SJ, Bradley LA, Jensen I, Spangfort E, Sundell L. The secondary prevention of low back pain: A controlled study with follow-up. *Pain* 1989 Feb; 36(2):197–207.

155. Manniche C, Hesselsoe G, Bentzen L, Christensen I, Lundberg E. Clinical trial of intensive muscle training for chronic low back pain. *Lancet* 1988 Dec 24–31; 2(8626–8627):1473–1476.

156. MelzacL R, Vetere P, Finch L. Transcutaneous electrical nerve stimulation for low back pain. A comparison of TENS and massage for pain and range of motion. *Phys Ther* 1983 Apr,63(4):489–443.

157. Deyo RA, Walsh NE, Mamn DC, Schoenfeld LS, Ramamurthy S. A controlled trial of transcutaneous electrical nerve stimulation (TENS) and exercise for chronic low back pain [see comments]. *N Engl J Med* 1990 Jun 7; 322(23):1627–1634.

158. Gemignani G, Olivieri I, Ruju G, Pasero G. Transcutaneous electrical nerve stimulation in ankylosing spondylitis: A double-blind study [letter]. *Arthritis Rheum* 1991 Jun; 34(6):788–789.

159. Graff-Radford SB, Reeves JL, Baker RL, Chiu D. Effects of transcutaneous electrical nerve stimulation on myofascial pain and trigger point sensitivity. *Pain* 1989; 37:1–5.

160. Hackett GI, Seddon D, Kaminski D. Electroacupuncture compared with paracetamol for acute low back pain. *Practitioner* 1988 Feb 22; 232(1443):1634.

161. Lehmann TR, Russell DW, Spratt KF. The impact of patients with nonorganic physical findings on a controlled trial of transcutaneous electrical nerve stimulation and electroacupuncture. *Spine* 1983 Sep; 8(6):625–634.

162. Lehmann TR, Russell DW, Spratt KF, Colby H, Liu YK, Fairchild ML, Christensen S. Efficacy of electroacupuncture and TENS in the rehabilitation of chronic low back pain patients. *Pain* 1986 Sep; 26(3): 277–290.

163. Thorsteinsson G, Stonnington HH, Stillwell GK, Elveback LR. Transcutaneous electrical stimulation: A double-blind trial of its efficacy for pain. *Arch Phys Med Rehabil* 1977 Jan; 58:8–13.

164. Thorsteinsson G, Stonnington HH, Stillwell GK, Elveback LR. The placebo effect of transcutaneous electrical stimulation. *Pain* 1978; 5:3141.

165. Basford TR, Smith MA. Shoe insoles in the workplace. *Orthopedics* 1988 Feb; 11(2):285–288.

166. Batlié MC, Bigos SJ, Fisher LD, Spengler DM, Hansson TH, Nachemson AL, Wortley MD. The role of spinal flexibility in back pain complaints within industry. A prospective study. *Spine* 1990 Aug; 15(8):768–773.

167. Horal J. The clinical appearance of low back disorders in the city of Gothenburg, Sweden. Comparisons of incapacitated probands with matched controls. *Acta Orthop Scand* 1969; 118 (Suppl):15–23, 68–73.

168. Hult L. Cervical, dorsal and lumbar spinal syndromes. *Acta Orthop Scand* 1954; 16 (Suppl):7–73.

169. Reddell CR, Congleton JJ, Huchingson RD, Montgomery JF. An evaluation of a weightlifting belt and back injury prevention training class for airline baggage handlers. *Applied Ergonomics* 1992; 23(5):319–329.

170. Walsh NE, Schwartz RK. The influence of prophylactic orthoses on abdominal strength and low back injury in

the workplace [see comments]. *Am J Phys Med Rehabil* 1990 Oct; 69(5):245–250.

171. Million R, Haavik Nilsen K, Jayson MN, Baker RD. Evaluation of low back pain and assessment of lumbar corsets with and without back supports. *Ann Rheum Dis* 1981; 40:449–454.

172. Larsson U, Chöler U, Lidström A, Lind G, Nachemson A, Nilsson B, Roslund J. Auto-traction for treatment of lumbago-sciatica. A multicentre controlled investigation. *Acta Orthop Scand* 1980 Oct; 51(5):791–798.

173. Mathews JA, Hickling J. Lumbar traction: A double-blind controlled study for sciatica. *Rheumatol Rehabil* 1975; 14:222–225.

174. Pal B, Mangion P, Hossain MA, Diffey BL. A controlled trial of continuous lumbar traction in the treatment of back pain and sciatica. *Br J Rheumatol* 1986 May; 25(2):181–183.

175. Weber H, Ljunggren AE, Walker L. Traction therapy in patients with herniated lumbar intervertebral discs. *J Oslo City Hosp* 1984 Jul–Aug; 34(7–8):61–70.

176. Haskvitz EM, Hanten WP. Blood pressure response to inversion traction. *Phys Ther* 1986 Sep; 66(9):13614.

177. Asfour SS, Khalil TM, Waly SM, Goldberg ML, Rosomoff RS, Rosomoff HL. Biofeedback in back muscle strengthening. *Spine* 1990 Jun; 15(6):510–513.

178. Bush C, Ditto B, Feuerstein M. A controlled evaluation of paraspinal EMG biofeedback in the treatment of chronic low back pain. *Health Psychol* 1985; 4(4):307–321.

179. Flor H, Haag G, Turk DC, Koehler H. Efficacy of EMG biofeedback, pseudotherapy, and conventional medical treatment for chronic rheumatic back pain. *Pain* 1983 Sep; 17(1):21–31.

180. Nouwen A. EMG biofeedback used to reduce standing levels of paraspinal muscle tension in chronic low back pain. *Pain* 1983 Dec; 17(4):353–360.

181. Flor H, Haag G, Turk DC. Long-term efficacy of EMG biofeedback for chronic rheumatic back pain. *Pain* 1986 Nov; 27(2):195–202.

182. Stuckey SJ, Jacobs A, Goldfarb J. EMC biofeedback training, relaxation training, and placebo for the relief of chronic back pain. *Percept Mot Skills* 1986 Dec; 63(3):1023–1036.

183. Bourne IH. Treatment of chronic back pain. Comparing corticosteroid lignocaine injections with lignocaine alone. *Practitioner* 1984 Mar; 228(1389):333–338.

184. Frost FA, Jessen B, Siggaard-Andersen J. A control, double-blind comparison of mepivacaine injection versus saline injection for myofascial pain. *Lancet* 1980 Mar 8; 8167:499–501.

185. Garvey TA, Marks MR, Wiesel SW. A prospective, randomized. double blind evaluation of trigger-point injection therapy for low-back pain. *Spine* 1989 Sep; 14(9):962–964.

186. Collée G, Dijkmans BAC, Vandenbroucke JP, Cats A. Iliac crest pain syndrome in low back pain. A double blind, randomized study of local injection therapy. *J Rheumatol* 1991; 18(7):1060–1063.

187. Ongley MJ, Klein RG, Dorman TA, Eek BC, Hubert LJ. A new approach to the treatment of chronic low back pain. *Lancet* 1987 Jul 18; 2(8551):143–146.

188. Sonne M, Christensen K, Hansen SE, Jensen EM. Injection of steroids and local anaesthetics as therapy for low-back pain. *Scand J Rheumatol* 1985; 14(4):343–345.

189. Sullivan JGB. The anesthesiologist's approach to back pain. In: Herkowitz HN, Garfin SR, Balderston RA, Eismont FJ, Bell GR, Wiesel SW (eds.). *The spine*. 3rd ed.

Philadelphia: W.B. Saunders,1992:1945–1961.

190. Wilkinson HA. Alternative therapies for the failed back syndrome. In: Frymoyer JW (ed.). *The adult spine: Principles and practice*. New York: Raven Press,1991: 2069–2091.

191. Jackson RP. The facet syndrome. Myth or reality? *Clin Orthop Rel Res* 1992 Jun; 279:110–121

192. Carette S, Marcoux S, Truchon R, Grondin C, Gagnon J, Allard Y, Latulippe M. A controlled trial of corticosteroid injections into facet joints for chronic low back pain. *N Engl J Med* 1991 Oct 3; 325(14):1002–1007.

193. Lilius G, Laasonen EM, Myilynen P, Harilainen A, Grtinlund G. Lumbar facet joint syndrome. A randomised clinical trial. *J Bone Joint Surg [Br]* 1989 Aug; 71(4):6814.

194. Marks RC, Houston T, Thulbourne T. Facet joint injection and facet nerve block: A randomised comparison in 86 patients with chronic low back pain. *Pain* 1992; 49:325–328.

195. Nash TP. Facet joints—intra-articular steroids or nerve block? *Pain Clinic* 1990; 3(2):77–82.

196. Thomson SJ, Lomax DM, Collett BJ. Chemical: Meningism after lumbar facet joint block with local anaesthetic and steroids. *Anaesthesia* 1991 Jul; 45(7):563–564.

197. Warfield CA. Facet syndrome and the relief of low back pain. *Hosp Pract [Off]* 1988 Oct 30; 23(10A):41-247–248.

198. Mooney V. Injection studies. Role in pain definition. In: Frymoyer JW (ed.). *The adult spine: Principles and practice*. New York: Raven Press, 1991:527–540.

199. White AH. Injection techniques for the diagnosis and treatment of low back pain. *Orthop Clin North Am* 1983 Jul; 14(3):553–567.

200. Breivik H, Hesla PE, Molnar I, Lind B. Treatment of chronic low back pain and sciatica: Comparison of caudal epidural injections of bupivacaine and methylprednisolone with bupivacaine followed by saline. *Adv Pain Res Ther* 1976; 1:927–932.

201. Bush K, Hillier S. A controlled study of caudal epidural injections of triamcinolone plus procaine for the management of intractable sciatica. *Spine* 1991; 16(5):572–575.

202. Cuckler JM, Bernini PA, Wiesel SW, Booth RE Jr, Rothman RH, Pickens GT. The use of epidural steroids in the treatment of lumbar radicular pain. A prospective, randomized double-blind study. *J Bone Joint Surg [Am]* 1985 Jan; 67(1):63–66.

203. Dallas TL, Lin RL, Wu WH, Wolskee P. Epidural morphine and methylprednisolone for low-back pain. *Anesthesiology* 1987 Sep; 67(3):408–411.

204. Dilke TF, Burry HC, Grahame R. Extradural corticosteroid injection in management of lumbar nerve root compression. *Br Med J* 1973 Jun 16; 2(867):635–637.

205. Klenerman L, Greenwood R, Davenport KT, White DC, Peskett S. Lumbar epidural injections in the treatment of sciatica. *Br J Rheumatol* 1984; 23(1):35–38.

206. Ridley MG, Kingsley GH, Gibson T, Grahame R. Outpatient lumbar epidural corticosteroid injection in the management of sciatica. *Br J Rheumatol* 1988; 27(4):295–299.

207. Snoek W, Weber H, Jorgensen B. Double blind evaluation of extradural methyl prednisolone for herniated lumbar discs. *Acta Orthop Scand* 1977; 48:635–641.

208. Kepes ER, Duncalf D. Treatment of backache with spinal injections of local anesthetics. spinal and systemic steroids. A review. *Pain* 1985 May; 22(1):3347.

209. Rocco AG, Frank E, Kaul AF, Lipson SJ, Gallo JP. Epidural steroids, epidural morphine and epidural steroids com-

bined with morphine in the treatment of post-laminectomy syndrome. *Pain* 1989 Mar; 36(3):297–303.

210. Coan RM, Wong G, Ku SL, Chan YC, Wang L, Ozer FT, Coan PL. The acupuncture treatment of low back pain: A randomized controlled trial. *Am J Clin Med* 1980; 8(2):181–189.

211. Edelist G, Gross AE, Langer F. Treatment of low back pain with acupuncture. *Can Anaesth Soc J* 1976 May; 23(3):303–306.

212. Ghia TN, Mao W, Toomey TC, Gregg JM. Acupuncture and chronic pain mechanisms. *Pain* 1976; 2:285–299.

213. Gunn CC, Milbrandt WE. Tenderness at motor points. A diagnostic and prognostic aid for low-back injury. *J Bone Joint Surg [Am]* 1976 Sep; 58(6):815–825.

214. Mendelson G, Kidson MA, Loh ST, Scott DF, Selwood TS, Kranz H. Acupuncture analgesia for chronic low back pain. *Clin Exp Neurol* 1978; 15:182–185.

215. Mendelson G, Selwood TS, Kranz H, Loh TS, Kidson MA, Scott DS. Acupuncture treatment of chronic back pain. A double-blind placebo controlled trial. *Am J Med* 1983 Jan; 74(1):49–55.

216. ter Riet G, Kleijnen J, Knipschild P. Acupuncture and chronic pain: A criteria-based meta-analysis. *J Clin Epidemiol* 1990; 43(11):1191–1199.

217. Kent G, Brondum J, Keenlyside RA, Lafazia LM, Scott HD. A large outbreak of acupuncture-associated hepatitis B. *Am J Epidemiol* 1988; 127(3):591–598.

218. Lee MHM, Liao S, Kottke FJ, Lehmann JF. *Krusen's handbook of physical medicine and rehabilitation.* Philadelphia: W.B. Saunders,1990. Chapter 16, Acupuncture in physiatry.

219. Willms D. Possible complications of acupuncture (letter). *West J Med* 1991; 154(6):736–737.

220. Wright R, Kupperman TL, Liebhaber MI. Bilateral tension pneumothoraces after acupuncture. *West J Med* 1991; 154(1):102–103.

221. Chaffin DB. A biomechanical strength model for use in industry. *Appl Ind Hyg* 1988 Mar; 3(3):79–86.

222. Damkot DK, Pope MH, Lord J, Frymoyer JW. The relationship between work history, work environment and low back pain in men. *Spine* 1984; 9:395–399.

223. Drury CG. Influence of restricted space on manual materials handling. *Ergonomics* 1985 Jan; 28(1):167–175.

224. Dul J, Hilderbrandt VH. Ergonomic guidelines for the prevention of low back pain at the workplace. *Ergonomics* 1987 Feb; 30(2):419–429.

225. Garg A, Moore JS. Epidemiology of low-back pain in industry. *Occup Med* 1992 Oct–Dec; 7(4):593–608.

226. Nachemson AL. Disc pressure measurements. *Spine* 1981 Jan/Feb; 6(1):93–97.

227. National Institute for Occupational Safety and Health (NIOSH). *Work practices guide for manual lifting.* US Department of Health and Human Services, National Institute for Occupational Safety and Health. Cincinnati, OH: March 1981. NIOSH Technical Report No. 81-122.

228. Waters TR, Putz-Anderson V, Garg A, Fine U. Revised NIOSH equation for the design and evaluation of manual lifting tasks. *Ergonomics* 1993; 36(7):749–776.

229. Deyo RA, Diehl AK, Rosenthal M. How many days of bed rest for acute low back pain? A randomized clinical trial. *N Engl J Med* 1986 Oct 23; 315(17):1064–1070.

230. Gilbert JR, Taylor DW, Hildebrand A, Evans C. Clinical trial of common treatments for low back pain in family practice. *Br Med J [Clin Res]* 1985 Sep 21; 291(6498): 791–794.

231. Bortz WM. The disuse syndrome. *West J Med* 1984 Nov; 141(5):691–694.

232. Deyo RA. Non-operative treatment of low back disorders. Differentiating useful from useless therapy. In: Frymoyer JW (ed.). *The adult spine: Principles and practice.* New York: Raven Press,1991:1567–1580.

233. Buswell J. Low back pain: A comparison of two treatment programmes. *N Z J Physiother* 1982 Aug; 10(2):13–17.

234. Davies JE, Gibson T, Tester L. The value of exercises in the treatment of low back pain. *Rheumatol Rehabil* 1979; I8:243–247.

235. Donelson R, Grant W, Kamps C, Medcalf R. Pain response to sagittal end range spinal motion. A prospective, randomized, multicentered trial. *Spine* 1991 Jun; 16(6 Suppl):S206–S212.

236. Gundewall B, Liljeqvist M, Hansson T. Primary prevention of back symptoms and absence from work. A prospective randomized study among hospital employees. *Spine* 1993; 18(5):587–594.

237. Kellett KM, Kellett DA, Nordholm LA. Effects of an exercise program on sick leave due to back pain. *Phys Ther* 1991 Apr; 71(4):283–291; discussion 291–293.

238. Kendall PH, Jenkins JM. Exercises for backache: A double-blind controlled trial. *Physiotherapy* 1968; 54: 154–157.

239. Lidström A, Zachrisson M. Physical therapy on low back pain and sciatica. An attempt at evaluation. *Scand J Rehab Med* 1970; 2:37–42.

240. McCain GA, Bell DA, Mai FM, Halliday PD. A controlled study of the effects of a supervised cardiovascular fitness training program on the manifestations of primary fibromyalgia. *Arthritis Rheum* 1988 Sep; 31(9):1135–1141.

241. Reilly K, Lovejoy B, Williams R, Roth H. Differences between a supervised and independent strength and conditioning program with chronic low back syndromes. *J Occup Med* 1989 Jun; 31(6):547–550.

242. Turner JA, Clancy S, McQuade KT, Cardenas DD. Effectiveness of behavioral therapy for chronic low back pain: A component analysis. *J Consult Clin Psychol* 1990 Oct; 58(5):573–579.

243. Zylbergold RS, Piper MC. Lumbar disc disease: Comparative analysis of physical therapy treatments. *Arch Phys Med Rehabil* 1981 Apr; 62:176–179.

244. Andersson GBJ. Posture and compressive spine loading: Intradiscal pressures, trunk myoelectric activities, intraabdominal pressures, and biochemical analyses. *Ergonomics* 1985; 28(1):91–93.

245. Andersson GBJ, Örtengren R, Nachemson AL, Elstrtöm G, Broman H. The sitting posture: An electromyographic and discometric study. *Orthop Clin North Am* 1975 Jan; 6(1):105–120.

246. Fordyce WE, Brockway JA, Bergman JA, Spengler D. Acute back pain: A control-group comparison of behavioral vs traditional management methods. *J Behav Med* 1986 Apr,9(2):127–140.

247. Nachemson A. Towards a better understanding of low-back pain: A review of the mechanics of the lumbar disc. *Rheumatol Rehabil* 1975; 14:129–143.

248. Nachemson AL. The lumbar spine. An orthopaedic challenge. *Spine* 1W6 Mar; 1(1):59–71.

249. Nachemson A, Elfsröm G. Intravital dynamic pressure measurements in lumbar discs. A study of common movements, maneuvers and exercises. *Scand J Rehab Med* 1970; 1 (Suppl):1–40.

250. Nordin M, Örtengren R, Andersson GBJ. Measurements of trunk movements during work. *Spine* 1984; 9(5):465–469.

251. Sachs BL, Ahmad SS, LaCroix M, Olimpio D, Heath R, David JA, Scala AD. Objective assessment for exercise treatment on the B-200 isostation as part of work tolerance rehabilitation. A random prospective blind evaluation with comparison control population. *Spine* 1994 Jan 1; 19(1):49–52.

252. Schultz AB, Andersson GBJ. Analysis of loads on the lumbar spine. *Spine* 1981 Jan–Feb; 6(1):76–82.

253. Schultz AB, Andersson GBJ, Örtengren R, Haderspeck K, Nachemson A. Loads on the lumbar spine. Validation of a biomechanical analysis by measurements of intradiscal pressures and myoelectric signals. *J Bone Joint Surg [Am]* 1982; 64:713–720.

254. Aiello I, Serra G, Tugnoli V, Cristofori MC, Migliore A, Roccella P, Rosati G. Electrophysiological findings in patients with lumbar disc prolapse. *Electromyogr Clin Neurophysiol* 1984 May; 24(4):313–320.

255. Arena JG, Sherman RA, Bruno GM, Young TR. Electromyographic recordings of low back pain subjects and non-pain controls in six different positions: Effect of pain levels. *Pain* 1991 Apr; 45(1):23–28.

256. Braddom RI, Johnson EW. Standardization of H-reflex and diagnostic use in S1 radiculopalhy. *Arch Phys Med Rehabil* 1974 Apr; 55:161–166.

257. Kthatri BO, Baruah J, McQuillen MP. Correlation of electromyography with computed tomography in evaluation of lower back pain. *Arch Neurol* 1984 Jun; 41(6):594–597.

258. Sihvonen T, Partanen J, Hänninen O, Soimakallio S. Electric behavior of low back muscles during lumbar pelvic rhythm in low back pain patients and healthy controls. *Arch Phys Med Rehabil* 1991 Dec; 72:1080–1087.

259. Stolov WC, Slimp JC. Dermatomal somatosensory evoked potentials in lumbar spinal stenosis. Am Assoc Electromyography and Electrodiagnosis. *Am Electrencephalography Soc Joint Symp* 1988; 17–22.

260. Young A, Getty J, Jackson A, Kinslan E, Sullivan M, Parry CW. Variations in the pattern of muscle innervation by the L5 and S1 nerve roots. *Spine* 1983 Sep; 8(6):616–624.

261. Ahern DK, Follick MJ, Council R, Laser-Worston N, Litchman H. Comparison of lumbar paravertebral EMG patterns in chronic low back pain patients and non-patient controls. *Pain* 1988 Aug; 34(2):153–160.

262. Esdaile JM, Rosenthall L, Terkeltaub R, Kloiber R. Prospective evaluation of sacroiliac scintigraphy in chronic inflammatory back pain. *Arthritis Rheum* 1980 Sep; 23(9):998–1003.

263. Lowe J, Schachner E, Hirschberg E, Shapiro Y, Libson E. Significance of bone scintigraphy in symptomatic spondylolysis. *Spine* 1984 Sep; 9(6):653–655.

264. Miron SD, Khan MA, Wiesen ET, Kushner I, Bellon EM. The value of quantitative sacroiliar scintigrophy in detection of sacroiliitis. *Clin Rheumatol* 1983 Dec; 2(4):407–414.

265. Schütte HE, Park WM. The diagnostic value of bone scintigraphy in patients with low back pain. *Skeletal Radiol* 1983; 10(1):14.

266. Whalen JL, Brown ML, McLeod R, Fitzgerald RH Jr. Limitations of indium leukocyte imaging for the diagnosis of spine infections. *Spine* 1991 Feb; 16(2):193–197.

267. Mills GH, Davies GK, Getty CJM, Conway J. The evaluation of liquid crystal thermography in the investiga-

tion of nerve root compression due to lumbosacral lateral spinal stenosis. *Spine* 1986 Jun; 11(5):427–432.

268. Hoffman RM, Kent DL, Deyo RA. Diagnostic accuracy and clinical utility of thermography for lumbar radiculopathy. A meta-analysis. *Spine* 1991 Jun; 16(6):623–628.

269. Chafetz N, Wexler CE, Kaiser JA. Neuromuscular thermography of the lumbar spine with CT correlation. *Spine* 1988 Aug; 13(8):922–925.

270. Harper CM Jr, Low PA, Fealey RD, Chelimsky TC, Proper CJ, Gillen DA. Utility of thermography in the diagnosis of lumbosacral radiculopathy. *Neurology* 1991 Jul; 41(7):1010–1014.

271. Perelman RB, Adler D, Humphreys M. Electronic infrared thermography. A clinical comparison with computerized tomography of the lumbosacral spine. *J Neurol Orthop Med Surg* 1985 Apr; 6(1):7–12.

272. o YT, Aminoff MT, Olney RK. The role of thermography in the evaluation of lumbosacral radiculopathy [see comments]. *Neurology* 1989 Sep; 39(9):1154–1158.

273. Boden SD, Davis DO, Dina TS, Patronas NJ, Wiesel SW. Abnormal magnetic-resonance scans of the lumbar spine in asymptomatic subjects. *J Bone Joint Surg [Am]* 1990:72(3):403–408.

274. Hilselberger WE, Witten RM. Abnormal myelograms in asymptomatic patients. *J Neurosurg* 1968; 28:204–206.

275. Wiesel SW, Tsourmas N, Feffer HL, Citrin CM, Patronas N. A study of computer-assisted tomography. I. The incidence of positive CAT scans in an asymptomatic group of patients. *Spine* 1984 Sep; 9(6):549–551.

276. Biering-Sorensen F, Hansen FR, Schroll M, Runeborg O. The relation of spinal x-ray to low-back pain and physical activity among 60-year-old men and women. *Spine* 1985 Jun; 10(5):445–451.

277. Bigos SJ, Hansson T, Castillo RN, Beecher PJ, Wortley MD. The value of preemployment roentgenographs for predicting acute back injury claims and chronic back pain disability. *Clin Orthop Rel Res* 1992 Oct; 283:124–129.

278. Deyo RA, Diehl AK. Lumbar spine films in primary care current use and effects of selective ordering criteria. *J Gen Intern Med* 1986 Jan–Feb; 1(1):20–25

279. Fullenlove TM, Williams AJ. Comparative roentgen findings in symptomatic and asymptomatic backs. *Radiology* 1957; 68:572–574.

280. Grubb SA, Lipscomb HJ, Guilford WB. The relative value of lumbar roentgenograms, metrizamide myelography, and discography in the assessment of patients with chronic low-back syndrome. *Spine* 1987 Apr; 12(3):282–286.

281. Hansson T, Bigos S, Beecher P, Wortley M. The lumbar lordosis in acute and chronic low-back pain. *Spine* 1985 Mar; 10(2):154–155.

282. Kaplan DM, Knapp M, Romm FJ, Velez R. Low back pain and x-ray films of the lumbar spine: A prospective study in primary care. *South Med J* 1986 Jul; 79(7):8114.

283. LaRocca H, Macnab I. Value of pre-employment radiographic assessment of the lumbar spine. *Can Med Assoc J* 1969 Oct 4; 101:49–54.

284. LaRocca H, Macnab I. Value of pre-employment radiographic assessment of the lumbar spine. *Indus Med* 1970 Jun; 39(6):253–258.

285. Leboeuf C, Kimber D, White K. Prevalence of spondylolisthesis, transitional anomalies and low intercrestal line in a chiropractic patient population. *J Manipulative Physiol Ther* 1984 Jun; 12(3):200–204.

286. Libson E, Bloom RA, Dinari G. Symptomatic and

asymptomatic spondylolysis and spondylisthesis in young adults. *Int Orthop* 1982; 6:259–261.

287. Libson E, Bloom RA, Dinari G, Robin GC. Oblique lumbar spine radiographs: Importance in young patients. *Radiology* 1984 Apr; 151(l):89–90.

288. Magora A, Schwartz A. Relation between the low back pain syndrome and x-ray findings. 1. Degenerative osteoarthritis. *Scand J Rehab Med* 1976; 8:115–125.

289. Magora A, Schwartz A. Relation between the low back pain syndrome and x-ray findings. 3. Spina bifida occulta. *Scand J Rehab Med* 1980; 12(1):9–15.

290. Magora A, Schwartz A. Relation between low back pain and x-ray changes. 4. Lysis and olisthesis. *Scand J Rehab Med* 1980; 12(2):47–52.

291. Paajanen H, Erkintalo M, Dahlsbbm S, Kuusela T, Svedström E, Kormano M. Disc degeneration and lumbar instability. Magnetic resonance examination of 16 patients. *Acta Orthop Scand* 1989 Aug; 60(4):375–378.

292. Splithoff CA. Lumbosacral junction: Roentgenographic comparison of patients with and without backaches. *JAMA* 1953 Aug 22; 152(17):1610–1613.

293. Swärd L, Hellström M, Jacobsson B, Peterson L. Back pain and radiologic changes in the thoraco-lumbar spine of athletes. *Spine* 1990 Feb; 15(2):124–129.

293. Torgerson WR, Dotter WE. Comparative roentgenographic study of the asymptomatic and symptomatic lumbar spine. *J Bone Joint Surg* 1976 Sep; 58(6):850–853.

295. Boxall D, Bradford DS, Winter RB, Moe JH. Management of severe spondylolisthesis in children and adolescents. *J Bone Joint Surg [Am]* 1979 June; 6l-A(4):479–495.

296. Hall FM. Back pain and the radiologist. *Radiology* 1980 Dec; 137(3):861–63.

297. Kent DL, Haynor DR, Larson EB, Deyo RA. Diagnosis of lumbar spinal stenosis in adults: A metaanalysis of the accuracy of CT, MR, and myelography. *Am J Roentgenol* 1992 May; 158:1135–1144.

298. Fries JW, Abodeely DA, Vijungco JG, Yeager VL, Gaffey WR. Computed tomography of herniated and extruded nucleus pulposus. *J Comput Assist Tomogr* 1982 Oct; 6(5):874–887.

299. Gillström P, Ericsson K, Hindmarsh T. A comparison of computed tomography and myelography in the diagnosis of lumbar disc herniation. *Arch Orthop Trauma Surg* 1986; 106(1):12–14.

300. Haughton VM, Eldevik OP, Magnaes B, Amundsen P. A prospective comparison of computed tomography and myelography in the diagnosis of herniated lumbar disks. *Neuroradiology* 1982 Jan; 142(1):103–110.

301. Hirsch C, Nachemson A. The reliability of lumbar disk surgery. *Clin Orthop* 1963; 29:189.

302. Jackson RP, Cain TE, Jacobs RR, Cooper BR, McManus GE. The neuroradiographic diagnosis of lumbar herniated nucleus pulposus: I. A comparison of computed tomography (CT), myelography, CT-myelography, discography, and CT-discography. *Spine* 1989; 14(12):1356–1360.

303. Jackson RP, Cain JE, Jacobs RR, Cooper BR, McManus GE. The neuroradiographic diagnosis of lumbar herniated nucleus pulposus: II. A comparison of computed tomography (CT), myelography, CT-myelography, and magnetic resonance imaging. *Spine* 1989; 14(12):1362–1367.

303. Ketonen L, Gyldensted C. Lumbar disc disease evaluated by myelography and postmyelography spinal computed tomography. *Neuroradiology* 1986; 28(2):144–149.

305. Masaryk TJ, Ross JS, Modic MT, Boumphrey F, Bohlman H, Wilber G. High-resolution MR imaging of sequestered lumbar intervertebral disc. *Am J Roentgenol* 1988 May; 150:1155–1162.

306. Modic MT. Hasaryk T, Boumphrey F, Goorm; Lstic M, Bell G. Lumbar herniated disk disease and canal stenosis: Prospective evaluation by surface coil MR, CT, and myelography. *AJR* 1986 Oct; 147(4):757–765.

307. Moufarrij NA, Hardy RW, Weinstein UA. Computed tomographic, myelographic, and operative findings in patients with suspected herniated lumbar discs. *Neurosurgery* 1983 Feb; 12(2):184–188.

308. Schipper J, Kardaun JW, Braakman R, van Dongen KJ, Blaauw G. Lumbar disk herniation: Diagnosis with CT or myelography. *Radiology* 1987 Oct; 165(1):227–231.

309. Slebus FG, Braakman R, Schipper J, van Dongen KJ, Westendorpde Serière M. Non-corresponding radiological and surgical diagnoses in patients operated for sciatica. *Acta Neurochir* 1988; 94:137–143.

310. Szypryt EP, Twining P, Wilde GP, Mulholland RC, Worthington BS. Diagnosis of lumbar disc protrusion. A comparison between magnetic resonance imaging and radiculography. *J Bone Joint Surg [Br]* 1988 Nov; 70(5): 717–722.

311. Sackett DL, Haynes RB, Guyatt GH, TugweU P. *Clinical epidemiology: A basic science for clinical medicine.* 2nd ed. Boston: Little, Brown, 1991.

312. Bell GR, Rothman RH, Booth RE, Cuckler JM, Garfin S, Herkowitz H, Simeone FA, Dolinskas C, Han SS. A study of computer-assisted tomography. II. Comparison of metrizamide myelography and computed tomography in the diagnosis of herniated lumbar disc and spinal stenosis. *Spine* 1984; 9(6):552–556.

313. Bolender NF, Schönström NSR, Spengler DM. Role of computed tomography and myelography in the diagnosis of central spinal stenosis. *J Bone Joint Surg* 1985 Feb; 67A(2):240–246.

314. Epstein NE, Epstein JA, Carras R, Hyman RA. Far lateral lumbar disc herniations and associated structural abnormalities. An evaluation in 60 patients of the comparative value of CT, MRI, and myelo-CT in diagnosis and management *Spine* 1990 Jun; 15(6):534–539.

315. Herkowitz HN, Gafin SR, Bell GR, Bumphrey F, Rothman RH. The use of computerized tomography in evaluating non-visualized vertebral levels caudad to a complete block on a lumbar myelogram. *J Bone Joint Surg* 1987 Feb; 69A(2):218–224.

316. Modic MT, Pavlicek W, Weinstein MA, Boumphrey F, Ngo F, Hardy R, Duchesneau PM. Magnetic resonance imaging of intervertebral disk disease. *Radiology* 1984 Ju1; 152(1):103–111.

317. Schnebel B, Kingston S, Watkins R, Dillin W. Comparison of MRI to contrast CT in the diagnosis of spinal stenosis. *Spine* 1989 Mar; 14(3):332–337.

318. Schönström NSR, Bolender NF, Spengler DM. The pathomorphology of spinal stenosis as seen on CT scans of the lumbar spine. *Spine* 1985; 10(9):806–811.

319. Stockley I, Getty CJM, Dixon AK, Glaves I, Euinton HA, Banington NA. Lumbar lateral canal entrapment: Clinical, radiculographic and computed tomographic findings. *Clin Radiol* 1988; 39:144–149.

320. Voelker JL, Mealey J Jr, Eskridge JM, Gilmor RL. Metrizamide-enhanced computed tomography as an adjunct in metrizamide myelography in the evaluation

of lumbar disc herniation and spondylosis. *Neurosurgery* 1987 Mar; 20(3):379–384.

321. Zlatkin MB, Lander PH, Hadjipavlou AG, Levine JS. Paget disease of the spine: CT with clinical correlation. *Radiology* 1986 Ju1; 160(1):155–159.

322. Powell MC, Wilson M, Szypryt P, Symonds EM, Worthington BS. Prevalence of lumbar disc degeneration observed by magnetic resonance in symptomless women. *Lancet* 1986 Dec 13; 2(8520):1366–1367.

323. Weinreb JC, Wolbarsht LB, Cohen JM, Brown CE, Maravilla KR. Prevalence of lumbosacral intervertebral disk abnormalities on MR images in pregnant and asymptomatic nonpregnant women. *Radiology* 1989 Jan:170(1 Pt l):125–128.

324. Colhoun E, McCall IW, Williams L, Cassar Pullicino VN. Provocation discography as a guide to planning operations on the spine. *J Bone Joint Surg [Br]* 1988 Mar; 70(2):267–271.

325. Gill K, Jackson RP. CT-discography. In: Frymoyer TW (ed.). *The adult spine: Principles and practice.* New York: Raven Press, 1991:443–456.

326. Holt EP. The question of lumbar discography. *J Bone Joint Surg [Am]* 1968 Jun; 50(4):720–726.

327. Walsh TR, Weinstein M, Spratt KF, Lehmann TR, Aprill C, Sayre H. Lumbar discography in normal subjects. A controlled, prospective study. *J Bone Joint Surg [Am]* 1990 Aug; 72(7):1081–1088.

328. Crawshaw C, Frazer AM, Merriam WF, Mulholland RC, Webb JK. A comparison of surgery and chemonucleolysis in the treatment of sciatica. A prospective randomized trial. *Spine* 1984 Mar; 9(2):195–198.

329. Ejeskär A, Nachemson A, Hers P, Lysell E, Andersson G, Irstam L, Peterson LE. Surgery versus chemonucleolysis for herniated lumbar discs. A prospective study with random assignment. *Clin Orthop* 1983 Apr; (174):236–242.

330. Fraser RD. Chymopapain for the treatment of intervertebral disc herniation: A preliminary report of a double-blind study. *Spine* 1982; 7:608–612.

331. Fraser RD. Chymopapain for the treatment of intervertebral disc herniation. The final report of a double-blind study. *Spine* 1984 Nov–Dec; 9(8):815–818.

332. Gogan WJ, Fraser RD. Chymopapain. A 10-year, double-blind study. *Spine* 1992; 17(4):388–394.

333. Javid MJ, Nordby EL, Ford LT, Hejna W3, Whisler WW, Burton C, Millett DK, Wiltse L, Widell EH Jr, Boyd RJ, Newton SE, Thisted R. Safety and efficacy of chymopapain (Chymodiactin) in herniated nucleus pulposus with sciatica. Results of a randomized, double-blind study. *JAMA* 1983 May 13; 249(18):2:89–94.

334. Revel M, Payan C, Vallee C, et al. Automated percutaneous lumbar discectomy versus chemonucleolysis in the treatment of sciatica. *Spine* 1993; 8(1):1–7.

335. Tullberg T, Isacson J, Weidenhielm L. Does microscopic removal of lumbar disc herniation lead to better results than the standardized procedure? Results of a one-year randomized study. *Spine* 1993; 18(1):17–20.

336. van Alphen HAM, Braakman R, Bezemer PD, Broere G, Berfelo MW. Chemonucleolysis versus discectomy: A randomised multicenter trial. *J Neurosurg* 1989 Jun; 70(6):869–875.

337. Watters WC 3d, Mirkovic S, Boss J. Treatment of the isolated lumbar intervertebral disc herniation: Microdiscectomy versus chemonucleolysis *Spine* 1988 Mar; 13(3):360–362.

338. Weber H. The effect of delayed disc surgery on muscular paresis. *Acta Orthop Scand* 1975:46:531–542.

339. Weber H. Lumbar disc herniation. A controlled, prospective study with ten years of observation. *Spine* 1983 Mar; 8(2):131–140.

340. Hoffman RM, Wheeler KJ, Deyo RA. Surgery for herniated lumbar discs: A literature synthesis. *J Gen Intern Med* 1993 Sept; 8:487–496.

341. Agre K, Wilson RR, Brim M, McDermott DJ. Chymodiactin postmarketing surveillance. Demographic and adverse experience data in 29,075 patients. *Spine* 1984 Jul–Aug; 9(5):479–485.

342. Alexander AH, Burkus JK, Mitchell JB, Ayers WV. Chymopapain chemonucleolysis versus surgical discectomy in a military population. *Clin Orthop* 1989 Jul; (244): 158–165.

343. Bouillet R. Treatment of sciatica. A comparative survey of complications of surgical treatment and nucleolysis with chymopapain. *Clin Orthop* 1990 Feb; (251):144–152.

344. Deeb ZL, Schimel S, Daffner RH, Lupetin AR, Hryshko FG, Blakley JB. Intervertebral disk-space infection after chymopapain injection. *Am J Neuroradiol* 1985; 6(1):55–58.

345. Deyo RA, Cherkin DC, Loeser JD, Bigos SJ, Ciol M. Morbidity and mortality in association wilh operations on the lumbar spine. The influence of age, diagnosis, and procedure. *J Bone Joint Surg [Am]* 1992; 74-A(4):536–543.

346. Herkowitz HN, Kurz LT. Degenerative lumbar spondylolisthesis with spinal stenosis. *J Bone Joint Surg [Am]* 1991 July; 73-A(6):802–808.

347. Johnsson KE, Rosén I, Udén A. The natural course of lumbar spinal stenosis. *Acta Orthop Scand* 1990; 61(Suppl 1):237:24.

348. Katz JM, Lipson SJ, Larson MG, McInnes JM, Fossel AH, Liang MH. The outcome of decompressive laminectomy for degenerative lumbar stenosis. *J Bone Joint Surg [Am]* 1991 July; 73-A(6):809–816.

349. Lee CK, deBari A. Lumbosacral spinal fusion with Knodt distraction rods. *Spine* 1986 May; l1(4):373–375.

350. White AH, von Rogov P, Zucherman J, Heiden D. Lumbar laminectomy for herniated disc: A prospective controlled comparison with internal fixation fusion. *Spine* 1987 Apr; 12(3):305–307.

351. Tumer JA, Ersek M, Herron L, H; L,elkorn J, Kent D, Ciol MA, Deyo R. Patient outcomes after lumbar spinal fusions. *JAMA* 1992 Aug 19; 268(7):907–911.

352. Bigos SJ, Battié MC, Spengler DM, Fisher LD, Fordyce WE, Hansson TH, Nachemson AL, Zeh J. A longitudinal, prospective study of industrial back injury reporting. *Clin Orthop* 1992 Jun; (279):21–34.

353. Eie N. Comparison of the results in patients operated upon for ruptured lumbar discs with and without spinal fusion. *Acta Neurochir* 1978; 41:107–113.

354. Frymoyer JW, Hanley E, Howe J, Kuhlmann D, Matteri R. Disc excision and spine fusion in the management of lumbar disc disease. *Spine* 1978 Mar; 3(1):1–6.

355. Schofferman J, Anderson D, Hines R, Smith G, White A. Childhood psychological trauma correlates with unsuccessful lumbar spine surgery. *Spine* 1992 Jun; 17(6S):S138–S144.

356. Vaughan Pk Malcolm BW, Maistrelli GL. Results of L4/5 disc excision alone versus disc excision and fusion. *Spine* 1988 Jun; 13(6):690–695.

357. Waddell G. Biopsychosocial analysis of low back pain. *Baillieres Clin Rheumatol* 1992 Oct; 6(3):523–557.

358. Bigos SJ, Battié MC, Spengler DM, Fisher LD, Fordyce WE, Hansson TH, Nachemson AL, Wortley MD. A prospective study of work perceptions and psychosocial factors affecting the report of back injury. *Spine* 1991; 16(1):1–6

359. Skovron ML, Szpalski M, Nordin M, Melot C, Cukier D. Sociocultural factors and back pain. A population-based study in Belgian adults. *Spine* 1994 Jan 15; 19(2):129–137.

360. Wiltse LL, Rocchio PD. Preoperative psychological tests as predictors of success of chemonucleolysis in the treatment of the low-back syndrome. *J Bone Joint Surg [Am]* 1975 Jun; 57(4):478–483.

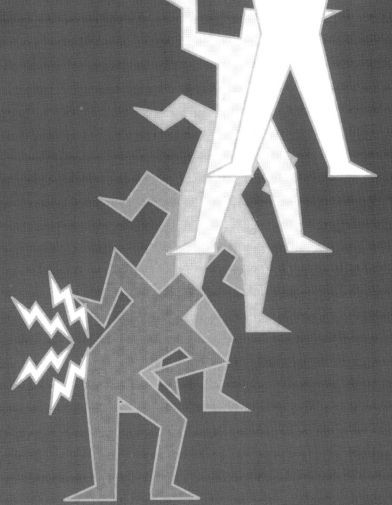

Quick Reference Guide for Clinicians

Number 14

# Acute Low Back Problems in Adults: Assessment and Treatment

Clinical Practice Guideline

Acute Low Back Problems in Adults

**U.S. Department of Health and Human Services**
Public Health Service
Agency for Health Care Policy and Research

## Attention Clinicians:

The Clinical Practice Guideline on which this Quick Reference Guide for Clinicians is based was developed by a multidisciplinary, private-sector panel comprising health care professionals and a consumer representative sponsored by the Agency for Health Care Policy and Research (AHCPR). Panel members were:

Stanley J. Bigos, MD (Chair)
Reverend O. Richard Bowyer
G. Richard Braen, MD
Kathleen C. Brown, PhD, RN
Richard A. Deyo, MD, MPH
Scott Haldeman, MD, PhD, DC
John L. Hart, DO
Ernest W. Johnson, MD
Robert B. Keller, MD
Daniel K. Kido, MD
Matthew H. Liang, MD, MPH
Roger M. Nelson, PhD, PTT

Margareta Nordin, Dr. Med. Sc.
Bernice D. Owen, PhD, RN
Malcolm H. Pope, Dr. Med. Sc., PhD
Richard K. Schwartz, MS, OTR
Donald H. Stewart, Jr., MD
Jeffrey L. Susman, MD
John J. Triano, DC, MA
Lucius Tripp, MD, MPH
Dennis Turk, PhD
Clark Watts, MD, JD
James Weinstein, DO

Special consultants to the panel were: Michele Battié, PT, PhD; Claire Bombardier, MD; Nortin Hadler, MD; Alf Nachemson, MD, PhD; Gordon Waddell, MD. John Holland, MD, MPH and John Webster, MD served as project directors. Project methodologists were David Schriger, MD, MPH and Paul Shekelle, MD,MPH.

An explicit, science-based methodology was employed along with expert clinical judgment to develop specific statements on patient assessment and management on acute low back problems. Extensive literature searches were conducted and critical reviews and syntheses were used to evaluate empirical evidence and significant outcomes. Peer review and pilot testing were undertaken to evaluate the validity, reliability, and utility of the guideline in clinical practice.

This *Quick Reference Guide for Clinicians* presents a clinical strategy for applying the statements and recommendations from the *Clinical Practice Guideline.* The latter provides a description of the guideline development process, thorough analysis and discussion of the available research, critical evaluation of the assumptions and knowledge of the field, more complete information for health care decisionmaking, consideration for patients with special needs, and references. Decisions to adopt particular recommendations from either publication must be made by practitioners in light of available resources and circumstances presented by the individual patient.

AHCPR invites comments and suggestions from users for consideration in development and updating of future guidelines.

**Quick Reference Guide for Clinicians**

**Number 14**

# Acute Low Back Problems in Adults: Assessment and Treatment

## Purpose and Scope

Low back problems affect virtually everyone at some time during their life. Surveys indicate a yearly prevalence of symptoms in 50 percent of working age adults; 15-20 percent seek medical care. Low back problems rank high among the reasons for physician office visits and are costly in terms of medical treatment, lost productivity, and nonmonetary costs such as diminished ability to perform or enjoy usual activities. In fact, for persons under age 45, low back problems are the most common cause of disability.

Acute low back problems are defined as activity intolerance due to lower back or back-related leg symptoms of less than 3 months' duration. About 90 percent of patients with acute low back problems spontaneously recover activity tolerance within 1 month. The approach to a new episode in a patient with a recurrent low back problem is similar to that of a new acute episode.

The findings and recommendations included in the *Clinical Practice Guideline* define a paradigm shift away from focusing care exclusively on the pain and toward helping patients improve activity tolerance. The intent of this *Quick Reference Guide* is to bring to life this paradigm shift. The guide provides information on the detection of serious conditions that occasionally cause low back symptoms (conditions such as spinal fracture, tumor, infection, cauda equina syndrome, or non-spinal conditions). However, treatment of these conditions is beyond the scope of this guideline. In addition, the guideline does not address the care of patients younger than 18 years or those with chronic back problems (back-related activity limitations of greater than 3 months' duration).

## Initial Assessment

■ Seek potentially dangerous underlying conditions.

■ In the absence of signs of dangerous conditions, there is no need for special studies since 90 percent of patients will recover spontaneously within 4 weeks.

A focused medical history and physical examination are sufficient to assess the patient with an acute or recurrent limitation due to low back symptoms of less than 4 weeks duration. Patient responses and findings on the history and physical examination, referred to as "red flags" (Table 1), raise suspicion of serious underlying spinal conditions. Their absence rules out the need for special studies during the first 4 weeks of symptoms when spontaneous recovery is expected. The medical history and physical examination can also alert the clinician to non-spinal pathology (abdominal, pelvic, thoracic) that

1

can present as low back symptoms. Acute low back symptoms can then be classified into one of three working categories:

■ **_Potentially serious spinal condition_**—tumor, infection, spinal fracture, or a major neurologic compromise, such as cauda equina syndrome, suggested by a red flag.

■ **_Sciatica_**—back-related lower limb symptoms suggesting lumbosacral nerve root compromise.

■ **_Nonspecific back symptoms_**—occurring primarily in the back and suggesting neither nerve root compromise nor a serious underlying condition.

## Table 1. Red flags for potentially serious conditions

| Possible fracture | Possible tumor or infection | Possible cauda equina syndrome |
|---|---|---|
| **From medical history** | | |
| Major trauma, such as vehicle accident or fall from height.<br><br>Minor trauma or even strenuous lifting (in older or potentially osteoporotic patient). | Age over 50 or under 20.<br><br>History of cancer.<br><br>Constitutional symptoms, such as recent fever or chills or unexplained weight loss.<br><br>Risk factors for spinal infection: recent bacterial infection (e.g., urinary tract infection); IV drug abuse; or immune suppression (from steroids, transplant, or HIV).<br><br>Pain that worsens when supine; severe nighttime pain. | Saddle anesthesia.<br><br>Recent onset of bladder dysfunction, such as urinary retention, increased frequency, or overflow incontinence.<br><br>Severe or progressive neurologic deficit in the lower extremity. |
| **From physical examination** | | |
| | | Unexpected laxity of the anal sphincter.<br><br>Perianal/perineal sensory loss.<br><br>Major motor weakness: quadriceps (knee extension weakness); ankle plantar flexors, evertors, and dorsiflexors (foot drop). |

2

## Medical History

In addition to detecting serious conditions and categorizing back symptoms, the medical history establishes rapport between the clinician and patient. The patient's description of present symptoms and limitations, duration of symptoms, and history of previous episodes defines the problem. It also provides insight into concerns, expectations, and nonphysical (psychological and socioeconomic) issues that may alter the patient's response to treatment. Assessment tools such as pain drawings and visual analog pain-rating scales may help further document the patient's perceptions and progress.

A patient's estimate of personal activity intolerance due to low back symptoms contributes to the clinical assessment of the severity of the back problem, guides treatment, and establishes a baseline for recommending daily activities and evaluating progress.

Open-ended questions, such as those listed below, can gauge the need for further discussion or specific inquiries for more detailed information:

■ *What are your symptoms?*

Pain, numbness, weakness, stiffness?

Located primarily in back, leg, or both?

Constant or intermittent?

■ *How do these symptoms limit you?*

How long can you sit, stand, walk?

How much weight can you lift?

■ *When did the current limitations begin?*

How long have your activities been limited? More than 4 weeks?

Have you had similar episodes previously?

Previous testing or treatment?

■ *What do you hope we can accomplish during this visit?*

## Physical Examination

Guided by the medical history, the physical examination includes:

■ General observation of the patient.

■ A regional back exam.

■ Neurologic screening.

■ Testing for sciatic nerve root tension.

The examination is mostly subjective since patient response or interpretation is required for all parts except reflex testing and circumferential measurements for atrophy.

3

## Addressing Red Flags

Physical examination evidence of severe neurologic compromise that correlates with the medical history may indicate a need for immediate consultation. The examination may further modify suspicions of tumor, infection, or significant trauma. A medical history suggestive of non-spinal pathology mimicking a back problem may warrant examination of pulses, abdomen, pelvis, or other areas.

## Observation and Regional Back Examination

Limping or coordination problems indicate the need for specific neurologic testing. Severe guarding of lumbar motion in all planes may support a suspected diagnosis of spinal infection, tumor, or fracture. However, given marked variations among persons with and without symptoms, range-of-motion measurements of the back are of limited value.

Vertebral point tenderness to palpation, when associated with other signs or symptoms, may be suggestive of but not specific for spinal fracture or infection. Palpable soft-tissue tenderness is, by itself, an even less specific or reliable finding.

## Neurologic Screening

The neurologic examination can focus on a few tests that seek evidence of nerve root impairment, peripheral neuropathy, or spinal cord dysfunction. Over 90 percent of all clinically significant lower extremity radiculopathy due to disc herniation involves the L5 or S1 nerve root at the L4-5 or L5-S1 disc

level. The clinical features of nerve root compression are summarized in Figure 1.

- ■ *Testing for Muscle Strength.* The patient's inability to toe walk (calf muscles, mostly S1 nerve root), heel walk (ankle and toe dorsiflexor muscles, L5 and some L4 nerve roots), or do a single squat and rise (quadriceps muscles, mostly L4 nerve root) may indicate muscle weakness. Specific testing of the dorsiflexor muscles of the ankle or great toe (suggestive of L5 or some L4 nerve root dysfunction), hamstrings and ankle evertors (L5-S1), and toe flexors (S1) is also important.

- ■ *Circumferential Measurements.* Muscle atrophy can be detected by circumferential measurements of the calf and thigh bilaterally. Differences of less than 2 cm in measurements of the two limbs at the same level may be a normal variation. Symmetrical muscle bulk and strength are expected unless the patient has a neurologic impairment or a history of lower extremity muscle or joint problem.

- ■ *Reflexes.* The ankle jerk reflex tests mostly the S1 nerve root and the knee jerk reflex tests mostly the L4 nerve root; neither tests the L5 nerve root. The reliability of reflex testing can be diminished in the presence of adjacent joint or muscle problems. Up-going toes in response to stroking the plantar footpad (Babinski or plantar

4

response) may indicate upper motor-neuron abnormalities (such as myelopathy or demyelinating disease) rather than a common low back problem.

■ ***Sensory Examination.*** Testing light touch or pressure in the medial (L4), dorsal (L5), and lateral (S1) aspects of the foot (Figure 1) is usually sufficient for sensory screening.

## Figure 1. Testing for lumbar nerve root compromise.

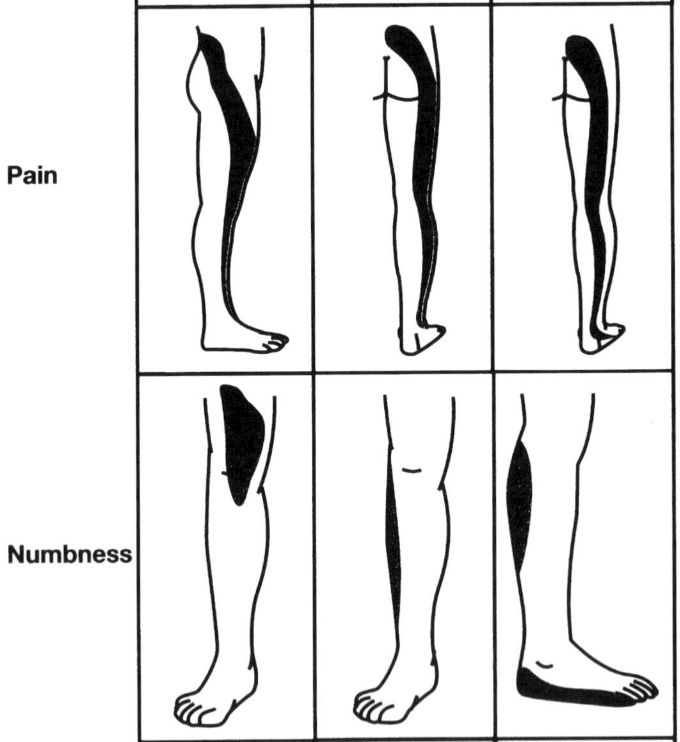

| Nerve root | L4 | L5 | S1 |
|---|---|---|---|
| Pain | | | |
| Numbness | | | |
| Motor weakness | Extension of quadriceps. | Dorsilflexion of great toe and foot. | Plantar flexion of great toe and foot. |
| Screening exam | Squat & rise. | Heel walking. | Walking on toes. |
| Reflexes | Knee jerk diminished. | None reliable. | Ankle jerk diminished. |

5

# Clinical tests for sciatic tension

***The straight leg raising (SLR) test*** (Figure 2) can detect tension on the L5 and/or S1 nerve root. SLR may reproduce leg pain by stretching nerve roots irritated by a disc herniation.

## Figure 2. Instructions for the Straight Leg Raising (SLR) Test

(1) Ask the patient to lie as straight as possible on a table in the supine position.

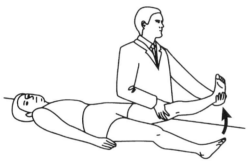

(2) With one hand placed above the knee of the leg being examined, exert enough firm pressure to keep the knee fully extended. Ask the patient to relax.

(3) With the other hand cupped under the heel, slowly raise the straight limb. Tell the patient, "If this bothers you, let me know, and I will stop."

4) Monitor for any movement of the pelvis before complaints are elicited. True sciatic tension should elicit complaints before the hamstrings are stretched enough to move the pelvis.

(5) Estimate the degree of leg elevation that elicits complaint from the patient. Then determine the most distal area of discomfort: back, hip, thigh, knee, or below the knee.

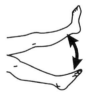

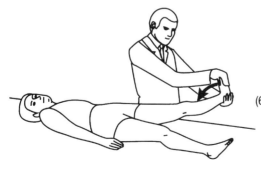

(6) While holding the leg at the limit of straight leg raising, dorsiflex the ankle. Note whether this aggravates the pain. Internal rotation of the limb can also increase the tension on the sciatic nerve roots.

6

Pain below the knee at less than 70 degrees of straight leg raising, aggravated by dorsiflexion of the ankle and relieved by ankle plantar flexion or external limb rotation, is most suggestive of tension on the L5 or S1 nerve root related to disc herniation. Reproducing back pain alone with SLR testing does not indicate significant nerve root tension.

***Crossover pain*** occurs when straight raising of the patient's well limb elicits pain in the leg with sciatica. Crossover pain is a stronger indication of nerve root compression than pain elicited from raising the straight painful limb.

***Sitting knee extension*** (Figure 3) can also test sciatic tension. The patient with significant nerve root irritation tends to complain or lean backward to reduce tension on the nerve.

## Figure 3. Instructions for sitting knee extension test.

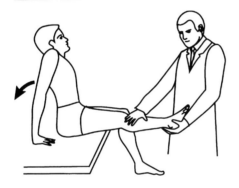

With the patient sitting on a table, both hip and knees flexed at 90 degrees, slowly extend the knee as if evaluating the patella or bottom of the foot. This maneuver stretches nerve roots as much as a moderate degree of supine SLR.

7

# Inconsistent Findings and Pain Behavior

The patient who embellishes a medical history, exaggerates pain drawings, or provides responses on physical examination inconsistent with known physiology can be particularly challenging. A strongly positive supine straight leg raising test without complaint on sitting knee extension and inconsistent responses on examination raise a suspicion that nonphysical factors may be affecting the patient's responses. "Pain behaviors" (verbal or nonverbal communication of distress or suffering) such as amplified grimacing, distorted gait or posture, moaning, and rubbing of painful body parts may also cloud medical issues and even evoke angry responses from the clinician.

Interpreting inconsistencies or pain behaviors as malingering does not benefit the patient or the clinician. It is more useful to view such behavior and inconsistencies as the patient's attempt to enlist the practitioner as an advocate, a plea for help. The patient could be trapped in a job where activity requirements are unrealistic relative to the person's age or health. In some cases, the patient may be negotiating with an insurer or be involved in legal actions. In patients with recurrent back problems, inconsistencies and amplifications may simply be habits learned during previous medical evaluations. In working with these patients, the clinician should attempt to identify any psychological or socioeconomic pressures that might be influenced in a positive manner. The overall goal should always be to facilitate the patient's recovery and avoid the development of chronic low back disability.

8

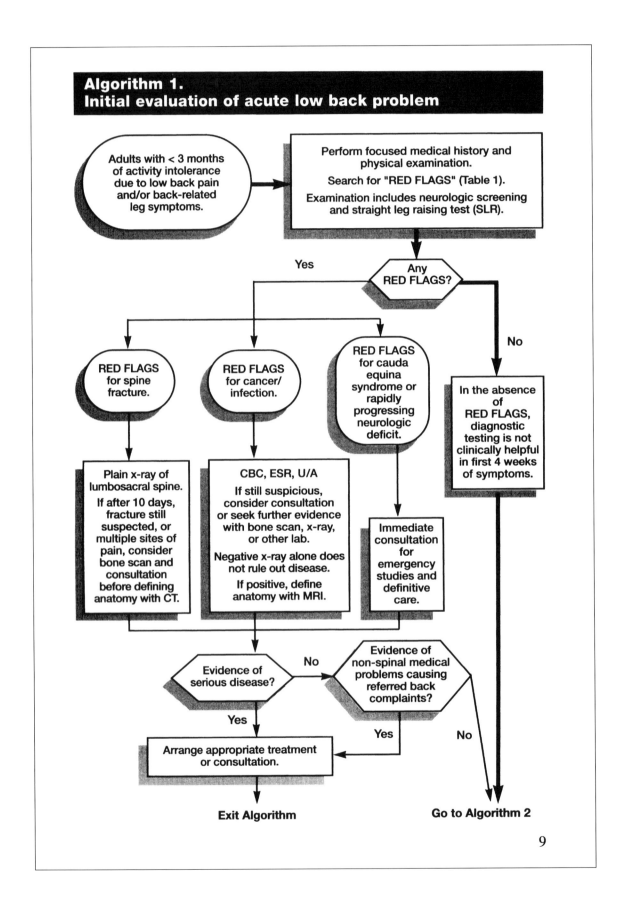

**Algorithm 1.**
**Initial evaluation of acute low back problem**

Adults with < 3 months of activity intolerance due to low back pain and/or back-related leg symptoms.

Perform focused medical history and physical examination.

Search for "RED FLAGS" (Table 1).

Examination includes neurologic screening and straight leg raising test (SLR).

Any RED FLAGS?

Yes

No

RED FLAGS for spine fracture.

RED FLAGS for cancer/infection.

RED FLAGS for cauda equina syndrome or rapidly progressing neurologic deficit.

In the absence of RED FLAGS, diagnostic testing is not clinically helpful in first 4 weeks of symptoms.

Plain x-ray of lumbosacral spine.

If after 10 days, fracture still suspected, or multiple sites of pain, consider bone scan and consultation before defining anatomy with CT.

CBC, ESR, U/A

If still suspicious, consider consultation or seek further evidence with bone scan, x-ray, or other lab.

Negative x-ray alone does not rule out disease.

If positive, define anatomy with MRI.

Immediate consultation for emergency studies and definitive care.

Evidence of serious disease?

No

Evidence of non-spinal medical problems causing referred back complaints?

Yes

Yes

No

Arrange appropriate treatment or consultation.

**Exit Algorithm**

**Go to Algorithm 2**

## Initial Care

■ Education and assurance.

■ Patient comfort.

■ Activity alterations.

## Patient Education

If the initial assessment detects no serious condition, assure the patient that there is "no hint of a dangerous problem" and that "a rapid recovery can be expected." The need for education will vary among patients and during various stages of care. An obviously apprehensive patient may require a more detailed explanation. Patients with sciatica may have a longer expected recovery time than patients with nonspecific back symptoms and thus may need more education and reassurance. Any patient who does not recover within a few weeks may need more extensive education about back problems and the reassurance that special studies may be considered if recovery is slow.

## Patient Comfort

Comfort is often a patient's first concern. Nonprescription analgesics will provide sufficient pain relief for most patients with acute low back symptoms. If treatment response is inadequate, as evidenced by continued symptoms and activity limitations, prescribed pharmaceuticals or physical methods may be added. Comorbid conditions, side effects, cost, and provider/patient preference should guide the clinician's choice of recommendations. Table 2 summarizes comfort options.

## Oral Pharmaceuticals

The safest effective medication for acute low back problems appears to be acetaminophen. Nonsteroidal anti-inflammatory drugs (NSAIDs), including aspirin and ibuprofen, are also effective although they can cause gastrointestinal irritation/ulceration or (less commonly) renal or allergic problems. Phenylbutazone is not recommended due to risks of bone marrow suppression. Acetaminophen may be used safely in combination with NSAIDs or other pharmacologic or physical therapeutics, especially in otherwise healthy patients.

Muscle relaxants seem no more effective than NSAIDs for treating patients with low back symptoms, and using them in combination with NSAIDs has no demonstrated benefit. Side effects including drowsiness have been reported in up to 30 percent of patients taking muscle relaxants.

Opioids appear no more effective than safer analgesics for managing low back symptoms. Opioids should be avoided if possible and, when chosen, used only for a short time. Poor patient tolerance and risks of drowsiness, decreased reaction time, clouded judgment, and potential misuse/-dependence have been reported in up to 35 percent of patients. Patients should be warned of these potentially debilitating problems.

10

## Table 2.  Symptom control methods

| Recommended | | |
|---|---|---|
| **Nonprescription analgesics** | | |
| Acetaminophen (safest)<br>NSAIDs (Aspirin,[1] Ibuprofen[1]) | | |
| **Prescribed pharmaceutical methods** | **Prescribed physical methods** | |
| **Nonspecific low back symptoms and/or sciatica** | **Nonspecific low back symptoms** | **Sciatica** |
| Other NSAIDs[1] | Manipulation<br>(in place of medication or a shorter trial if combined with NSAIDs) | |
| Options | | |
| **Nonspecific low back symptoms and/or sciatica** | **Nonspecific low back symptoms** | **Sciatica** |
| Muscle relaxants[2,3,4]<br><br>Opioids[2,3,4] | Physical agents and modalities[2]<br>(heat or cold modalities for home programs only)<br><br>Shoe insoles[2] | Manipulation (in place of medication or a shorter trial if combined with NSAIDs)<br><br>Physical agents and modalities[2]<br>(heat or cold modalities for home programs only)<br><br>Few days' rest[4]<br><br>Shoe insoles[2] |

[1]Aspirin and other NSAIDs are not recommended for use in combination with one another due to the risk of GI complications.
[2]Equivocal efficacy.
[3]Significant potential for producing drowsiness and debilitation; potential for dependency.
[4]Short course (few days only) for severe symptoms.

11

## Physical Methods

■ *Manipulation,* defined as manual loading of the spine using short or long leverage methods, is safe and effective for patients in the first month of acute low back symptoms without radiculopathy. For patients with symptoms lasting longer than 1 month, manipulation is probably safe but its efficacy is unproven. If manipulation has not resulted in symptomatic and functional improvement after 4 weeks, it should be stopped and the patient reevaluated.

■ *Traction* applied to the spine has not been found effective for treating acute low back symptoms.

■ *Physical modalities* such as *massage, diathermy, ultrasound, cutaneous laser treatment, biofeedback,* and *transcutaneous electrical nerve stimulation (TENS)* also have no proven efficacy in the treatment of acute low back symptoms. If requested, the clinician may wish to provide the patient with instructions on self-application of heat or cold therapy for temporary symptom relief.

■ *Invasive techniques* such as *needle acupuncture* and *injection procedures* (injection of trigger points in the back; injection of facet joints; injection of steroids, lidocaine, or opioids in the epidural space) have no proven benefit in the treatment of acute low back symptoms.

■ *Other miscellaneous therapies* have been evaluated. No evidence indicates that *shoe lifts* are effective in treating acute low back symptoms or limitations, especially when the difference in lower limb length is less than 2 cm. Shoe insoles are a safe and inexpensive option if requested by patients with low back symptoms who must stand for prolonged periods. Low back corsets and back belts, however, do not appear beneficial for treating acute low back symptoms.

12

## Activity Alteration

To avoid both undue back irritation and debilitation from inactivity, recommendations for alternate activity can be helpful. Most patients will not require bed rest. Prolonged bed rest (more than 4 days) has potential debilitating effects, and its efficacy in the treatment of acute low back problems is unproven. Two to four days of bed rest are reserved for patients with the most severe limitations (due primarily to leg pain).

### Avoiding undue back irritation.

Activities and postures that increase stress on the back also tend to aggravate back symptoms. Patients limited by back symptoms can minimize the stress of lifting by keeping any lifted object close to the body at the level of the navel. Twisting, bending, and reaching while lifting also increase stress on the back. Sitting, although safe, may aggravate symptoms for some patients. Advise these patients to avoid prolonged sitting and to change position often. A soft support placed at the small of the back, armrests to support some body weight, and a slight recline of the chair back may make required sitting more comfortable.

### Avoiding debilitation.

Until the patient returns to normal activity, aerobic (endurance) conditioning exercise such as walking, stationary biking, swimming, and even light jogging may be recommended to help avoid debilitation from inactivity. An incremental, gradually increasing regimen of aerobic exercise (up to 20 to 30 minutes daily) can usually be started within the first 2 weeks of symptoms. Such conditioning activities have been found to stress the back no more than sitting for an equal time period on the side of the bed. Patients should be informed that exercise may increase symptoms slightly at first. If intolerable, some exercise alteration is usually helpful.

Conditioning exercises for trunk muscles are more mechanically stressful to the back than aerobic exercise. Such exercises are not recommended during the first few weeks of symptoms, although they may later help patients regain and maintain activity tolerance.

There is no evidence to indicate that back-specific exercise machines are effective for treating acute low back problems. Neither is there evidence that stretching of the back helps patients with acute symptoms.

## Work Activities

When requested, clinicians may choose to offer specific instructions about activity at work for patients with acute limitations due to low back symptoms. The patient's age, general health, and perceptions of safe limits of sitting, standing, walking or lifting (noted on initial history) can help provide reasonable starting points for activity recommendations. Table 3 provides a guide for recommendations about sitting and lifting. The clinician should make clear to patients and employers that:

■ Even moderately heavy unassisted lifting may aggravate back symptoms.

■ Any restrictions are intended to allow for spontaneous recovery or time to build activity tolerance through exercise.

Activity restrictions are prescribed for a short time period only, depending upon work requirements (no benefits apparent beyond 3 months).

| Table 3. Guidelines for sitting and unassisted lifting | | | | | | | |
|---|---|---|---|---|---|---|---|
| | Symptoms | | | | | | |
| | Severe | → | Moderate | → | Mild | → | None |
| Sitting[1] | 20 min | → | → | → | → | → | 50 min |
| Unassisted lifting[2] | | | | | | | |
| Men | 20 lbs | → | 20 lbs | → | 60 lbs | → | 80 lbs |
| Women | 20 lbs | → | 20 lbs | → | 35 lbs | → | 40 lbs |

[1]Without getting up and moving around.
[2]Modification of NIOSH Lifting Guidelines, 1981, 1993. Gradually increase unassisted lifting limits to 60 lbs (men) and 35 lbs (women) by 3 months even with continued symptoms. Instruct patient to limit twisting, bending, reaching while lifting and to hold lifted object as close to navel as possible.

14

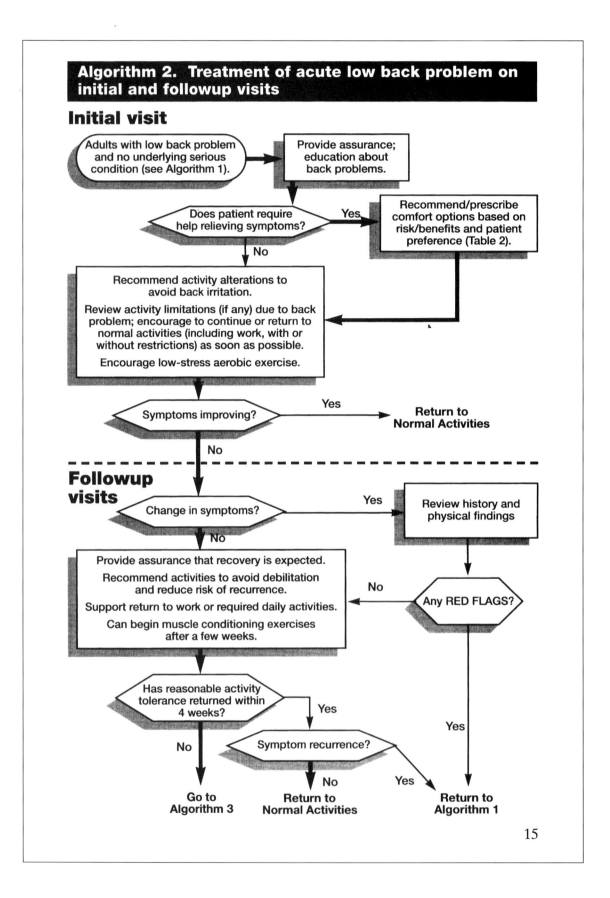

**Algorithm 2. Treatment of acute low back problem on initial and followup visits**

**Initial visit**

Adults with low back problem and no underlying serious condition (see Algorithm 1).

Provide assurance; education about back problems.

Does patient require help relieving symptoms?

Yes — Recommend/prescribe comfort options based on risk/benefits and patient preference (Table 2).

No

Recommend activity alterations to avoid back irritation.

Review activity limitations (if any) due to back problem; encourage to continue or return to normal activities (including work, with or without restrictions) as soon as possible.

Encourage low-stress aerobic exercise.

Symptoms improving? — Yes → **Return to Normal Activities**

No

**Followup visits**

Change in symptoms? — Yes → Review history and physical findings

No

Provide assurance that recovery is expected.

Recommend activities to avoid debilitation and reduce risk of recurrence.

Support return to work or required daily activities.

Can begin muscle conditioning exercises after a few weeks.

Any RED FLAGS?

No

Has reasonable activity tolerance returned within 4 weeks?

Yes — Symptom recurrence?

No

**Go to Algorithm 3**          **Return to Normal Activities**          Yes → **Return to Algorithm 1**

Yes (RED FLAGS) → **Return to Algorithm 1**

15

## Special Studies and Diagnostic Considerations

Routine testing (laboratory tests, plain x-rays of the lumbosacral spine) and imaging studies are not recommended during the first month of activity limitation due to back symptoms except when a red flag noted on history or examination raises suspicion of a dangerous low back or non-spinal condition. If a patient's limitations due to low back symptoms do not improve in 4 weeks, reassessment is recommended. After again reviewing the patient's activity limitations, history, and physical findings, the clinician may then consider further diagnostic studies, and discuss these with the patient.

### Timing and Limits of Special Studies

Waiting 4 weeks before considering special tests allows 90 percent of patients to recover spontaneously and avoids unneeded procedures. This also reduces the potential confusion of falsely labeling age-related changes on imaging studies (commonly noted in patients older than 30 without back symptoms) as the cause of the acute symptoms. In the absence of either red flags or persistent activity limitations due to continuous limb symptoms, imaging studies (especially plain x-rays) rarely provide information that changes the clinical approach to the acute low back problem.

### Selection of Special Studies

Prior to ordering imaging studies the clinician should have noted either of the following:

■ The emergence of a red flag.

■ Physiologic evidence of tissue insult or neurologic dysfunction.

Physiologic evidence may be in the form of definitive nerve findings on physical examination, electrodiagnostic studies (when evaluating sciatica), and a laboratory test or bone scan (when evaluating nonspecific low back symptoms). Unquestionable findings that identify specific nerve root compromise on the neurologic examination (see Figure 1) are sufficient physiologic evidence to warrant imaging. When the neurologic examination is less clear, however, further physiologic evidence of nerve root dysfunction should be considered before ordering an imaging study. Electromyography (EMG) including H-reflex tests may be useful to identify subtle focal neurologic dysfunction in patients with leg symptoms lasting longer than 3-4 weeks. Sensory evoked potentials (SEPs) may be added to the assessment if spinal stenosis or spinal cord myelopathy is suspected.

Laboratory tests such as erythrocyte sedimentation rate (ESR), complete blood count (CBC), and urinalysis (UA) can be useful to screen for nonspecific medical diseases (especially infection and tumor) of the low back. A bone scan can detect physiologic reactions to suspected spinal tumor, infection, or occult fracture.

Should physiologic evidence indicate tissue insult or nerve impairment, discuss with a consultant selection of an imaging test to define

16

a potential anatomic cause (CT for bone, MRI for neural or other soft tissue). Anatomic definition is commonly needed to guide surgery or specific procedures. Selection of an imaging test should also take into consideration any patient allergies to contrast media (myelogram) or concerns about claustrophobia (MRI) and costs. A discussion with a specialist on selection of the most clinically valuable study can often assist the primary care clinician to avoid duplication. Table 4 provides a general comparison of the abilities of different techniques to identify physiologic insult and define anatomic defects. Missing from the table is discography, which is not recommended for assessing patients with acute low back symptoms.

In general, an imaging study may be an appropriate consideration for the patient whose limitations due to consistent symptoms have persisted for 1 month or more:

■ When surgery is being considered for treatment of a specific detectable loss of neurologic function.

■ To further evaluate potentially serious spinal pathology.

Reliance upon imaging studies alone to evaluate the source of low back symptoms, however, carries a significant risk of diagnostic confusion, given the possibility of falsely identifying a finding that was present before symptoms began.

## Table 4. Ability of different techniques to identify and define pathology

| Technique | Identify physiologic insult | Define anatomic defect |
|---|---|---|
| History | + | + |
| Physical examination: Circumference measurements | + | + |
| Reflexes | ++ | ++ |
| Straight leg raising (SLR) | ++ | + |
| Crossed SLR | +++ | ++ |
| Motor | ++ | ++ |
| Sensory | ++ | ++ |
| Laboratory studies (ESR, CBC, UA) | ++ | 0 |
| Bone scan[1] | +++ | ++ |
| EMG/SEP | +++ | ++ |
| X-ray[1] | 0 | + |
| CT[1] | 0 | ++++[2] |
| MRI | 0 | ++++[2] |
| Myelo-CT[1] | 0 | ++++[2] |
| Myelography[1] | 0 | ++++[2] |

[1]Risk of complications (radiation, infection, etc.): highest for myelo-CT, second highest for myelography, and relatively less risk for bone scan, x-ray, and CT.

[2]False-positive diagnostic findings in up to 30 percent of people without symptoms at age 30.

**Note:** Number of plus signs indicates relative ability to identify or define.

17

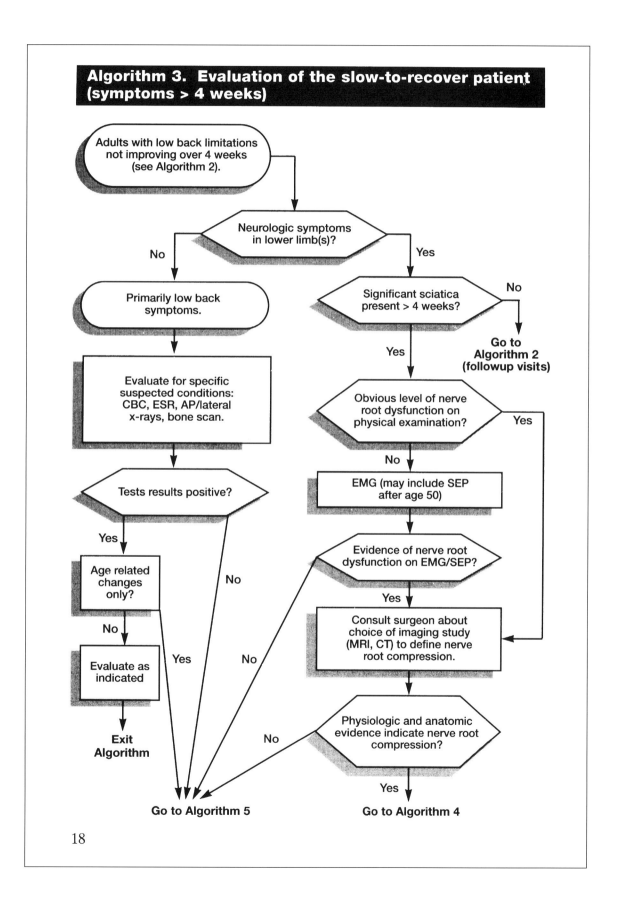

## Algorithm 3. Evaluation of the slow-to-recover patient (symptoms > 4 weeks)

Adults with low back limitations not improving over 4 weeks (see Algorithm 2).

Neurologic symptoms in lower limb(s)?

No — Primarily low back symptoms.

Evaluate for specific suspected conditions: CBC, ESR, AP/lateral x-rays, bone scan.

Tests results positive?

Yes — Age related changes only?

No — Evaluate as indicated

**Exit Algorithm**

No — **Go to Algorithm 5**

Yes — Significant sciatica present > 4 weeks?

No — **Go to Algorithm 2 (followup visits)**

Yes — Obvious level of nerve root dysfunction on physical examination?

Yes

No — EMG (may include SEP after age 50)

Evidence of nerve root dysfunction on EMG/SEP?

Yes — Consult surgeon about choice of imaging study (MRI, CT) to define nerve root compression.

No — **Go to Algorithm 5**

Physiologic and anatomic evidence indicate nerve root compression?

No — **Go to Algorithm 5**

Yes — **Go to Algorithm 4**

18

## Management Considerations After Special Studies

Definitive treatment for serious conditions (see Table 1) detected by special studies is beyond the scope of this guideline. When special studies fail to define the exact cause of symptoms, however, no patient should receive an impression that the clinician thinks "nothing is wrong" or that the problem could be "in their head." Assure the patient that a clinical workup is highly successful in detecting serious conditions, but does not reveal the precise cause of most low back symptoms.

### Surgical Considerations

Within the first 3 months of acute low back symptoms, surgery is considered only when serious spinal pathology or nerve root dysfunction obviously due to a herniated lumbar disc is detected. A disc herniation, characterized by protrusion of the central nucleus pulposus through a defect in the outer annulus fibrosis, may trap a nerve root causing irritation, leg symptoms and nerve root dysfunction. The presence of a herniated lumbar disc on an imaging study, however, does not necessarily imply nerve root dysfunction. Studies of asymptomatic adults commonly demonstrate intervertebral disc herniations that apparently do not entrap a nerve root or cause symptoms.

Therefore, nerve root decompression can be considered for a patient if all of the following criteria exist:

■ Sciatica is both severe and disabling.

■ Symptoms of sciatica persist without improvement for longer than 4 weeks or with extreme progression.

■ There is strong physiologic evidence of dysfunction of a specific nerve root with intervertebral disc herniation confirmed at the corresponding level and side by findings on an imaging study.

Patients with acute low back pain alone, without findings of serious conditions or significant nerve root compression, rarely benefit from a surgical consultation.

Many patients with strong clinical findings of nerve root dysfunction due to disc herniation recover activity tolerance within 1 month; no evidence indicates that delaying surgery for this period worsens outcomes. With or without an operation, more than 80 percent of patients with obvious surgical indications eventually recover. Surgery seems to be a luxury for speeding recovery of patients with obvious surgical indications but benefits fewer than 40 percent of patients with questionable physiologic findings. Moreover, surgery increases the chance of future procedures with higher complication rates. Overall, the incidence of first-time disc surgery complications, including infection and bleeding, is less than 1 percent. The figure increases dramatically with older patients or repeated procedures.

19

**Direct and indirect nerve root decompression for herniated discs.** Direct methods of nerve root decompression include laminotomy (expansion of the interlaminar space for access to the nerve root and the offending disc fragments), microdiscectomy (laminotomy using a microscope), and laminectomy (total removal of laminae). Methods of indirect nerve root decompression include chemonucleolysis, the injection of chymopapain or other enzymes to dissolve the inner disc. Such chemical treatment methods are less efficacious than standard or microdiscectomy and have rare but serious complications. Any of these methods is preferable to percutaneous discectomy (indirect, mechanical disc removal through a lateral disc puncture).

**Management of spinal stenosis.** Usually resulting from soft tissue and bony encroachment of the spinal canal and nerve roots, spinal stenosis typically has a gradual onset and begins in older adults. It is characterized by nonspecific limb symptoms, called *neurogenic claudication* or *pseudoclaudication,* that interfere with the duration of comfortable standing and walking. The symptoms are commonly bilateral and rarely associated with strong focal findings on examination.

Neurogenic claudication, however, can be confused or coexist with *vascular claudication,* in which leg pain also limits walking. The symptoms of vascular insufficiency can be relieved by simply standing still while relief of neurogenic claudication symptoms usually require the patient to flex the lumbar spine or sit.

The surgical treatment for spinal stenosis is usually complete laminectomy for posterior decompression. Offending soft tissue and osteophytes that encroach upon nerve roots in the central spinal canal and foramen are removed. Fusion may be considered to stabilize a degenerative spondylolisthesis with motion between the slipped vertebra and adjacent vertebrae. Elderly patients with spinal stenosis who tolerate their daily activities usually need no surgery unless they develop new signs of bowel or bladder dysfunction. Decisions on treatment should take into account the patient's preference, lifestyle, other medical problems, and risks of surgery. Surgery for spinal stenosis is rarely considered in the first 3 months of symptoms.

Except for cases of trauma-related spinal fracture or dislocation, fusion alone is not usually considered in the first 3 months following onset of low back symptoms.

20

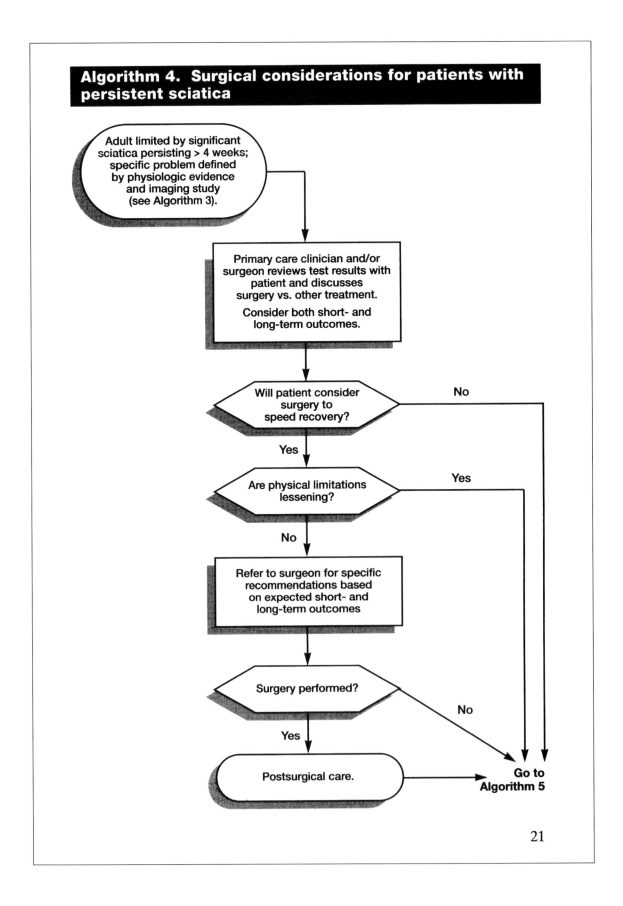

**Algorithm 4. Surgical considerations for patients with persistent sciatica**

Adult limited by significant sciatica persisting > 4 weeks; specific problem defined by physiologic evidence and imaging study (see Algorithm 3).

Primary care clinician and/or surgeon reviews test results with patient and discusses surgery vs. other treatment.

Consider both short- and long-term outcomes.

Will patient consider surgery to speed recovery?

No → Yes

Are physical limitations lessening?

Yes → No

Refer to surgeon for specific recommendations based on expected short- and long-term outcomes

Surgery performed?

No → Yes

Postsurgical care. → **Go to Algorithm 5**

21

# Further Management Considerations

Following diagnostic or surgical procedures, the management of most patients becomes focused on improving physical conditioning through an incrementally increased exercise program. The goal of this program is to build activity tolerance and overcome individual limitations due to back symptoms. At this point in treatment, symptom control methods are only an adjunct to making prescribed exercises more tolerable.

■ Begin with low-stress aerobic activities to improve general stamina (walking, riding a bicycle, swimming, and eventually jogging).

■ Exercises to condition specific trunk muscles can be added a few weeks after. The back muscles may need to be in better condition than before the problem occurred. Otherwise, the back may continue to be painful and easily irritated by even mild activity. Following back surgery, recovery of activity tolerance may be delayed until protective muscles are conditioned well enough to compensate for any remaining structural changes.

■ Finally, specific training to perform activities required at home or work can begin. The objective of this program is to increase the patient's tolerance in carrying out actual daily duties.

When patients demonstrate difficulty regaining the ability to tolerate the activities they are required (or would like) to do, the clinician may pose the following diagnostic and treatment questions:

■ Could the patient have a serious, undetected medical condition? A careful review of the medical history and physical examination is warranted.

■ Are the patient's activity goals realistic? Exploring briefly the patient's expectations, both short- and long-term, of being able to perform specific activities at home, work, or recreation may help the patient assess whether such activity levels are actually achievable.

■ If for any reason the achievement of activity goals seems unlikely, what are the patient's remaining options? To answer this question, the patient is often required to gather specific information from family, friends, employers, or others. If, on followup visits, the patient has made no effort to gather such information, the clinician has the opportunity to point out that low back symptoms alone rarely prevent a patient from addressing questions so important to his or her future. This observation can lead to an open, nonjudgmental discussion of common but complicated psychosocial problems or other issues that often can interfere with a patient's recovery from low back problems. The clinician can then help the patient address or arrange further evaluation of any specific problem limiting the patient's progress. This can usually be accomplished as the patient continues, with the clinician's encouragement, to build activity tolerance through safe, simple exercises.

22

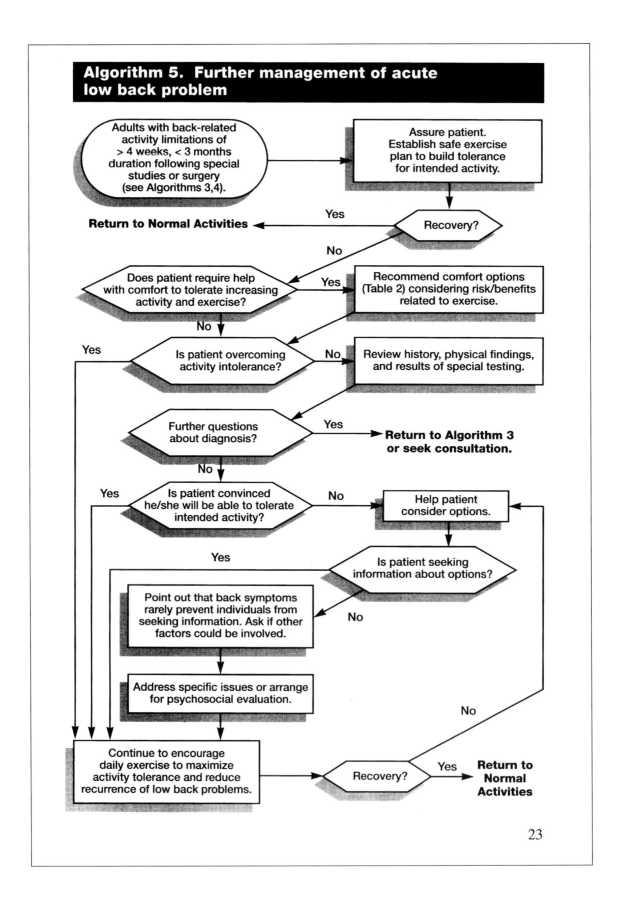

## Algorithm 5. Further management of acute low back problem

Adults with back-related activity limitations of > 4 weeks, < 3 months duration following special studies or surgery (see Algorithms 3,4).

Assure patient. Establish safe exercise plan to build tolerance for intended activity.

Recovery?

**Return to Normal Activities** ← Yes

No

Does patient require help with comfort to tolerate increasing activity and exercise?

Yes → Recommend comfort options (Table 2) considering risk/benefits related to exercise.

No

Is patient overcoming activity intolerance?

No → Review history, physical findings, and results of special testing.

Yes

Further questions about diagnosis?

Yes → **Return to Algorithm 3 or seek consultation.**

No

Is patient convinced he/she will be able to tolerate intended activity?

No → Help patient consider options.

Yes

Is patient seeking information about options?

Yes

Point out that back symptoms rarely prevent individuals from seeking information. Ask if other factors could be involved.

No

Address specific issues or arrange for psychosocial evaluation.

Continue to encourage daily exercise to maximize activity tolerance and reduce recurrence of low back problems.

Recovery? Yes → **Return to Normal Activities**

No

23

# Table 5.  Summary of Guideline Recommendations

The ratings in parentheses indicate the scientific evidence supporting each recommendation according to the following scale:

A = strong research-based evidence (multiple relevant and high-quality scientific studies).

B = moderate research-based evidence (one relevant, high-quality scientific study or multiple adequate scientific studies).

C = limited research-based evidence (at least one adequate scientific study in patients with low back pain).

D = panel interpretation of evidence not meeting inclusion criteria for research-based evidence.

The number of studies meeting panel review criteria is noted for each category.

| | Recommend | Option | Recommend against |
|---|---|---|---|
| **History and physical exam** 34 studies | Basic history (B). History of cancer/ infection (B). Signs/symptoms of cauda equina syndrome (C). History of significant trauma (C). Psychosocial history (C). Straight leg raising test (B). Focused neurological exam (B). | Pain drawing and visual analog scale(D). | |
| **Patient education** 14 studies | Patient education about low back symptoms (B). Back school in occupational settings (C). | Back school in non-occupational settings (C). | |
| **Medication** 23 studies | Acetaminophen (C). NSAIDs (B). | Muscle relaxants (C). Opioids, short course (C). | Opioids used >2 wks (C). Phenylbutazone (C). Oral steroids (C). Colchicine (B). Antidepressants (C). |
| **Physical treatment methods** 42 studies | Manipulation of low back during first month of symptoms (B). | Manipulation for patients with radiculopathy (C). Manipulation for patients with symptoms >1 month (C). Self-application of heat or cold to low back. Shoe insoles (C). Corset for prevention in occupational setting (C). | Manipulation for patients with undiagnosed neurologic deficits (D). Prolonged course of manipulation (D). Traction (B). TENS (C). Biofeedback (C). Shoe lifts (D). Corset for treatment (D). |
| **Injections** 26 studies | | Epidural steroid injections for radicular pain to avoid surgery (C). | Epidural injections for back pain without radiculopathy (D). Trigger point injections (C). Ligamentous injections (C). Facet joint injections (C). Needle acupuncture (D). |

24

| | Recommend | Option | Recommend against |
|---|---|---|---|
| **Bed rest**<br>4 studies | | Bed rest of 2-4 days for severe radiulopathy (D). | Bed rest > 4 days (B). |
| **Activities and exercise**<br>20 studies | Temporary avoidance of activities that increase mechanical stress on spine (D).<br>Gradual return to normal activities (B).<br>Low-stress aerobic exercise (C).<br>Conditioning exercises for trunk muscles after 2 weeks (C).<br>Exercise quotas (C). | | Back-specific exercise machines (D).<br>Therapeutic stretching of back muscles (D). |
| **Detection of physiologic abnormalities**<br>14 studies | If no improvement after 1 month, consider:<br>Bone scan (C).<br>Needle EMG and H-reflex tests to clarify nerve root dysfunction (C).<br>SEP to assess spinal stenosis (C). | | EMG for clinically obvious radiculopathy (D).<br>Surface EMG and F-wave tests (C).<br>Thermography (C). |
| **X-rays of L-S spine**<br>18 studies | When red flags for fracture present (C).<br>When red flags for cancer or infection present (C). | | Routine use in first month of symptoms in absence of red flags (B).<br>Routine oblique views (B). |
| **Imaging**<br>18 studies | CT or MRI when cauda equina, tumor, infection, or fracture strongly suspected (C).<br>MRI test of choice for patients with prior back surgery (D).<br>Assure quality criteria for imaging tests (B). | Myelography or CT-myelography for preoperative planning (D). | Use of imaging test before one month in absence red flags (B).<br>Discography or CT-discography (C). |
| **Surgical considerations**<br>14 studies | Discuss surgical options with patients with persistent and severe sciatica and clinical evidence of nerve root compromise after 1 month of conservative therapy (B).<br>Standard discectomy and microdiscectomy of similar efficacy in treatment of herniated disc (B).<br>Chymopapain, used after ruling out allergic sensitivity, acceptable but less efficacious than discectomy to treat herniated disc (C). | | Disc surgery in patients with back pain alone, no red flags, and no nerve root compression (D).<br>Percutaneous discectomy less efficacious than chymopapain (C).<br>Surgery for spinal stenosis within the first 3 months of symptoms (D).<br>Stenosis surgery when justified by imaging test rather than patient's functional status (D).<br>Spinal fusion during the first 3 months of symptoms in the absence of fracture, dislocation, complications of tumor or infection (C). |
| **Psychosocial factors** | Social, economic, and psychological factors can alter patient response to symptoms and treatment (D). | | Referral for extensive evaluation/treatment prior to exploring patient expectations or psychosocial factors (D). |

25

**Patient Guide**

# Understanding Acute Low Back Problems

**Acute Low Back Problems in Adults**

**Consumer Version
Clinical Practice Guideline
Number 14**

## About the Back and Back Problems

The human spine (or backbone) is made up of small bones called vertebrae. The vertebrae are stacked on top of each other to form a column. Between each vertebra is a cushion known as a disc. The vertebrae are held together by ligaments, and muscles are attached to the vertebrae by bands of tissue called tendons.

Openings in each vertebra line up to form a long hollow canal. The spinal cord runs through this canal from the base of the brain. Nerves from the spinal cord branch out and leave the spine through the spaces between the vertebrae.

The lower part of the back holds most of the body's weight. Even a minor problem with the bones, muscles, ligaments, or tendons in this area can cause pain when a person stands, bends, or moves around. Less often, a problem with a disc can pinch or irritate a nerve from the spinal cord, causing pain that runs down the leg, below the knee called sciatica.

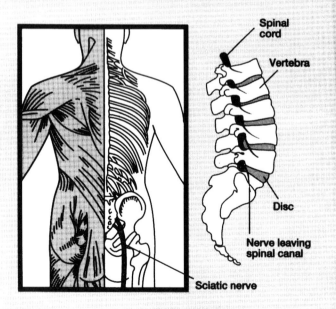

**Figure 1. Muscles of the back and the spine**

# Understanding Acute Low Back Problems

## Purpose

This booklet is about acute low back problems in adults. If you have a low back problem, you may have symptoms that include:

■ Pain or discomfort in the lower part of the back.

■ Pain or numbness that moves down the leg (sciatica).

Low back symptoms can keep you from doing your normal daily activities or doing things that you enjoy.

> A low back problem may come on suddenly or gradually. It is **acute** if it lasts a short while, usually a few days to several weeks. An episode that lasts longer than 3 months is not acute.

If you have been bothered by your lower back, you are not alone. Eight out of ten adults will have a low back problem at some time in their life. And most will have more than one episode of acute low back problems. In between episodes, most people return to their normal activities with little or no symptoms.

This booklet will tell you more about acute low back problems, what to do, and what to expect when you see a health care provider.

## Causes of Low Back Problems

Even with today's technology, the exact reason or cause of low back problems can be found in very few people. Most times, the symptoms are blamed on poor muscle tone in the back, muscle tension or spasm, back sprains, ligament or muscle tears, joint problems. Sometimes nerves from the spinal cord (see Figure 1) can be irritated by "slipped" discs causing buttock or leg pain. This may also cause numbness, tingling, or weakness in the legs.

People who are in poor physical condition or do work that includes heavy labor or long periods of sitting or standing are at greater risk for low back problems. These people also get better more slowly. Emotional stress or long periods of inactivity may make back symptoms seem worse.

Low back problems are often painful. But the good news is that very few people turn out to have a major problem with the bones or joints of the back or a dangerous medical condition.

## Things To Do About Low Back Problems

### Seeing a health care provider

Many people who develop mild low back discomfort may not need to see a health care provider right away. Often, within a few days, the symptoms go away without any treatment.

A visit to your health care provider is a good idea if:

- Your symptoms are severe.

- The pain is keeping you from doing things that you do every day.

- The problem does not go away within a few days.

If you also have problems controlling your bowel or bladder, if you feel numb in the groin or rectal area, or if there is extreme leg weakness, call your health care provider right away.

Your health care provider will check to see if you have a medical illness causing your back problem (chances are you will not). Your health care provider can also help you get some relief from your symptoms.

Your health care provider will:

- Ask about your symptoms and what they keep you from doing.

- Ask about your medical history.

- Give you a physical exam.

## Talking about your symptoms

Your health care provider will want to know about your back problem. Here are some examples of the kinds of questions he or she may ask you. You can write down the answers in the space below each question:

When did your back symptoms start?

_____

_____

_____

Which of your daily activities are you not able to do because of your back symptoms?

_____

_____

_____

Is there anything you do that makes the symptoms better or worse?

_____

_____

_____

_____

Have you noticed any problem with your legs?

_____

_____

Around the time your symptoms began, did you have a fever or symptoms of pain or burning when urinating?

_____

_____

## Talking about your medical history

Be sure to tell your health care provider about your general health and about illnesses you have had in the past. Here are some questions your health care provider may ask you about your medical history. You can write your answers in the space below each question:

Have you had a problem with your back in the past? If so, when?

_____

_____

_____

What medical illnesses have you had (for example, cancer, arthritis, or diseases of the immune system)?

_____

_____

Which medicines do you take regularly?

_____

_____

_____

_____

_____

Have you ever used intravenous (IV) drugs?

_____

_____

Have you recently lost weight without trying?

_____

_____

You should also tell your health care provider about anything you may be doing for your symptoms: medicines you are taking, creams or ointments you are using, and other home remedies.

## Having a physical exam

Your health care provider will examine your back. Even after a careful physical examination, it may not be possible for your health care provider to tell you the exact cause of your low back problem. But you most likely will find out that your symptoms are not being caused by a dangerous medical condition. Very few people (about 1 in 200) have low back symptoms caused by such conditions. You probably won't need special tests (page 11) if you have had low back symptoms for only a few weeks.

## Getting Relief

Your health care provider will help you get relief from your pain, discomfort, or other symptoms. A number of medicines and other treatments help with low back symptoms. The good news is that most people start feeling better soon.

## Proven treatments

**Medicine** often helps relieve low back symptoms. The type of medicine that your health care provider recommends depends on your symptoms and how uncomfortable you are.

■ If your symptoms are mild to moderate, you may get the relief you need from an over-the-counter (non-prescription) medicine such as acetaminophen, aspirin, or ibuprofen. These medicines usually have fewer side effects than prescription medicines and are less expensive.

■ If your symptoms are severe, your health care provider may recommend a prescription medicine.

For most people, medicine works well to control pain and discomfort. But any medicine can have side effects. For example, some people cannot take aspirin or ibuprofen because it can cause stomach irritation and even ulcers. Many medicines prescribed for low back pain can make people feel drowsy. These medicines should not be taken if you need to drive or use heavy equipment. Talk to your health care provider about the benefits and risks of any medicine recommended. If you develop side effects (such as nausea, vomiting, rash, dizziness), stop taking the medicine, and tell your health care provider right away.

Your health care provider may recommend one or more of the following to be used alone or along with medicine to help relieve your symptoms.

■ **Heat or cold applied to the back.** Within the first 48 hours after your back symptoms start, you may want to apply a cold pack (or a bag of ice) to the painful area for 5 to 10 minutes at a time. If your symptoms last longer than 48 hours, you may find that a heating pad or hot shower or bath helps relieve your symptoms.

■ **Spinal manipulation.** This treatment (using the hands to apply force to the back to "adjust" the spine) can be helpful for some people in the first month of low back symptoms. It should only be done by a professional with experience in manipulation. You should go back to your health care provider if your symptoms have not responded to spinal manipulation within 4 weeks.

*Keep in mind that everyone is different. You will have to find what works best to relieve your own back symptoms.*

## Other treatments

A number of other treatments are sometimes used for low back symptoms. While these treatments may give relief for a short time, none have been found to speed recovery or keep acute back problems from returning. They may also be expensive. Such treatments include:

- Traction.
- TENS (transcutaneous electrical nerve stimulation).
- Massage
- Biofeedback.
- Acupuncture.
- Injections into the back.
- Back corsets.
- Ultrasound.

## Physical activity

Your health care provider will want to know about the physical demands of your life (your job or daily activities). Until you feel better, your health care provider may need to recommend some changes in your activities. You will want to talk to your health care provider about your own personal situation. In general, when pain is severe, you should avoid:

- Heavy lifting.
- Lifting when twisting, bending forward, and reaching.
- Sitting for long periods of time.

**The most important goal is for you to return to your normal activities as soon as it is safe.** Your health care provider and (if you work) your employer can help you decide how much you are able to do safely at work. Your schedule can be gradually increased as your back improves.

## Bed rest

If your symptoms are severe, your health care provider may recommend a short period of bed rest. However, bed rest should be limited to 2 or 3 days. Lying down for longer periods may weaken muscles and bones and actually slow your recovery. If you feel that you must lie down, be sure to get up every few hours and walk around—even if it hurts. Feeling a little discomfort as you return to normal activity is common and does not mean that you are hurting yourself.

## About Work and Family

Back problems take time to get better. If your job or your normal daily activities make your back pain worse, it is important to communicate this to your family, supervisor, and coworkers. Put your energy into doing those things at work and at home that you are able to do comfortably. Be productive, but be clear about those tasks that you are not able to do.

## Things You Can Do Now

While waiting for your back to improve, you may be able to make yourself more comfortable if you:

- Wear comfortable, low-heeled shoes.

- Make sure your work surface is at a comfortable height for you.

- Use a chair with a good lower back support that may recline slightly.

- If you must sit for long periods of time, try resting your feet on the floor or on a low stool, whichever is more comfortable.

- If you must stand for long periods of time, try resting one foot on a low stool.

- If you must drive long distances, try using a pillow or rolled-up towel behind the small of your back. Also, be sure to stop often and walk around for a few minutes.

- If you have trouble sleeping, try sleeping on your back with a pillow under your knees, or sleep on your side with your knees bent and a pillow between your knees.

## Exercise

A gradual return to normal activities, including exercise, is recommended. Exercise is important to your overall health and can help you to lose body fat (if needed). Even if you have mild to moderate low back symptoms, the following things can be done without putting much stress on your back:

- Walking short distances.

- Using a stationary bicycle.

- Swimming.

It is important to start any exercise program slowly and to gradually build up the speed and length of time that you do the exercise. At first, you may find that your symptoms get a little worse when you exercise or become more active. Usually, this is nothing to worry about. However, if your pain becomes severe, contact your health care provider. Once you are able to return to normal activities comfortably, your health care provider may recommend further aerobic and back exercises.

## If You Are Not Getting Better

Most low back problems get better quickly, and usually within 4 weeks. If your symptoms are not getting better within this time period, you should contact your health care provider.

### Special tests

Your health care provider will examine your back again and may talk to you about getting some special tests. These may include x-rays, blood tests, or other special studies such as an MRI (magnetic resonance imaging) or CT (computerized tomography) scan of your back. These tests may help your health care provider understand why you are not getting better. Your health care provider may also want to refer you to a specialist.

Certain things, such as stress (extra pressure at home or work), personal or emotional problems, depression, or a problem with drug or alcohol use can slow recovery or make back symptoms seem worse. If you have any of these problems, tell your health care provider.

## About Surgery

Even having a lot of back pain does not by itself mean you need surgery. Surgery has been found to be helpful in only 1 in 100 cases of low back problems. In some people, surgery can even cause more problems. This is especially true if your only symptom is back pain.

People with certain nerve problems or conditions such as fractures or dislocations have the best chance of being helped by surgery. In most cases, however, decisions about surgery do not have to be made right away. Most back surgery can wait for several weeks without making the condition worse.

If your health care provider recommends surgery, be sure to ask about the reason for the surgery and about the risks and benefits you might expect. You may also want to get a second opinion.

## Prevention of Low Back Problems

The best way to prevent low back problems is to stay fit. If you must lift something, even after your back seems better, be sure to:

- Keep all lifted objects close to your body.

- Avoid lifting while twisting, bending forward, and reaching.

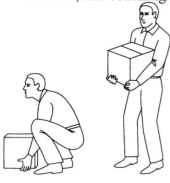

**Figure 2. Safe lifting and carrying positions**

You should continue to exercise even after your back symptoms have gone away. There are many exercises that can be done to condition muscles of your body and back. You should talk to your health care provider about the exercises that would be best for you.

## When Low Back Symptoms Return

More than half of the people who recover from a first episode of acute low back symptoms will have another episode within a few years. Unless your back symptoms are very different from the first episode, or you have a new medical condition, you can expect to recover quickly and fully from each episode.

## While Your Back is Getting Better

It is important to remember that even though you are having a problem with your back now, most likely it will begin to feel better soon. It is important to keep in mind that you are the most important person in taking care of your back and in helping to get back to your regular activities.

It may also help you to remember that:

- Most low back problems last for a short amount of time and the symptoms usually get better with little or no medical treatment.

- Low back problems can be painful. But pain rarely means that there is serious damage to your back.

- Exercise can help you to feel better faster and prevent more back problems. A regular exercise program adds to your general health and may help you get back to the things you enjoy doing.

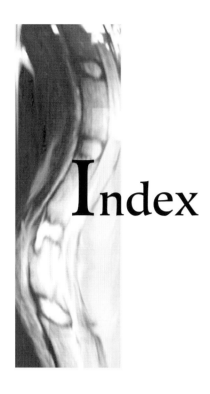

# Index

*Page numbers followed by f indicate an illustration; those followed by t indicate a table.*